ORTHOPEDIC DISEASES

PHYSIOLOGY–PATHOLOGY–RADIOLOGY

BY

Ernest Aegerter, M.D.

Professor of Pathology and Director of the Department of Pathology, Temple University Medical Center and School of Medicine; Professor of Orthopedic Pathology, University of Pennsylvania Graduate School of Medicine; Chief in Pathology, Philadelphia General Hospital; Consultant in Pathology, Frankford Hospital, United States Naval Hospital and Veterans Administration Hospitals, Philadelphia

AND

John A. Kirkpatrick, Jr., M.D.

Radiologist, St. Christopher's Hospital for Children; Assistant Professor of Radiology, Temple University Medical Center; Radiologist, Children's Heart Hospital; Attending (Radiology), Veterans Administration Hospital, Philadelphia

W. B. SAUNDERS COMPANY

Philadelphia   1958   London

Preface

THE "BASIC SCIENCE" aspect of bone disease has lagged behind that of other systems, not from lack of need or interest, but largely perhaps because of the very nature of bone, which until recently has defied investigation on the cellular and intracellular level. The rigors of salt removal by acid so distort the fine morphologic detail of cytoplasm and nucleus that conclusions have depended, until recently, mostly on interpretation of artefacts. Abnormal variations in mineralization were impossible to appreciate when the mineral had to be removed before the tissue could be examined. Knowledge of the healing of human bone was derived from that acquired by animal experimentation since even today we are denied serial sampling of the process as it occurs in our patients. Biopsies are usually relatively difficult and taxing to the donor so that the course of a disease process must be extrapolated from one or two known points in time.

Today there is feverish activity in the fields of bone morphology and function. New techniques and tools have become available. Histochemistry, immunologic chemistry and radioactive isotopes have allowed us to probe within the cell membrane. The ability to section undemineralized bone, microradiography and x-ray diffraction are telling us something of the tissue in its natural state. Phase, ultraviolet and electron microscopy reveal aspects of cell composition that heretofore were undreamed of. These new tools have set the anatomists, the chemists, the physicists and the physiologists to work hacking out new trails which will eventually converge in precise knowledge of the skeletal tissue cells, what they are and what they are doing in health and disease.

All this sound and fury has bewildered the busy physician who must correlate the new material with one hand while he administers his knowledge with the other. It will take many books to sift the facts, to concentrate the verbiage, to reduce the product to the level of practicability. This book is meant as a starter. It looks at bone disease from the standpoint of its altered morphology and physiology, yet it tries to interpret these in terms of symptomatology and roentgenography. Diseases must be understood if they are to be successfully treated. This book is concerned with the understanding of the diseases which affect the musculoskeletal system. The diagnosis of orthopedic diseases necessitates an understanding of the pathology and physiology of bone; from these disciplines arise the clinical manifestations and the radiographic and laboratory findings.

Very little original material is recorded here. Almost all of it can be found in published papers if the searcher will spend the time and energy. The virtue of this volume, if such it has, is in the availability of this material. A consuming interest in the subject for nearly twenty years has given the authors the opportunity of selecting what they think the physician should know. There is no pretense at completeness, for such would remove it from the field of practical usage. It is intended for the clinician who wants to increase his diagnostic efficiency, for the radiologist who is perplexed by the meaning of an overwhelming array of radiographic nuances, for the pathologist who is distraught by his inability to interpret what he sees through his microscope, for the young specialist who wants to pass his board examinations and for the medical student who must acquire a certain amount of knowledge of orthopedic diseases in order to graduate.

The first four chapters are intended as a review of the complicated anatomy and physiology of the tissues of the skeleton. It is difficult to imagine how one can understand the disease process until one understands the normal. The fifth chapter is a simple histology of the tissues involved in orthopedic diseases. It is meant for the orthopedist and the radiologist who have forgotten rudimentary structural components of bone. It is not meant for the pathologist who reviews these basic principles in the first month of his residency. Chapter Six is a primer of bone radiology intended for the pathologist and the orthopedist who must know the fundamentals of radiology if they are to appreciate gross bone pathology. The remaining chapters are divided into three sections, each section grouping the skeletal diseases in a manner which should make them easier to find and to remember. Classification is stressed, perhaps overstressed, with the deliberate intention of presenting a concept of the whole before attempting the specific. There is no truer maxim in diagnostic medicine than "Before one can name the entity, one must know the possibilities."

When one attempts to acknowledge the help which is so important in writing any medical book, it is difficult to know where to start and where to end. First, perhaps, there were all our colleagues in other fields who unselfishly supplied cases and patiently instructed us in the fundamentals of their specialties. Principal of these is Dr. John Royal Moore, Chief of the Departments of Orthopedics at Temple Medical Center, Philadelphia Shriner's Hospital and St. Christopher's Hospital for Children. Most of the material in this book is derived from patients from his services. Many of the radiographs are from the Department of Radiology of Temple Medical Center and we are indebted to Dr. W. E. Chamberlain and his staff for permission to use them. Dr. Howard Steel read the entire manuscript and kept us thinking in terms of the patient.

Then there are our friends in our own specialties. Dr. James Arey of St. Christopher's Hospital read manuscript and offered many valuable suggestions. Dr. William Ehrich of Philadelphia General Hospital, Dr. E. B. D. Neuhauser of Children's Medical Center, Boston, and Dr. John Hope of the Children's Hospital of Philadelphia supplied unusual and hard-to-come-by cases. Grateful thanks are given our assistants in pathology and radiology, too many to list here, who did our work while we wrote.

Credit for the technique of the photomicrographs goes to Dr. E. S. Gault and for the rest of the illustrative material to Mr. William Taylor, both of Temple. Whatever faults there are in this field must be blamed on the authors who sacrificed perfection for punctuality.

An author gets the credit, favorable or adverse, for the words he puts down, but for every hour he writes, someone must spend at least an equal amount of time in transcribing it to a readable state. The authors happen to have the most talented, efficient and cheerful secretaries in the world. To them, Mrs. Hildegard Kates and Mrs. Dorothy McKee, this book rightfully should be dedicated. Our sincere thanks go to Jane Kirkpatrick, co-worker on the text, and to John A. Duross who skillfully arranged the index.

Finally, we owe a debt of gratitude to those wonderful institutions which housed us, nourished us, taught us and endured us while we worked, Temple Medical Center and its pediatric unit, St. Christopher's Hospital for Children. If any good comes of this labor let it reflect bountifully upon them.

ERNEST AEGERTER
JOHN A. KIRKPATRICK, JR.

Contents

Section II

DISTURBANCES IN SKELETAL DEVELOPMENT

Section IV

TUMORS AND TUMOR-LIKE PROCESSES

A General Consideration
of Connective Tissues

Cellular Components
of Connective Tissue

Factors in Cell Differentiation

The various components of the connective tissues, i.e., fat, fibrous tissue, cartilage and bone, arise as differentiated elements from the primitive mesoderm. Differentiation of a cell from those of the totipotent cell mass to become the highly specialized unit of tissue structure is the result of a number of influencing factors some of which are as yet poorly understood. It is presently believed that the mechanism by which a mature cell reproduces by mitotic division resides in the chromatin constituents of the nucleus. This substance, largely desoxyribose nucleic acid, is supplied by the cytoplasm and, therefore, conditioned by enzymatic processes which take place in the cytoplasm of the cell. As long as the cytoplasmic metabolic processes are stable it may be assumed that the nuclear hereditary constituents will remain constant and reproduction may continue indefinitely, each cell a faithful duplicate, in both morphology and function, of its predecessor. We may call the combined agents which govern this exact duplication the primary heredity factor.

Obviously this type of exact reproduction can take place only among cells which are completely differentiated, i.e., cells whose enzymatic constituents are mature and stable, and in an environment which is absolutely unchanging. Thus the chondroblast may give rise to identical chondroblasts, osteoblasts to identical osteoblasts, and so on, as long as the medium in which they exist remains the same. If we introduce new elements into the cell environment, we may force the cytoplasmic metabolism to change and conceivably produce a

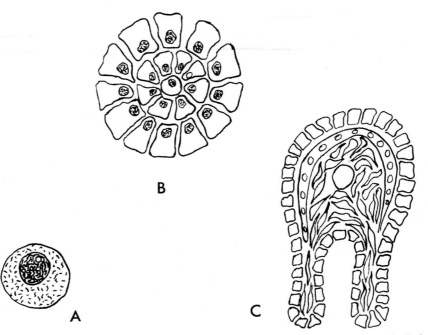

FIG. 1.   Schematic drawing to illustrate cell differentiation. *A,* The unicellular organism ingests what it needs from its environment, processes it to form the plasmagenes in the cytoplasm and passes on the refined product, mostly desoxyribonucleic acid, to the nucleus. It discharges its wastes into its environment. *B,* In the multicellular organism the surface cells still have access to environmental resources but the central cells must accommodate their metabolism to the materials that can penetrate between the surface cells. These materials are contaminated by the catabolic products of the surrounding cells. *C,* The more complex the organism becomes, the greater the possibilities for differentiation. This drawing illustrates the effects of the secondary heredity factor upon the deep cells.

change in the molecular constituency or arrangement of the nuclear heredity apparatus. We may designate the environmental influence on a cell its secondary or somatic heredity factor.

It is probable that this latter factor is a potent agent in what we know as cell differentiation. It is obvious that in the development of a multicellular organism the environment of cells must change until a stage of stable maturity is reached. When the embryonic form consists of a single cell or a small group of cells each with at least some free surface, the cell may choose from its environment what it needs and discharge its metabolic refuse as it likes. As the organism grows and the early cells become surrounded by other cells (Fig. 1) the resources of the deep cells become more and more limited, since the environmental substances must penetrate between surrounding cells to reach them and in doing so must be conditioned by the catabolic products of the surrounding cells. So the environment of the deep cell is changed and thus its metabolic pattern must change if the cell is to survive. Changes in the intracytoplasmic chemistry may result in changes in the nuclear hereditary apparatus and thus, by means of the somatic hereditary factor, differentiation and specialization are achieved to the point of stable maturity.

When the state of maturation is complete we may expect a cell to faithfully reproduce its kind in the normal, physiologic repair of necrobiosis. However, if its environmental resources are altered by changes in blood supply or changes in the selective dispersion of its surrounding, intercellular supportive components, one may find alterations in its heredity mechanism which result in offspring which differ from the mother cell. These differences may be forecalculated when the environmental changes are known. When the heredity alteration is reversible we call this change in morphology and function "metaplasia," a physiologic or near-physiologic process. Disturbances in cell health and growth patterns sufficient to induce tissue changes constitute the lesions of disease. It is the understanding of these lesions, a recognition of their morphologic and functional characteristics, that is the field of interest of the pathologist.

The Development of Cells

The primitive mesoderm is a pleomorphic tissue substance which arises in the very early stages of embryologic development. As one examines it through the microscope one sees a mound of stellate and reticulated cells in a gel matrix (Fig. 2). As the celomic cavity develops, the cells on the cavity surface, and thus the cells which come to line the cavity, swell and line up in a single layer. Their rounded free surfaces characterize their cell type which we may designate as primitive mesothelium. It is of interest that wherever mesodermal tissue or one of its derivatives borders on a natural space or cavity, such as the lumina of blood vessels, the pericardial, pleural or peritoneal cavities or the joint or tendon spaces, they tend to take this shape. These are known generally in their mature, differentiated state as endothelial or simply mesothelial cells. In the vessels they retain their name of endothelial cells. Lining the major body cavities they are called serosal cells and when they face joint and tendon spaces they are designated synovial cells (Fig. 57, page 76).

The reticulated portion of the mesoderm forms a syncytium. Deposits of this syncytium are best seen in the mature organism in the spleen, the lymph nodes and scattered lymph follicles, and in the bone marrow. Apparently the differences of environment condition its morphology and function, for though there are similarities, the functions particularly of marrow, spleen and lymph node reticulum appear to

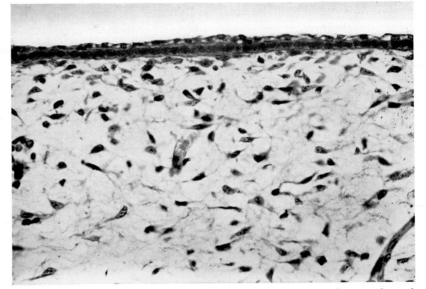

FIG. 2.   A section through the wall of the celomic cavity of an early embryo. The clear area above represents celomic cavity. There is a mound of primitive mesodermal cells. They are spindled and stellate, connected by a cobweb tracery of fibrillae in a gel ground substance. This substance condenses and the cells differentiate into the various mesenchymal derivatives. The cells which abut on an enclosed space (the celomic cavity in this illustration) thicken and flatten to form mesothelial cells. Depending upon the space which they enclose they become endothelial (vessel), serosal (peritoneum and pleura) or synovial (joint) cells. In an edematous (myxomatous) environment the various derivatives in postnatal life may revert back to the primitive mesenchyme morphology.

differ. One of the functions of reticulum is the production of motile cells. Those of the myelogenous reticulum, that of the bone marrow, concern the orthopedic pathologist (Fig. 52, page 72).

From the reticulated cells of the primitive mesoderm comes a multipotent cell which gives rise to derivatives other than the mesothelium and reticulum (Fig. 3). These cells form a primitive, reticulated, widely disseminated tissue which is known as mesenchyme. Its cells soon differentiate, depending upon their position and environment, into a variety of forms and these, the mesenchymal derivatives, that is, bone, cartilage, connective tissue, muscle and fat, make up the bulk of tissue which concerns those interested in orthopedic pathology.

The metabolic processes of some of these cells result in the accumulation of respiratory pigment known as myoglobin. The cells elongate and form intercellular fibrillae. Some develop cross striations and form skeletal muscle cells while others fail to form striations and mature into involuntary muscle.

Others of this same stem cell type begin to accumulate droplets of lipid material. These droplets coalesce to form a solid accumulation which distends the cell membrane and pushes the nucleus to one side, eventually flattening it against the cell wall. These cells usually form in aggregates and eventually the cytoplasmic membranes of many rupture and lakes of neutral fat are formed between the cells. Thus fat deposits are formed throughout the body, these deposits acting as storehouses of energy. These aggregates of fat cells fill in the angles and crevices, especially of moving parts such as muscles and tendons. Within the medullary areas of bone the fat cells take over the regions previously occupied by the marrow as it progressively shrinks during the aging process. Within the long bones, however, these fat cells retain their conversion potentialities and, under certain conditions of functional marrow destruction, may supply the bed for new marrow

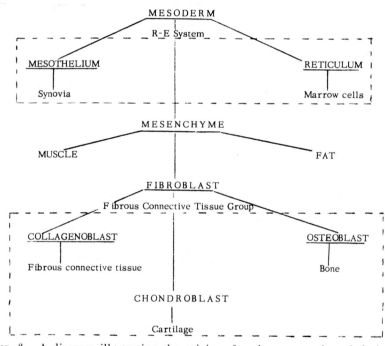

FIG. 3.   A diagram illustrating the origins of various mesenchymal derivatives. From the mesoderm comes the mesothelium which, depending upon its environment, differentiates into endothelium, serosa or synovial lining cells (Fig. 2). From it also comes the reticulum which persists in postnatal life in most body tissues but is concentrated in certain stations—the bone marrow and the lymph nodes, spleen and intestinal lymph follicles. The specialization of other forms depends upon their locations. Marrow reticulum gives rise to the myelogenous series of cells producing principally leukocytes and red cells. Mesenchyme comes from the primitive mesoderm and differentiates to produce a number of forms: muscle, both striated and nonstriated, fat and a group, the intercellular matrix of which is composed largely of fibers. This groups evolves by way of a cell which, because of this matrix, is best called the fibroblast. The morphology of the mature cell is related to the type of matrix, the collagenoblast (usually called fibroblast) in collagen, the chondroblast in hyalin and the osteoblast in osteoid.

proliferation. The available, unneeded neutral fat of the dietary intake certainly plays an important role in the aggregate number of the lipo-blasts (eventually, the lipocytes) but the distribution of the fat deposits is controlled, apparently to some extent, by endocrine influence.

The Fibroblast and Its Derivatives

A more differentiated form of the mesenchyme remains throughout the life of the organism. The cells of this stage of mesenchymal development seem to have no generally recognized name though the name best suited to them is "fibroblast." This term suggests that they are fiber-producing and, indeed, this is the most important character common to each of the three mature cell types, the collagen-producing fibrocyte (collagenoblast), the bone-producing osteocyte and the cartilage-producing chondrocyte, which come from them. This cell, the fibroblast, is a remarkably labile form which apparently differentiates into any one of three directions, each of the three resultant specialized forms constituting one of the components of what we know as connective tissue. These are fibrous connective tissue, cartilage and bone. It is of great importance that any one of the early or blast forms of these cell types may, upon alteration of its environmental circumstance, undergo conversion to any of the other forms within the fibrous tissue group, and perhaps outside the group they may change to fat, reticular and mesothelial forms and possibly even to non-striated muscle, though conversion to fat and especially muscle is denied by many histologists.

The cells of this basic fiber-producing group vary considerably in size but their average diameter is about that of the ordinary macrophage (Fig. 29, page 52). Their nuclei resemble those of macrophages and they, too, are motile in a liquid medium. They may phagocytize particulate matter. Indeed, but for the degree of their motility and phagocytic activity it is doubtful if they can be differentiated from macrophages (Fig. 25, page 50), and there is reason to believe that any differences that exist are those of environmental influence rather than genetic background.

The collagenoblast, that is, the collagen-producing cell usually called fibroblast, can be differentiated from the fibrous tissue blast form only when there is production of collagen about it. As this cell ages it elongates to a thin spindle with pointed ends to each of which is attached a long, fine argentophilic fibril (Fig. 30, page 53). As it multiplies and matures it comes to lie in a more or less homogeneous (at ordinary microscope magnification) matrix (Fig. 31, page 53). Its growth pattern suggests either that the matrix is formed by the maturing fibroblasts or at least that these cells are instrumental in its production. The nucleus becomes elongated and pyknotic until eventually it becomes a thick, short black line with hematoxylin staining. The cytoplasmic borders are lost in the collagen matrix. The latter stains a buff to a strong pink with eosin, brown with colloidal silver, green with trichrome and blue with Mallory's stain. It should be emphasized that the mature fibrocyte is a fully differentiated, distinctive form but that its young, blast form cannot be differentiated from the young forms of the chondroblast and osteoblast except by the presence of collagen.

The chondroblast separates itself from the pool of undifferentiated fibroblasts and can be identified at first only by the hyalin which is laid down in its proximity and by the blue-gray tint it acquires with hematoxylin staining. The nature of this staining reaction has been investigated by Lillie[1] who has shown that it is probably due to the presence of considerable amounts of ribose nucleic acid. As it matures it swells and comes to lie in a space (the lacuna) within the hyalin matrix. The space is actually an artefact since the cell is so exceedingly fragile that ordinary processing for microscopic examination causes it to shrink away from the more durable hyalin walls. The microscopist rarely has an opportunity of studying the cytologic detail of the chondrocyte because of this distortion. As the hyalin is being laid down, the cell multiplies so that clusters of two, three, four or more cells are found caught in the matrix (Fig. 36, page 56). Hyalin with ordinary magnification has a glassy or powdery, homogeneous appearance with a pale to medium blue color when stained with hematoxylin. The blue color with hematoxylin is apparently due to its chief constituent, chondroitin sulfate.

The osteoblast in the resting stage likewise cannot be differentiated from the young forms of the other two types of connective tissue (Fig. 40, page 60). In enchondral bone formation the cells line up in a single row along the face of a calcified hyalin bar and then usually become cuboidal in shape (Fig. 41, page 61). As they swell their cytoplasm takes on a gray blue tint with hematoxylin. Follis[2] has investigated this phenomenon and by special staining technique has concluded that it is due to an unusually high component of ribose nucleic acid. He points out that since chondroblasts and osteoblasts are involved in the production of the intercellular substances, hyalin and osteoid, which are composed largely of proteins, the cytoplasmic ribose nucleic acid may be significant and vital to this function. He has noted that this staining reaction disappears in scurvy[3] and osteogenesis imperfecta, conditions in which there is failure of osteoid production.

A band of homogeneous material appears between the hyalin bar and the row of cells. This is osteoid, called an osteoid seam, and but for its tendency to take a somewhat deeper eosin stain its appearance is that of collagen until it is mineralized.

From the above cell descriptions it might be assumed that the blast cell of connective tissue, the fibroblast, is merely the resting form of the young fibrocyte, chondrocyte and osteocyte, and perhaps the lipocyte and reticulum cell, and that it awaits only the proper environmental stimulus to start it on its path of differentiation. Such may well be the case, but one must be careful about assuming that because cells are morphologically identical they are, therefore, functionally and genetically the same. Until we have more accurate and detailed methods of studying intracytoplasmic metabolism, we must consider the matter unsettled.

REFERENCES

1. Lillie, R. D.: Anat. Rec., *103*:611, 1949.
2. Follis, R. H.: Bull. Johns Hopkins Hosp., *85*:281, 1949.
3. Follis, R. H.: Bull. Johns Hopkins Hosp., *89*:9, 1951.

2

Intercellular Components of Connective Tissue

The cells that make up the connective tissues of the body are morphologically identical in their young forms. As they mature and differentiate, each of the three types of cells is identified by the intercellular substance which is laid down in its proximity. The collagenoblast (fibroblast) is identified with collagen, the chondroblast with hyalin and the osteoblast with osteoid.

In their early stages the intercellular substances are quite similar in appearance with ordinary magnification and their chemical components are almost the same with some variation in the relative amounts of various constituents. But, owing to certain factors in the maturation process, the physical characteristics of the three substances become quite different. Collagen is firm, fibrous and pliable. Hyalin is hard, resilient and usually not pliable. Mineralized osteoid is stony hard and rigid.

COLLAGEN

When examined by the electron microscope, collagen is found to be composed of four constituents, collagen fibers (Fig. 4), which make up the preponderant part, reticulin, elastin and ground substance.

The collagen fibers occur in bundles of parallel fibrils which can be seen with the ordinary microscope. With electronic magnification the fibrils are found to be long, slender and non-branching with periodic cross bars spaced at about 640 Ångström units.[1] The sub-

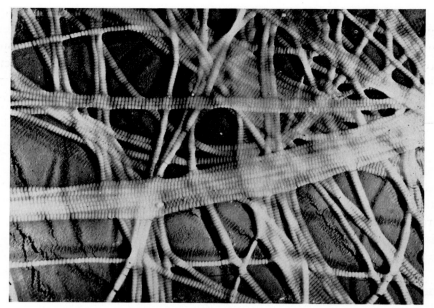

FIG. 4.   Collagen fibrils ($\times$ 18,300) taken with the electron microscope. They have been shadowed with chromium. (Courtesy of Drs. Gross and Schmitt, Massachusetts Institute of Technology.)

stance of collagen fibers is considered to be a fibrous protein; that is, it is composed of an arrangement of extended parallel polypeptide chains.[2] When heated in water it becomes soluble and forms a gel, in contrast to the corpuscular proteins found in serum albumin and globulin and hemoglobin which are denatured by heat and become less soluble. It is digested by collagenase such as that extracted from cultures of Type A Clostridium welchii but is not digested by trypsin and other proteolytic enzymes.

The reticulin components of collagen are much finer fibrils than the collagen fibers. In young collagen they appear as a network of wavy, branching argentophilic threads which are cross banded in approximately the same periodicity as collagen fibers. X-ray diffraction studies fail to reveal any essential chemical differences between reticulin and collagen fibers. Reticulin is abundant in young collagen but becomes increasingly more difficult to demonstrate as collagen ages. It has been suggested that reticulin is but the first stage of collagen fiber formation and that the former merges to form the latter.

The exact chemical properties of elastin, the third fibrillar constituent of collagen, are unknown. It is thought to have a molecular structure similar to that of rubber, and with the electron microscope it is found to appear as coarse filaments without periodic banding, supporting this theory.

The ground substance of collagen is composed of a group of mucopolysaccharides. These are made up principally of hexosamine and hexuronic acid. Of the three known mucopolysaccharides, chondroitin sulfate, hyaluronate and heparin, the first two have been identified in the ground substance. Of the several types of chondroitin sulfate perhaps four are found in various types of connective tissue. Chondroitin sulfate and hyaluronate are sugars in which a hydroxyl group is replaced by an amine group. They are chemically similar except that chondroitin sulfate contains ester sulfate groups while hyaluronate contains only the carboxyl group. The various types of mucopolysaccharides depend upon the type of sugar of which they are composed; for example, hyaluronate is a glucosamine and chondroitin sulfate, a galactosamine. The connective tissue mucopolysaccharides exist in a highly polymerized state. Hyaluronidase causes depolymerization.

The periodic acid–fuchsin reaction is currently regarded as the most practical method of demonstrating the presence of mucopolysaccharide in tissues. This test is sometimes referred to as the Hotchkiss-McManus stain or the periodic-Schiff reaction. This staining method depends upon the oxidation of a polysaccharide with periodic acid to yield an aldehyde. The product then gives a red to purple color when treated with the basic fuchsin reagent. Starch and glycogen may first be removed from the tissue by treating with amylase. Unfortunately, this reaction is apparently not specific for mucopolysaccharides and some tissues which are known to contain mucopolysaccharides do not stain with these reagents.

The phenomenon of metachromasia has also been used to demonstrate the presence of mucopolysaccharides, and particularly to define their state of polymerization. This test is sometimes called the Feulgen reaction. It depends upon the substitution of a methyl group for a hydrogen ion of an amino group. This change in chemical composition results in a change in color of certain absorbed dyes, usually from magenta to violet. Basic fuchsin is often used just as it is used in the last part of the Hotchkiss-McManus method. The term metachromasia is applied to the property of a tissue which causes this color change. Toluidine blue, also used, is changed to a reddish purple color by metachromatic substances. Depolymerized mucopolysaccharides are less metachromatic when stained with these dyes.

The Hale reaction is considered by some to be a more specific test than the two mentioned above. It depends upon the use of dialyzed iron which is bound to the amino acid groups. This iron will then give the Prussian blue reaction.

The ground substance of collagen varies considerably in its physical properties. It may take the form of a rather firm cement which acts as a binding substance for the endothelial cells of vessels, as a gel or as a liquid. These states apparently depend upon its water-binding properties. It appears that some portions of collagen ground substance may be in the gel state and other portions liquid but it is probable that the two are coextensive.[3] The mucopolysaccharides form the matrix substance which fills in the spaces between the various types of fibers.

Until relatively recent years the principal function ascribed to the connective tissues was that of support. With advances in our knowledge of the physical and chemical nature of collagen a completely new concept of collagen physiology evolves. The interest has been fired by the recognition of a group of clinical entities which have been called the connective tissue or collagen diseases. Out of the research related to these diseases has come much of our knowledge concerning the normal anatomy and activity of collagen.

Certainly one of its most important functions is that of dispersion. It must be remembered that almost all of our so-called parenchymal cells are supported and surrounded by collagen. While much attention has been paid to the condition of the finer ramifications of the vessels, capillary permeability, and the like, in considering the metabolic resources of parenchymal cells, little has been said about the collagen through which metabolic substances must pass before they reach these cells. It appears, without much factual evidence to support the thesis, that the ground substance is the dispersing agent which selectively protects and supplies the parenchymal cells it supports. Thus it becomes one of the important water-binding (and dispersing) agents in the body. Likewise it probably acts as an ion exchange resin which plays an important part in the control of electrolyte flow. When the calcium and phosphorus ions are considered it is apparent that collagen physiology is of utmost importance in the mineral metabolism of bone.

HYALIN

Hyalin, like collagen, is made up of collagen fibrils, reticulin, elastin and ground substance (Fig. 5). The principal differences between hyalin cartilage, fibrocartilage and elastic cartilage depend upon the relative amounts of these various components. Since hyalin cartilage is found almost exclusively in relation to bone growth and joint surfaces, the term cartilage or hyalin without qualification refers to hyalin cartilage.

The matrix of hyalin cartilage is seen most typically in the chon-dral plate of the unossified epiphysis. With the light microscope it is seen as a homogeneous, translucent matrix substance taking a pale blue stain with hematoxylin. With the electron microscope it is found to have a feltwork of fibers. The proportion of mucopolysaccharide ground substance is said to be much greater than in either collagen or osteoid. There are at least two types of chondroitin sulfate in hyalin.

The hyalin of articular cartilage and that at some distance from the epiphyseal line of the chondral plate is highly polymerized. As the epiphyseal plate is approached the hyalin becomes depolymerized and loses its metachromasia. This is the area of provisional calcifica-tion and it is thought that the calcium salt molecules have inactivated the bonds which formerly captured the dye.

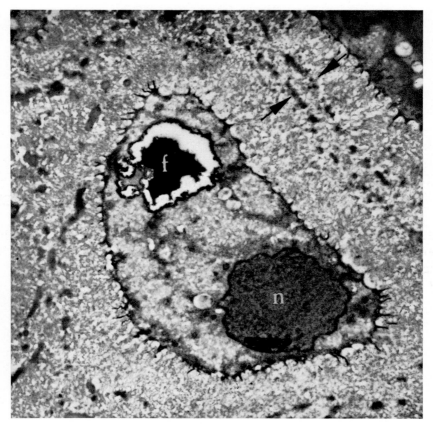

FIG. 5.   Electron micrograph of cartilage. The ovoid structure in the center is a chondrocyte with nucleus marked "n." Around this cell the cartilage matrix consists of a fine feltwork. Between the chondrocytes (the band between the two arrows) is a network of more dense substance ($\times$ 5000). (Courtesy of H. Sheldon and R. A. Robinson, Johns Hopkins University Medical School.)

OSTEOID

Through the ordinary microscope, osteoid is an eosin-staining, homogeneous substance which is morphologically identical with collagen. It is only its relationship to its osteoblasts or the advent of mineralization that distinguishes it with ordinary hematoxylin and eosin staining. Progress in the study of osteoid is much less advanced than for collagen and hyalin since mineralization follows close on the heels of normal osteoid production, thus interfering with study preparation. The demineralization processes are so rigorous that the application of data concerning decalcified bone to bone in its natural state is hazardous.

By piecing together the fragments of knowledge concerning the

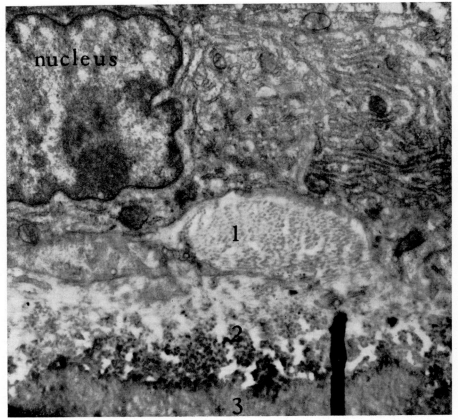

FIG. 6. *A*, Electron micrograph of a section of bone. The upper half of the photograph is an osteoblast with nucleus and cytoplasm. At 1 there is a bundle of collagen fibrils cut in cross section. At 2 the collagen fibrils are vested with an opaque coating which probably represents the earliest stage of accumulation of inorganic ions during calcification. This is the area of physiological osteoid. At 3 the osteoid is calcified ($\times$ 18,500). (From Sheldon, H. and Robinson, R. A.: J. Biophys. & Biochem. Cytol., vol. 13.)

chemical and physical properties of osteoid we may assume that they are much like those of hyalin and collagen, that is, that osteoid is made up of a feltwork of fibers in a ground substance (Fig. 6). It is reported that the ground substance is relatively less in amount and there is disagreement as to the presence of reticulin and especially elastin fibers.

Two other methods in addition to electron microscopy are being used to study the constituents of bone and the manner in which bone is laid down and mineralized. One of these, x-ray diffraction (Fig. 7), is a method whereby a beam of x-rays of less than 1 millimeter in diameter is passed through an object or solution and the pattern of diffraction recorded on a film. These patterns are highly characteristic within certain chemical groups when the spacings of the atoms are such as those seen in crystalline substances. Under these circumstances the diffraction pattern is characteristic of the chemical components of the material examined and offers a means of analysis of solid tissues without disruption of tissue structure.

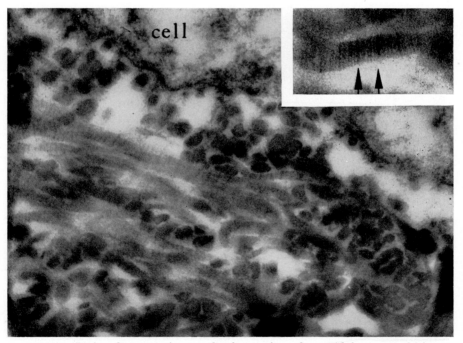

FIG. 6. *B*, An electron micrograph of a section of osteoid from a rachitic rat. At the upper right is pictured an osteoblast. Collagen fibrils are seen in the lower portion of the micrograph. The inset shows a greater magnification of a collagen fibril illustrating its periodic banding. The space between the arrows is about 640 Ångström units. Seven subbandings may be seen within the unit ($\times$ 60,000, inset $\times$ 100,000). (Courtesy of H. Sheldon and R. A. Robinson, Johns Hopkins University Medical School.)

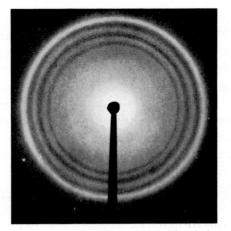

FIG. 7.   X-ray diffraction pattern of a piece of lamb bone. A very fine beam (less than 1 mm. in diameter) of x-rays is passed through an undemineralized section of bone. When the atomic constituents are arranged in space as they are in crystalline substances the chemical components can be read by the pattern of diffraction recorded on a film. (Courtesy of Drs. M. Spiegel-Adolf and G. Henny, Temple University Medical School.)

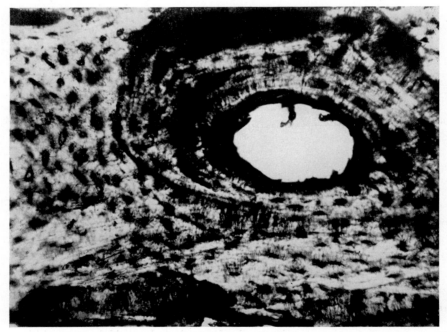

FIG. 8.   Microradiogram of an undemineralized bone section cut at about 70 microns. Lamellae are seen encircling the haversian canal with lacunae between them. The dark areas represent concentrations of opaque calcium salts. This method may be utilized to study relative mineral concentrations at the cellular level. ($\times$ 680.)

The other method is known as microradiography. A fine beam of
x-rays is passed through a section of undemineralized bone. These
sections are cut on a special microtome with an exceptionally heavy
blade of hardest steel. The films are then examined through the ordinary light microscope (Fig. 8) and when adjacent sections are used,
one prepared for microradiography and the other for routine staining,
the variations in opacity in the former reveal the pattern of lamellar
formation. By this method, relative densities can be appreciated which
are not demonstrable by transmitted light.

THE FORMATION OF INTERCELLULAR SUBSTANCE

Concerning the formation of connective tissue intercellular substance much has been written and little proven. Earlier writers, noting
that intercellular substance is found only in the presence of connective tissue cells, concluded that this material was produced and spun
out by the cells just as the substance of its web is secreted by the
spider. It became apparent, as tools for more detailed study became
available, that no such fiber production could be accorded with the
known facts of intracellular metabolism. Changing the course of investigation it was found that many of the factors of the intercellular
substance or the components which might be used in their synthesis
could be extracted from the proteins of the serum. It is thought, for
example, that normal ground substance is not formed in the ascorbic
acid deficiency state and that ground substance production begins
again when vitamin C is added. It has also been shown that hyalin
will not be normally produced in the absence of vitamin A.

The best guess seems to be that the various components of the
intercellular substance are built up as the result of molecular combinations which can occur only in the substrate provided by certain
chemical constituents perfusing from the blood stream and mingling
with the products secreted by the cells involved. Higgenbotham
believes that the fibroblasts ingest various mucopolysaccharides and
then elaborate certain constituents of the ground substance. Intensive
research is being carried on in this area at the present time and it is
hoped that within a short period definite information will be available.

THE DEPOSITION OF BONE SALTS

The mineral deposited in hyalin at the line of provisional calcification and in osteoid is not a simple chemical compound nor are
the chemical constituents constant in kind or amount. There appear

to be species differences, differences between members of the same species, between bones of the same organ and even between areas of the same bone. The chemical formula also differs with age and in bone disease. Whatever these differences may be, however, bone mineral always exists in the form of an apatite. An apatite is an arrangement in space of the various ions which make up the whole. Thus, if we attempt to write the formula for an apatite it would compare in a sense to the formula of a single room in a large building composed of numerous identical rooms. Four walls plus one ceiling plus one floor equals one room. However, this is not an independent structure for if one were able to remove a single room one would leave the six surrounding rooms incomplete. Thus, the structure of the crystals of bone mineral is made up of a lattice of ions in which one might find a representative area, but the removal of this area would destroy the integrity of the whole. A concept of this lattice structure is important in understanding the physiology of mineral metabolism.

Bone mineral is laid down in crystal form and the crystals maintain their individuality just as do the components of a brick wall. The crystals are thought to be flat and thin, approximating the shape of a hexagonal playing card. Though the exact relation of the mineral crystals to the various factors of the organic substance of bone is not definitely known as yet, it is thought that they are laid down within the ground substance, forming sheaths about the collagen fibers. Some mineral, in an amorphous state, may lie within the fibers themselves.

The formula for bone salt can best be approximated by that of a hydroxy apatite, thus: $3Ca_3(PO_4)_2 \cdot Ca(OH)_2$. It consists largely of Ca^{++}, $PO_4^{\equiv}$ and OH^- together with carbon dioxide, citrate and water. Other ions in trace amounts are Na^+, Mg^{++}, K^+, Cl^- and F^-.

The crystal configuration has been reviewed by Neuman and Neuman.[4] The constant and rapid turnover in normal bone explains the variability in composition at any given time. There appears to be a continuous interchange of ions between the crystal lattice and the fluid which bathes it. At times this may mean substitution of one mineral ion for another. Thus it becomes necessary to think of the rigid and seemingly permanent structure of bone as a dynamic system in a state of constant flux and, therefore, less static and fixed than the soft tissues which surround it.

In order to account for the facility with which ions are exchanged it is necessary to take into consideration the surface chemistry of the crystal lattice. If one chooses an area within the lattice in which there are represented all the ions in the proportions of the whole, we may call this area a unit. The crystal of bone salt is so thin that it is only a few of these units thick. A unit may exist within the depths of the lattice or in the surface and apparently the majority are in the latter position. Because of the unit structure of the crystalline component of bone, it has an immense surface area. Someone has estimated that the surface area of the mineral crystals in the skeleton of an average man probably exceeds a hundred acres. Since ions are apparently adsorbed on these surfaces and since the amount of fluid which bathes them is so relatively small that it must be a very thin layer indeed, it becomes easier to understand the remarkable facility with which the ionic composition of the lattice is kept in constant motion.

Of great importance to those interested in bone disease is the mechanism by which mineral salts are deposited in the organic matrix. Though the matter has been of major concern to a number of very able research workers, information which satisfies all of the known facts is still not available. Apparently several factors play a role in the mineralization of normal cartilage and bone. Much of the work has been done on in vitro specimens using the area of provisional calcification and the subchondral area of unmineralized osteoid of experimental rickets.

The pH of the area of mineral deposit is apparently of some importance. Mineralization will take place within the wide pH range of 6 to 8.5. On the alkaline side of pH 7.3 little is achieved by raising this figure. Change of the hydrogen ion concentration causes an increase in the phosphate ions but calcification in vitro is not enhanced, indicating that the pH itself is not critical.

The ion product of calcium and phosphate seems also of importance. However, the fact that it is not critical is shown by the same experiment and also by the fact that the ion concentration is considerably higher in the infant than in the adult, although, under proper conditions in the latter, mineral deposition proceeds unimpaired.

It was Robison[5] who first set forth the hypothesis that the alkaline phosphatase found in chondroblasts and osteoblasts is the local factor which results in the precipitation of calcium salt through the liberation of inorganic phosphate by the hydrolysis of phosphate ester. It is known that alkaline phosphatase brings about this result in the test tube. The idea was further enhanced by the description of the enzymatic degradation glycogenolysis that occurs in the mature chondrocytes as they approach the line of provisional calcification. It was necessary to abandon this theory when it was shown that glycogenolysis could not produce a substrate for the action of alkaline phosphatase and with the failure to demonstrate phosphate ester even in the absence of glycogenolysis. Then it was shown that calcification will take place in vitro, though apparently at a much slower rate, when all enzymes, including phosphatase, are inactivated. At present it is assumed that glycogenolysis must play some part in the process, though it may be no more specific than supplying the necessary energy. If phosphatase plays a role it may be in the production of the ground substance. Very little more of a definitive nature can be added at this time.

REFERENCES

1. Gross, J.: Structure and Biological Reactivity of Connective Tissue. In Ashford, M., Ed.: The Musculoskeletal System. New York, The Macmillan Co., 1952.
2. Shubert, M.: Chemistry of Connective Tissue. In Ashford, M., Ed.: The Musculoskeletal System. New York, The Macmillan Co., 1952.
3. McLean, F. C., and Urist, M. R.: Bone. Chicago, University of Chicago Press, 1955.
4. Neuman, W. F., and Neuman, M. W.: Chem. Rev., 53:1, 1953.
5. Robison, R.: Biochem. J., 17:256, 1923.

Normal Bone Production

At a very early time in embryonic development, fields of mesenchyme undergo condensation in the pattern of a model of the skeleton that is to be formed. The intercellular substance of the reticulated cell mass becomes increasingly more opaque until the skeletal pattern becomes distinct within the surrounding mesenchyme. The cells of this condensed mesenchyme then begin to swell and in a remarkably short time the whole apparatus takes on the appearance of a hyalin cartilage matrix in which are embedded young cartilage cells.

Transverse lines of division occur at intervals dividing the apparatus into bars, each of which represents the anlage of a future bone. The divisional lines represent the areas where joints will develop. At a certain period in the development of each bone a group of reticulated mesenchymal cells approximating the masses of primitive cartilage mature into fibroblasts. In the case of long bones this occurs as a collar about the middle of the hyalin bar (Fig. 9). Capillary buds from nearby vessels grow into this collar of fibroblasts and thus set up a focus of what is known as granulation tissue. Wherever an area of fibroblastic tissue becomes laced with a network of newly forming capillaries, whether it be in embryonic development or in the later repair of tissue injury, the resulting tissue is called granulation.

Granulation is simply highly vascularized young connective tissue. Wherever this highly vascularized tissue comes in contact with cartilage or bone, whether it be embryonic or quite mature, the cartilage and bone melt away before it. Thus, with the formation of a collar of granulation about the waist of the hyalin bar, the latter undergoes lysis and the granulation penetrates the bar from all points of its circumference until it forms a nucleus of fibroblasts and capillaries

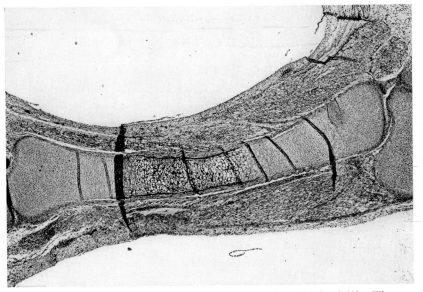

FIG. 9.   Low power photomicrograph of a bone in early fetal life. The mesenchymal tissue has thickened to form a cuff of periosteum about the mid-portion of
the cartilaginous bar. The underlying cartilage cells have become swollen with
glycogen in preparation for lysis and replacement with primitive fiberbone. ($\times$ 30.)

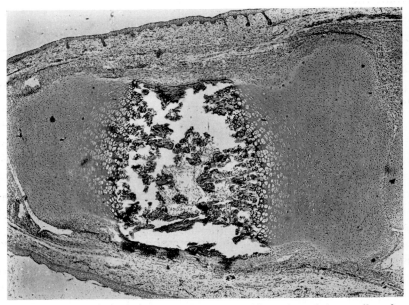

FIG. 10.   Primary center of ossification. The mid-portion of the cartilage bar has
ossified. A sphere of cartilage, the epiphysis, remains at each end. At the chondro-
osseous junction an epiphyseal line has formed. In the center of the bony portion,
the diaphysis, the bone is undergoing lysis and a few marrow cells are beginning to
appear. This embryonic bone now has all its component parts. ($\times$30.)

within its center. Even before completion of this activity the inter-fibroblastic substance in the wake of the advancing wedge becomes more dense and more eosinophilic and soon undergoes impregnation with bone salt. The fibroblasts of the vicinity take on the characteristics of osteoblasts and thus a cuff-like sheath of bone is laid down about the mid-portion of the cartilage bar. This sheath thickens and widens, extending out over the adjacent cartilage surfaces at either side. Thus is established the primary center of ossification (Fig. 10). At the same time the nucleus of vascularized fibroblastic tissue within the core is transformed into marrow reticulum. The structure now consists of a circle of bone surrounding a nucleus of marrow separating two masses of cartilage. About the whole structure the mesenchymal cells condense to form a thin fibrous capsule. Over the bone this fibrous tissue is called periosteum, over cartilage it is known as perichondrium.

Intramembranous Ossification

The periosteal tissue soon differentiates into two layers (Fig. 47, page 66). The outer and thicker layer is more dense and coarsely fibrillar, the inner is loose and more cellular. Where the cells of the inner layer, called the cambium, lie in contact with bone and cartilage, they soon become separated from them by a layer of pink-staining homogeneous substance which, because it soon becomes infiltrated with bone salt, one may call osteoid. Here and there these cells become caught in and surrounded by osteoid and then shrink to compact little cells with pyknotic nuclei within their cell space, the lacuna. They are now known as osteocytes. Successive layers of bone are laid down in concentric circles, each layer forming a lamina. Thus the compacta or the cortex of the diaphysis is formed. This manner of bone production, i.e., the formation of osteoid without a preformed hyalin scaffolding to shape the resultant osteoid mass, is known as intramembranous ossification. Since, in the mature skeleton, almost all of the compact bone of the shaft of long bones and nearly all of the flat bones have eventually come to be formed by this method, and since worn-out bone is so replaced in skeletal maintenance, intramembranous ossification accounts for the great bulk of the body's bone tissue.

Enchondral Ossification

The other manner of bone formation is known as enchondral ossification. Actually, it is essentially the same process, i.e., the transformation of fibroblasts into osteoblasts about which accumulates an

intercellular organic matrix of osteoid. But in enchondral bone formation the osteoid production is always guided by a pattern of preformed, calcified hyalin. Because the steps in the production of this
hyalin scaffolding are numerous, enchondral ossification is much more
complex.

In general it appears that bone mass is largely the result of intramembranous ossification whereas directional bone growth is accomplished principally by enchondral bone formation. The length growth
of cylindrical bones comes about through the latter and the width
or strength growth through the former.

Although similar, the two processes should be kept distinct. The
configuration of the skeleton, and thereby the conformity of the body,
are governed by the relative amounts of each type of growth. Moreover, some of the various diseases which affect skeletal formation,
growth and maintenance affect but one type of ossification. There
is also reason to believe that some of the various governing factors in
bone formation, particularly within the endocrine group, may affect
one or the other but not both mechanisms.

While the bone collar of primary ossification is forming, a frontier
of advancement is set up at either pole of the nucleus of marrow
tissue. This line is established at the junction of the marrow and the
spheroid masses of cartilage at either end of the structure. These
cartilage masses are now called the epiphyses, the line of junction is
called the epiphyseal line, the connecting cylinder of bone is known
as the diaphysis and the regions at either end of the diaphysis where
enchondral bone formation takes place to form cancellous tissue are
called the metaphyses.

The epiphysis is at first composed of a homogeneous body of
cartilage, with single chondroblasts, each in its lacuna, evenly dispersed
in a matrix of hyalin. Then the chondroblasts in the vicinity of the
epiphyseal line begin to enlarge, the lacuna is expanded, the cytoplasm takes on a basophilic staining quality with hematoxylin and
in it accumulates a substance which takes the glycogen stain. The
nucleus appears to imbibe water which breaks up the chromatin and
pushes it to the periphery beneath the nuclear membrane. In maturation the cytoplasm accumulates small globules of lipid. In enlarging,
the cell becomes flattened, its axis parallel to the epiphyseal line. This
widening of the cells and their surrounding lacunae appears to occur
at either side, in the direction of the cells closest by. The result is
that the cells interdigitate and come to lie in columns the axes of
which are perpendicular to the epiphyseal line (Fig. 35, page 56).
Between the columns the unaffected hyalin remains as an acellular

bar which separates or actually, in three dimensions, surrounds the columns.

Special techniques now will reveal the presence of enzymes, including alkaline phosphatase and succinic dehydrogenase,[1] within the cells, and at a certain point of maturation of the cartilage cells, i.e., at a certain level of the cell columns, bone salts begin to appear in the intervening hyalin bars. This is known as the line of provisional calcification. At this stage of maturation the glycogen disappears from the cytoplasm. Thus, it is assumed that it is utilized in some manner in the activity which results in the deposition of mineral salt. Each of the greatly enlarged cells, now known as mature chondrocytes, is separated from its neighbor cells on either side by a thin partition of hyalin. The lower margin of the lowest cells in the columns establishes the position of the epiphyseal line. The metaphyseal side of these cells are now exposed to the highly vascularized granulation at either pole of the marrow nucleus. The hyalin wall of the cells gives way, the chondrocyte is devoured by waiting phagocytes and granulation penetrates into the bay that is thus formed. Thus the granulation works its way up the column, cell after cell, the last intact cell establishing the level of the epiphyseal line. So the epiphyseal frontier advances, leaving in its wake in the metaphyseal area the intact calcified bars of hyalin which formerly separated (surrounded) the cellular columns, protruding into the granulation like parallel docks extending into a harbor.

It is apparent that unless fresh cartilage cells were added to the epiphysis the advancing epiphyseal line would soon spend the available supply and epiphyseal advancement would necessarily cease. New chondroblasts are supplied by division of the young chondroblasts in the depths of the epiphysis—interstitial proliferation—and by metaplasia of the fibroblasts in the deep layers of the surrounding perichondrium—appositional proliferation. As they mature they go through the same cycle as their predecessors. They swell with glycogen, take on enzymatic activity, their cytoplasm develops a blue color with hematoxylin and they columnate and apparently cause mineralization of the surrounding hyalin. Thus the epiphysis is continuously being replenished at one pole and dissipated at the other and length growth of the bone is accomplished by the chondroblastic addition.

The bars of mineralized hyalin which protrude into the metaphyseal granulation form the scaffolding upon which osteoid is to be laid. This is known as the hyalin lattice. With the appearance of these bars, the adjacent undifferentiated fibroblasts migrate to form a single layer covering the bars (Fig. 41, page 60). They change from a spindled to a cuboidal shape and alkaline phosphatase appears in their cytoplasm. Soon a layer of eosinophilic material appears between the cells and the hyalin bar. This is called the osteoid seam (Fig. 41, page 60). This seam surrounds the hyalin bar which becomes less deeply stained, then vacuolated and eventually disappears altogether. In the meantime, however, bone has been laid down to form a lacework of spicules, the primary spongiosa of the medullary area, in a matrix of marrow cells.

The bone of the primary spicules is coarsely fibrillar, the fibrillae run in undisciplined, patternless directions, and the numerous cells that are caught within their ramifications are young and plump. This material is known as primitive bone or coarse fiberbone (Fig. 43, page 63). As these spicules age they appear to dissolve, perhaps because of the lack of a stress stimulus which appears to be necessary for the persistence and health of all bone tissue. The resolving fragments, however, serve as the nidi for a new coat of osteoid laid down by more mature osteoblasts. This time the fibrillar structure is finer, the fibrillae are longer and run in parallel bundles in the trajectory lines of stress (Fig. 44, page 64). Fewer cells are trapped and they are smaller and more mature, now called osteocytes. These spicules form the secondary spongiosa.

Where the mass of bone necessary to withstand the stress to which it is exposed is greater than a few lamellae in thickness, the lamellae are laid down in concentric rings about a blood vessel, thus insuring a supply of blood to the contained osteocytes. The larger vessels travel in a longitudinal direction and thus their surrounding bone sheaths are oriented in the same direction except where a branch passes horizontally to connect two longitudinal vessels. The spaces carrying vessels (and accompanying nerves and supportive fibrous tissue) are known as haversian canals (Fig. 46, page 66) and the concentric laminae of bone, oriented with them, make up a haversian system. The tunnels carrying the connecting vessels are known as Volkmann's canals.

A cross section through the full thickness of the cortex (compacta) reveals numerous haversian canals (Fig. 50, page 70), circular hiatuses bearing the blood vessels and running longitudinally, parallel to the periosteal surface. These canals are formed by sheaths of bone appearing in cross section as circles and crescents. Each canal and its multilayered sheath of lamellae forms a haversian system. The irregular areas which fill in the regions between the haversian systems are also composed of lamellar bone but the concentric arrangement is lacking. These are known as interstitial lamellae. In most adult bone the major portion of the thickness of the lamellae is ensheathed by several lamellae which encircle the entire circumference of the shaft beneath the periosteum. In some bones one may find a sheath of several lamellae lining the inner cortical surface about the medullary canal.

At a certain period in the development and maturation of each bone a column of granulation invades the spheroid cartilaginous mass of the epiphysis from the perichondrium and penetrates into its very center. Here an aggregate of proliferating connective tissue cells is established just as in the wedge of granulation that resulted in the primary center of ossification. And in a like manner a nucleus of marrow cells surrounded by a shell of mineralized bone is formed. The chondroblasts in the depths of the epiphysis which are now adjacent to bone respond in the same manner as those along the epiphyseal line. They enlarge, flatten and columnate and set up a new zone of provisional calcification which in this case is a spheroid shell rather than a flat plate. This nucleus of bone is called the secondary center of ossification or the epiphyseal ossification center or, in practical usage, simply the center of ossification since the primary ossification center has long since disappeared. Radiologists are apt to refer to the secondary center of ossification as "the epiphysis." As this center grows it flattens, its broad surfaces facing the pole and the epiphyseal line. Thus, it tends to divide the original cartilaginous epiphysis into two plates of cartilage, one bounding the joint space called the articular plate and the other separating the osseous portion of the epiphysis from the diaphysis known as the epiphyseal or enchondral plate.

The time of the appearance of the secondary center of ossification is specific for each bone. It is present in the distal femoral epiphysis at birth but does not appear in some other bones until much later in skeletal growth.

Length growth of the cylindrical bones is thus accomplished by the apposition of new bone at the ends of the diaphysis. Frequently the rate of growth is not equal at both ends. The femur acquires most of its length growth by bone apposition at the distal end. The ulna and radius do the same. The proximal end is that of major growth in the humerus whereas the tibia has approximately equal growth at both ends.

As the time of completion of length growth is approached, the proliferation of chondroblasts in the epiphysis slows and eventually ceases. Thus in a short time the chondrocytes of the epiphyseal plate are exhausted and the epiphyseal line advances to the diaphyseal surface of the secondary center of ossification. When no cartilage remains separating the diaphysis from the bony epiphysis the center of ossification is said to be closed. From this point hence, length growth is at an end. A line of junction can be discerned on the roentgenogram for a considerable time but eventually this is obliterated by bony union.

The articular plate remains as a cap of hyalin cartilage covering the end of the bone. The time of closure for each epiphysis is specific. The condylar cartilage of the mandible is the last to ossify, normally in the late twenties. Thus, by mapping the time of appearance and ossification of the various secondary centers throughout the skeleton one can often calculate its age, if it be under twenty-five years, within a few months.

In a general way it may be stated that the human organism, in the course of his development, has three types of skeletons and that he changes these skeletons with growth just as does the crustacean who wears his skeleton on the outside. The first skeleton is composed of flexible cartilage, adequate in situations where coordinated movement is unimportant and where support is provided by the surrounding uterine walls. Since the skeleton is still moderately flexible at parturition, this flexibility lessens the danger of traumatic injury in the passage of the fetus through the narrow birth canal.

The second skeleton is composed of primitive fiberbone and this type of bone predominates throughout the first eighteen months of life. It is more rigid than cartilage and more resilient than adult bone. This type of bone is found in the marine vertebrates which must have coordinated movement but are supported by their environment. It is adequate for the infant who spends much of his time in the prone position.

When both support and movement are essential to the organism the primitive bone must be replaced by a more rigid structure laid down in the trajectory lines of stress. Thus, there is a gradual replacement of coarse fiberbone by the finer grained, oriented adult bone which is constructed along the pathways of greatest stress. In a sense, these changes in skeleton type constitute a phylogenetic recapitulation of the species.

Empirically, it may be said that the preponderance of bone mass and the cortical thickness of long bones are produced by intramembranous ossification. The length and shape of long bones are governed by enchondral ossification and the forces of stress. It is interesting that in certain skeletal diseases these two processes appear to rely upon different governing mechanisms.

REFERENCE

1. Follis, R. H., and Berthrong, M.: Bull. Johns Hopkins Hosp., 85:281, 1949.

4

Essential Factors in Normal Bone Production

Though enchondral bone formation is a continuing process, the various steps, which merge imperceptibly one into another often with considerable chronologic overlap, may be listed as follows:

1. Proliferation of epiphyseal chondroblasts to maintain normal thickness of the epiphyseal plate.

2. The formation of intercellular hyalin.

3. Maturation of chondroblasts with the acquisition of glycogen and enzymatic activity, enlargement and rearrangement into columns.

4. Mineralization of the hyalin bars to form the line of provisional calcification.

5. Invasion of the bases of the cartilage cell columns by the metaphyseal granulation.

6. Maturation of primitive fibroblastic cells to osteoblasts.

7. The production of the organic matrix of bone, osteoid.

8. The deposition of mineral salts within the osteoid.

9. The resolution of the hyalin cores of the spicules of the primary spongiosa.

10. The conversion of coarse fiberbone to adult bone to form the secondary spongiosa.

11. Modeling of young bones to attain the shape of the adult structure.

12. Bone maintenance, i.e., the replacement of bone which is being constantly eroded by normal catabolic activity.

It is apparent that these steps form a continuing chronologic chain and that a deviation at any link may result in an abnormal skeletal structure which one associates with bone disease. A great many of the factors which control normal skeleton formation, growth and maintenance are unknown, but it is evident that if one is to successfully prevent these deviations or to reverse them, once they are diagnosed, to a state of bone health an understanding of these factors is essential. The following is a résumé of what is known and what is assumed concerning some of these factors.

The discussion may be presented under three broad headings:

1. Factors related to the formation of the organic matrix of normal cartilage and bone.

2. Factors related to the deposition of mineral salt in the organic matrix of cartilage and bone.

3. Factors related to the normal lysis of cartilage and bone to allow for conversion from primitive to adult bone, modeling of young to mature bones and maintenance of adult bone to compensate for physiologic erosion.

Factors Related to the Formation of the Organic Matrix

DIET.   It has long been known that the level of the dietary caloric intake influences the ultimate skeletal stature. Presumptive evidence may be drawn from a comparison of averages of skeletal size in a race which is known to exist on a bare subsistence diet, such as those in certain parts of China and India, with a race whose caloric intake is adequate and above, such as the American. It is not inferred that an inadequate caloric intake affects the skeleton only. It is probable that skeletal growth is inhibited as a part of the general low metabolic state of all tissues.

In more specific instances the diet may lack certain essential food stuffs which are required for normal bone growth and maintenance. Among these, certain proteins probably head the list. It is interesting that the "essential amino acids" listed by the physiologic chemists as necessary for a state of body health have not been identified in cartilage and bone analysis. The amino acids which are involved in bone structure are abundant in ordinary diets. Never the less it is thought by most that the fastidious and often whimsical diets of the aged often constitute a factor in senile osteoporosis, and the leaching of skeletons of war populations in a state of chronic starvation (Fig. 11) may be due, at least in part, to qualitative dietary deficiencies.

It was Wolbach[1] who, in 1947, pointed out that a certain amount of vitamin A in one of its forms is necessary for normal epiphyseal cartilage cell growth, maturation, degeneration and bone modeling. It appears that chondroblasts do not mature properly nor calcified hyalin matrix normally resolve in the vitamin A deficiency state. It has also been shown that with inadequate amounts of this vitamin there is failure of normal resolution of bone, though surface apposition of bone is not impaired, so that normal modeling cannot take place. Since, in the experimental animal excessive vitamin A levels cause abnormal deossification, one is led to the conjecture that vitamin A may be a control factor in cartilage and bone lysis. Were this based in fact one might be led to further conjecture that certain conditions such as chondro-osteodystrophy (Morquio's disease), which appears to be a fault in chondroblastic maturation and fiberbone conversion, and osteopetrosis, which may be the result of excessive organic matrix production without compensating bone lysis, could be related to a congenital refractory state to vitamin A. Since other features of vitamin A deficiency have not been reported, if investigated, in these cases the conjecture is more interesting than practical.

In the experimental animal an ascorbic acid deficiency results in metabolic disturbances in the tissues of mesenchymal derivation. In the human the bleeding phenomena, inadequate scar formation in wound healing and deficiencies in organic bone matrix formation with

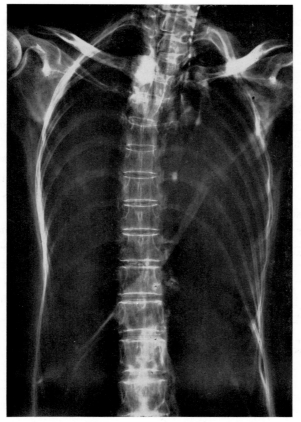

FIG. 11.   Roentgenogram of a patient showing severe starvation osteoporosis. This patient lived for months before her death on a daily ration of a few soda crackers and a cup of tea.

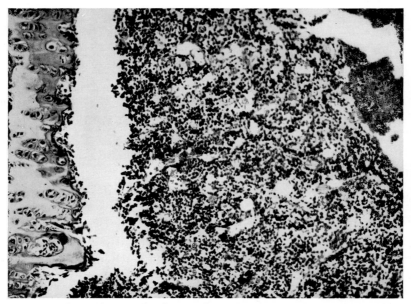

FIG. 12.   Photomicrograph of a section taken across the epiphyseal line in a case of scurvy. There is a complete lack of osteoid production and, therefore, no cancellous bone in the metaphysis. (× 200.)

low ascorbic acid blood levels suggest that this substance is essential for the formation of normal collagen and osteoid. The manifestations of childhood scurvy as seen in the skeleton can all be ascribed to hemorrhage and an inability of the osteoblasts to lay down osteoid (Fig. 12).

HORMONAL DISTURBANCES.   Disturbances in endocrine hormone secretion quite certainly can be incriminated in certain abnormal skeletal conditions. It has long been known that atrophy and destruction of the anterior lobe of the pituitary are frequently associated with various types of dwarfism, and an abnormal proliferation of eosinophilic cells has been seen in states of skeletal overgrowth, giantism and acromegaly. More recently a growth hormone has been isolated from the glandular portion of the hypophysis cerebri. To date insufficient quantities have been extracted and inadequate time has elapsed to fully evaluate this hormone, but it is known that there is cessation of bone growth without closure of the secondary ossification centers in the hypophysectomized animal and that growth may be restored with the growth hormone. It appears also that closure of the ossification centers may be delayed beyond the normal period with this hormone, the epiphyseal plate retaining its normal thickness. The exact point of influence is not known but it would seem at this writing that the growth hormone governs both chondroblastic and osteoblastic activity and, therefore, registers its effect on enchondral bone growth. It is not anticipated that the pituitary growth hormone will greatly reduce, by therapeutic use, the distressing consequences of pituitary dysfunction, since in most practical cases aberrations in eosinophilic cell secretion are accompanied by perversions of other pituitary hormone production.

Children born with inadequate thyroid secretory function fail to develop a normal skeletal stature and in cases of excessive thyroid secretion there is abnormal deossification of the bone that has already been formed. Again it is not known at which link in the complicated chain of bone growth the inadequacy is registered but the effect appears to be predominantly upon enchondral bone formation so that the stature is dwarfed. The result of inadequate thyroid function appears to be quite similar to that of deficient pituitary hormone secretion. The skeletal leaching which occurs in the severe and prolonged thyrotoxic state has been ascribed to a squandering of the essential proteins necessary for bone maintenance by the exaggerated basal metabolic rate. This explanation appears to be based purely upon assumption.

Concerning the steroid hormones elaborated by the gonads and the adrenal cortex, there is even less factual information and one is apt to find that a perusal of the reports available leads to contradictory findings. It is perhaps true that gonadal androgen stimulates both enchondral and intramembranous bone growth. Such has been ascribed to be the reason why the male skeleton is usually larger and heavier than that of the female.[2] The results of some studies suggest that the period of skeletal growth at which the abnormal gonadal function occurs is an important factor. If castration in the male is accomplished before puberty there may be an increase in long bone growth. In general, it is probably true that gonadal androgen stimulates both length and width growth in the bones of animals and the adolescent human.

The adrenal cortical androgen or so-called N hormone is generally regarded as the anabolic hormone for all protein-rich tissues. The effects of the sugar active hormones from the adrenal cortex which are supposed to produce deossification similar to that seen in Cushing's syndrome are thought by some to rob the stores of amino acids for neoglycogenesis, thus counteracting the effects of cortical androgen. Again these statements are largely hypothetical.

The so-called gonadotropic hormones from the trophoblastic cells of the placenta are said to have an androgenic effect upon bone growth. It is uncertain whether this effect is a direct action or mediated through the testis or adrenal cortex or both.

Concerning the granulosa cell secretion from the ovary (estrogen) there seems to be more conclusive evidence, at least on an experimental ground. It has been well established by a number of investigators that certain birds, principally pigeons, and some mammals will develop a measurable increase in the calcified spongiosa under the

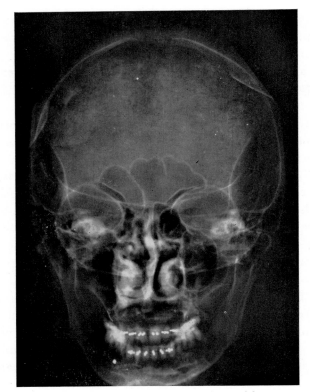

FIG. 13.   Roentgenogram of the skull of a patient with postmenopausal osteoporosis. The degree of osteoporosis is as severe in the skull as in other bones in
contrast to the deossification consequent to disuse atrophy.

influence of high estrogen levels. This increase may be reversed by
reducing the estrogen to normal. On the other hand, some of the
most severe cases of osteomalacia have developed in women who have
had numerous pregnancies in rapid succession with continuous lacta-
tion. Whether the bone softening is the result of an excessive drain
on the available calcium and protein or whether it is due to the increased estrogen level is debatable, but at any rate if the former is to
blame, the latter is not sufficient to maintain normal bone integrity.
Atrophy of the ovaries and, therefore, presumably a low estrogen level
have been thought to contribute to the cause of postmenopausal osteoporosis (Fig. 13). This may be true but therapy consisting of estrogen
alone in an attempt to build up the osteoporotic skeleton is apt to
be disappointing.

Factors Related to the Deposition of Mineral Salt in the Organic Matrix of Cartilage and Bone

Just as there is a critical caloric and protein dietary level for
organic matrix production so must there be an adequate supply of
calcium and phosphorus available for mineralization. Since both are

relatively ubiquitous materials found in a wide range of food substances, dietary inadequacy is almost unheard of in populations of average living standards. In China, where in some areas there is no milk, calcium deficiency may lead to bone disease. At least some of the infantile rickets seen in this country is probably due to a low protein diet and inadequate supplies of phosphorus.

More important to the availability of sufficient quantities of calcium and phosphorus for normal bone formation are factors which influence absorption through the gut wall. Apparently phosphorus absorption is obligatory and if adequate amounts are ingested they will reach the blood stream. The absorption of the calcium ion is more complicated. Insoluble soaps may be formed with large amounts of abnormal lipids produced as a result of celiac disease. Or the bowel wall may be the site of chronic and extensive disease which impairs the absorption function. This coupled with diarrhea may result in an inadequate absorption of calcium.

THE ACTION OF VITAMIN D.   More important than either the dietary amount or the state of the gut wall is the necessity for an adequate amount of vitamin D. It is now widely agreed that vitamin D is the principal governing factor in the absorption of calcium (Fig. 14). The actual mechanism of this function is still unknown, and whether it be at the level of the intestinal wall, in the humoral components of transport or within the index of receptiveness of the organic matrix

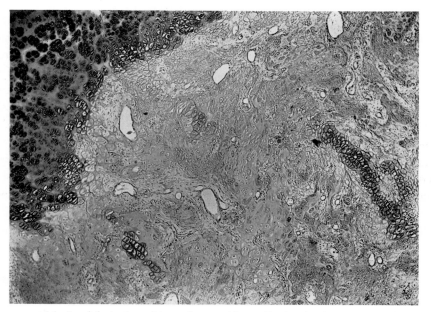

FIG. 14. In rickets there is ample osteoid production but a paucity of calcium salts for mineralization. At the upper left, one sees the cartilaginous epiphysis. In the metaphysis there are islands of cartilage surrounded by osteoid. This material remains soft and unmineralized. (×40.)

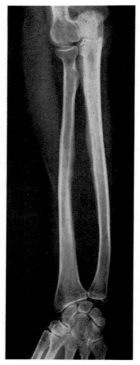

FIG. 15.   Roentgenogram of the forearm of a patient suffering from hypervitaminosis D. The entire skeleton reveals a loss of substance. Here the cortices
are abnormally thin.

cannot be stated at this time. Some patients appear to be refractory
to normal amounts of vitamin D and require many times the average
dosage to maintain normal skeletal growth. These cases have been
called vitamin D refractory rickets. It appears that the site of activity
of therapeutically large doses of the vitamin is not in the intestinal
mucosa, inducing it to absorb more calcium, but in the tubules of
the kidneys causing a conservation of phosphorus.

Besides its influence on the absorption of calcium through the gut
wall vitamin D has two other sites of action which may involve calcium
metabolism. Because huge amounts are necessary to elicit these actions
they are rarely encountered. The more important of these two is the
direct effect upon bone itself where it produces widespread deossification. The dosage must be large and continued over a long period,
and the eventual result may precisely mimic that of parathyroid adenoma. It usually can be differentiated by a higher serum phosphorus
level and of course by obtaining the history of excessive vitamin D
intake (Fig. 15).

The mechanism of the other action is more obscure. Albright
originally felt that large amounts of vitamin D acted very much like parathyroid hormone in causing phosphorus diuresis by blocking reab-

sorption through the kidney tubules. Several recent reports[3] by a number of authors indicate that vitamin D actually causes phosphate retention by increasing the absorption activity at the tubule level. Until more definitive data is available we must consider the matter in the realm of hypothesis. We do know that massive doses of vitamin D over a long period cause a clinical picture similar to that of hyperparathyroidism. The mechanism of deossification needs further investigation.

THE EFFECTS OF PARATHYROID HORMONE.   Even before Mandl first removed an enlarged parathyroid gland for demineralizing skeletal disease in 1925, there was considerable speculation concerning the relationship of the parathyroid hormone and bone calcification. Even then the matter was not wholly understood because there remained to be demonstrated the mechanism of the compensatory hyperplasia of the glands in states of chronic calcium loss. Ten years later Castleman and Mallory reviewed the pathology of parathyroid hyperplasia and parathyroid adenoma,[4] but the vagaries of morphology still haunt the pathologist in attempting to differentiate accurately the various physiologic disturbances which involve these glands.

It is now fairly generally agreed that the parathyroid is not responsible to any other gland secretion for its activity but rather it is governed by the serum calcium level. When the calcium serum content falls below a certain critical level the glands increase their secretory activity. One action is quite certain, that of the direct, demineralizing effect of parathormone upon bone. This has been shown experimentally by placing crystalline parathormone in contact with healthy bone. Such action also fits the facts which have emerged from the study of cases of parathyroid adenoma.

Concerning the possibility of another action of parathormone there has been more controversy. Albright and co-workers[5] believe one of the principal sites of action of the parathyroid hormone is upon the lining cells of the kidney tubules where it blocks reabsorption of phosphorus from the glomerular filtrate, inducing a phosphorus diuresis. Considerable work has been done in other quarters since the publication of their report and their findings have been generally corroborated. But the matter is not as simple as it sounds since Albright et al. reported cases of primary kidney disturbance in which excessive amounts of calcium are used as available base to substitute for the basic ions which the kidneys are unable to produce. This calcium utilization results in low serum levels and a stimulation of the parathyroids with production of excess hormone which causes deossification. The result is a confusion of cases of similar pathogenesis but different etiology. The tubular insufficiency mechanism is used by some to explain the circumstances of what is now known as Milkman's syndrome, a type of osteomalacia, which has until recently usually been classified as pseudohyperparathyroidism.

In hypoparathyroidism there is a failure of utilization of the skeletal calcium stores with lowering of the serum calcium level to cause tetany. Recently, a pseudohypoparathyroidism has been described in which the parathyroid glands are normal in appearance but if the hormone is secreted the skeleton apparently does not respond to its action.

KIDNEY FUNCTION.   Kidney function has been mentioned as a factor in the maintenance of a normal calcium balance. In Albright's "tubular-insufficiency-without-glomerular-insufficiency," in cases of high phosphate renal clearance and in those rare instances of Fanconi's syndrome in which an excessive production of organic acids requires the utilization of abnormal basic calcium ions, other kidney functions such as glomerular filtration are normal so that the principal action is calcium loss, phosphate loss or a combination, and the effect is upon the skeleton. The patient does not manifest a general nephritic symptomatology. However, in kidney disease severe enough to produce an acidosis over a long continued period without killing the patient the calcium stores are dissipated and the parathyroids are stimulated. Chronic low calcium levels eventually cause a secondary parathyroid hyperplasia and this condition must then be differentiated from parathyroid adenoma. The distinction may be difficult in some cases but usually the impaired kidney tubules are unable to respond to the excessive parathormone level and a failure of phosphorus diuresis results in high serum phosphorus levels. This in conjunction with the serum chemistry and symptoms of chronic uremia usually serves to differentiate renal rickets with secondary parathyroid hyperplasia from parathyroid adenoma.

Factors Related to the Normal Lysis of Bone and Cartilage

Finally, for normal skeletal growth, maturation and maintenance, the factors which govern conversion of coarse fiberbone to adult bone, modeling and the replenishment of physiologic erosion must be considered.

The stress stimulus is doubtless the most important of these. Throughout the skeleton, mechanical stress is apparently necessary to convert primitive bone to the adult type. Without it the lamellae remain unoriented and pressure causes distortion. These distortion effects are seen in several of the congenital, developmental disturbances in which there is an inability to convert fiberbone to adult bone, perhaps because the fiberbone is abnormal from the beginning.

The effect of the stress stimulus, or rather the lack of it, can be dramatically illustrated by the comparison of the roentgenogram of a normal extremity bone with that of the same bone after it has been immobilized in a cast for several weeks. If immobilization has been complete, severe deossification of the bone is apparent (Fig. 16). When considerable portions of the body are put in a cast and the patient is at bed rest, skeletal demineralization may be severe enough to cause a rise in serum calcium levels and even metastatic calcification of soft tissues and nephrolithiasis.

Modeling of bones is almost completely the result of the reorientation of the lamellae into haversian systems laid down in the trajectory lines of mechanical stress. Stress may be a matter of pressure or of tension but apparently either or an alternating of both may cause conversion from fiberbone to adult bone. This conversion results in a reshaping of the bone as a whole and this physiologic reshaping is known as modeling. Bone modeling may be graphically illustrated by superimposing the roentgenogram of an extremity bone of an adult over that of the same bone taken during early childhood (Fig. 17). It will be seen that the mid-portion of the earlier diaphysis has been expanded and thickened while the metaphyseal flare has undergone resorption to accommodate the silhouette of the longer shaft of the adult bone.

The principles of modeling can be understood by studying a longitudinal section through the secondary callus of a fracture site of a long

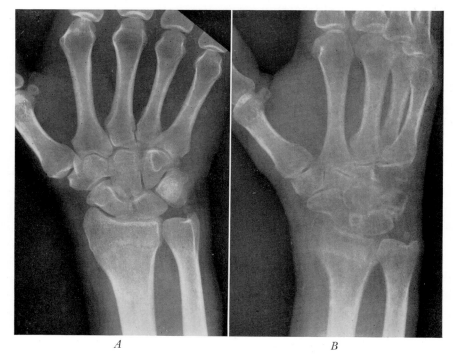

A   B

FIG. 16.   *A,* Roentgenogram of the carpal area shortly after fracture of the distal radius. The part was immobilized by plaster cast. *B,* Roentgenogram of the same area several weeks after immobilization. Note the disuse atrophy of the carpal bones.

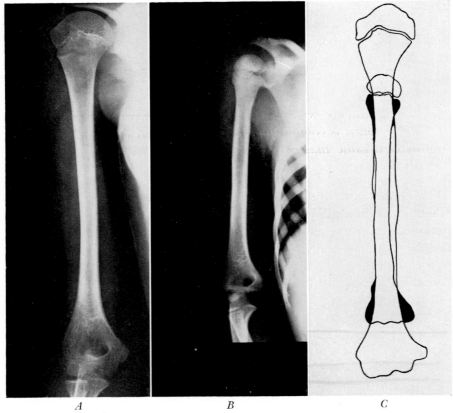

FIG. 17. *A*, Roentgenogram of the humerus of a twelve-year-old patient. *B*, Roentgenogram of the humerus of a five-year-old patient. *C*, Line drawing representing the silhouettes of the two bones illustrated in *A* and *B*. The blackened areas are the portions of the younger bone which must undergo lysis to form the shaft of the older bone. This is a part of the process of modeling.

bone in a case where alignment has not been good (Fig. 18). On the outer cortical surface representing the apex of angulation one will find subperiosteal, osteoclastic resorption of bone and on the inner cortical surface there will be a compensatory building up of bone by osteoblastic apposition. At the same level across the bone there will be bone absorption from the medullary surface and the laying down of new lamellae beneath the periosteum of the outer surface. Thus, there is accomplished a gradual reduction in angulation so that trajectory lines are straightened by a progressive shifting of the angulation area into a line with the epiphyses without interrupting tubulation.

The mechanism of pressure and tension changes in bone is not understood. It is agreed that stress in physiologic trajectory lines causes conversion of fiberbone to adult bone and stimulates osteoblasts to form sufficient osteoid to maintain the cortical thickness which would otherwise be diminished by normal catabolic activity in the mature skeleton. But if pressure is applied at right angles to the long axis of a cylindrical bone quite a different effect is seen. There is apt to be resorption of bone in the path of the stress. The explanation has been offered that the pressure interferes with the blood supply and that the impoverished bone wears away and is not replaced. This could scarcely be called a realistic explanation since elsewhere in the skeleton it is commonly observed that decreasing the vascularity stimulates organic matrix production and mineralization so that the bone becomes more dense.

It is possible that pressure causes bone erosion except where there is an interposition of a cartilage plate. This explanation holds at least for the initial changes which occur when the articular plate is destroyed by rheumatoid or osteoarthritis. At first there is resorp-

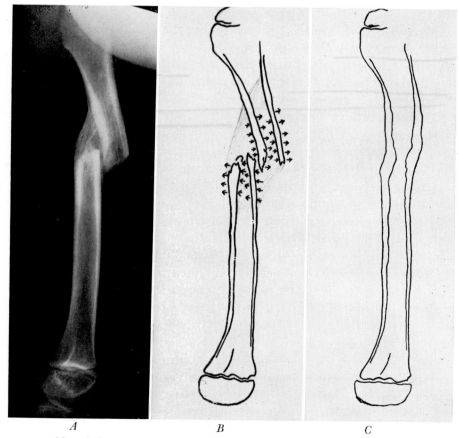

FIG. 18. *A*, Roentgenogram of a fractured femur showing angulation. *B*, Drawing of the bone shown in *A*. The arrows pointing away from the cortical surface indicate lysis. Those pointing toward the cortical surface indicate apposition. Under the influence of stress there is a gradual shifting and realignment without reducing bone mass or diminishing bone strength. *C*, Eventually alignment may be achieved due to bone shifting into the trajectories of stress.

tion of the bone end but then in the former there is bone production which may go on to ankylosis and in the latter there is a sealing of the eroded surface by excessive matrix production which results in eburnation.

It must be admitted, therefore, that the apparent paradoxical effects of vertical and longitudinal pressure remain an enigma, at least to the writer.

THE OSTEOCLAST.   Up to this point the function of the osteoclast has not been mentioned. Most observers contend that this cell causes deossification, that is, the disappearance of both organic matrix and its mineral content. This opinion is based largely on the facts that osteoclasts are usually found in large numbers where bone is undergoing resorption, they are often hard to find at sites where bone is predominantly building and they are found in Howship's lacunae, where it is supposed they have nibbled out the bone which they replace.

Some authors contend on the other hand that osteoclasts are merely scavenger cells which come in to phagocytize the debris produced by bone degeneration. But incriminatory evidence of bone fragments and minerals has not been demonstrated within their cytoplasm though other evidence of phagocytic activity has been noted.

The reports of Pommer[6] and von Kollicker[7] in earlier days of bone pathology were fraught with polemics but more recently the controversy has simmered with the admission on the part of most that neither the genesis nor function of the osteoclast is absolutely known.

Some facts and assumptions which are probably related to osteoclastic activity are summarized:

Though osteoid which has never been mineralized can be demonstrated, demineralized organic matrix is never seen in tissue section. Apparently the osteoid disintegrates first, thus releasing the mineral, or in the process of demineralization the matrix is simultaneously destroyed. The former seems the more plausible since in the laboratory the mineral may be removed in a variety of ways leaving an intact matrix. Thus the term "decalcified" or "demineralized" osteoid is loosely used. The exact term is "deossification."

The complete mechanism of calcium salt deposition is not known. It is believed by some that a local factor related to the chemistry of the mucopolysaccharide matrix is necessary. Perhaps a reversal of the change which invokes salt deposition may release it.

Hyalin ground substance undergoes depolymerization before mineral is deposited.

The fiber structure of collagen is destroyed by collagenase.

The mucoplysaccharide portion of the matrix is changed by hyaluronidase.

Calcium salts will go into solution by a lowering of the pH or be enticed from their crystal lattice by a chelating substance.

Parathormone, vitamin D and probably ascorbic acid have the ability of destroying bone on contact. It is not known whether this is a direct action, whether mediated by another agent produced by their action or whether they stimulate the production and activity of osteoclasts.

The origin of the osteoclast is not known. Some observers report a conversion of osteoblasts into osteoclasts and back to osteoblasts by raising and then lowering the estrogen level in pigeons and mice. Certain workers have felt that osteoclasts are formed by the simple merging of macrophages or histiocytes. Others have observed their formation from endothelial lining cells of budding capillaries.

The chemistry of intracytoplasmic metabolism of the osteoclast is not known.

Thus, it would appear that if the osteoclast is capable of destroying normal bone it must possess a factor or factors whose action is similar to that of hyaluronidase, collagenase and a calcium salt solvent.

Whether the osteoclast does or does not destroy bone is important to those interested in the physiology of that tissue. To the pathologist large numbers of osteoclasts mean bone destruction though the actual causative agents are varied, including alteration of blood supply, mechanical trauma, parathyroid hormone, vitamin D and a host of unknown forces working through such processes as Paget's disease, solitary cyst and neoplasia.

Additional light may be shed upon the activities of the osteoclast when we know more of its intracellular metabolism. As a working principle it is safe to say that in the presence of large numbers of osteoclasts, bone lysis is taking or has taken place. The reverse is not necessarily true in the absence of osteoclasts since it may be necessary to search numerous sections of normal bone before encountering a single osteoclast. The writing on the subject is an example of the futility and sometimes the damage which can result by the application of presumption dressed in the garb of fact.

REFERENCES

1. Wolbach, S. B.: J. Bone & Joint Surg., 29:171, 1947.
2. Gardner, W., and Pfeiffer, C.: Physiol. Rev., 23:139, 1943.
3. Zetterstrom, R.: Nature, 167:409, 1951.
4. Castleman, B., and Mallory, T. B.: Am. J. Path., 11:1, 1935.
5. Albright, F., Burnett, C. H., Parson, W., Reifenstein, E. C., and Roos, A.: Medicine, 25:4, 1946.
6. Pommer, G.: Virchows Arch. f. path. anat., 92:296, 1883.
7. von Kollicker, A.: Die normale Resorption des Knochengewebes, etc., F. C. W. Vogel, Leipzig, 1873.

5

Histology of the Musculoskeletal System

The chapters of this book subsequent to this one are intended for the clinician who encounters orthopedic diseases, the orthopedic surgeon, the radiologist and the pathologist. If the specialist of any but the last of these categories is interested in the microscopy of the musculoskeletal diseases (the interest of the pathologist is taken as a matter of faith), he may find some help in this, Chapter 5, for it is intended as a primer, of the most rudimentary type, of the histology of the tissue concerned. Since descriptions of cellular morphology make an almost unreadably dry text the material is presented largely in the form of a simple atlas. It is obvious that a very much more complete coverage can be found in any histology text, but since this book is devoted to the description of orthopedic diseases only, for the sake of oneness, it seems permissible to include only enough histology to allow the reader to appreciate the more detailed microscopy given later with the description of each disease entity.

It is assumed that the non-pathologist has forgotten most of anything he may have learned while peering through a microscope as a medical student. A considerable experience in teaching clinicians has impressed this fact upon the writer. Since any concept of morbid microscopic structure rests upon a comparison with normal structure, the following several pages bear illustrations of the latter.

This chapter should be read by the non-pathologist with a set of "bone slides" and a microscope at hand. The pathologist would do better not to read it at all.

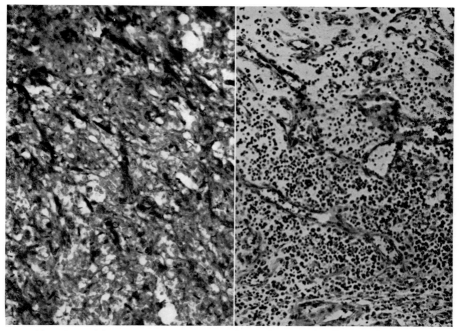

FIG. 19.   Organizing hematoma. (× 260.)   FIG. 20.   Granulation tissue. (× 130.)

FIGURE 19 represents an organizing hematoma. Soon after blood is extravasated into normal tissue, a network of fibrin is precipitated throughout the clot. Almost immediately, fibroblasts from the surrounding, viable tissue begin to proliferate and the young cells penetrate into the hematoma, climbing among the fibrin strands like sailors on a rigging. These fibroblasts form a network of their fibrils and as they mature they become fixed in this network. Their shape changes from polyhedral to fusiform and then to long spindles. Gradually collagen is laid down about them. In the illustration one can make out the pale, often disintegrating red cells in the background. The darker spindles seen throughout the section represent fibroblasts.

FIGURE 20 is a section of simple granulation tissue. In a hematoma or in an area where tissue has been injured, concomitant with the proliferation of fibroblasts, the tiny vessels in the contiguous tissue sprout into the affected area. These young vessels, consisting at first of simple tubes of endothelial cells, are supported by the networks of fibrin and fibroblastic fibrils. They penetrate all through the area, bringing the large supply of blood which is necessary for repair. As they age they develop supportive walls of fibrous tissue. About them are the exudative inflammatory cells and the edema which are consequent to the tissue injury. In the illustration one sees the sprouting vessels in an edematous matrix containing exudative inflammatory cells.

FIG. 21.   FIG. 22.

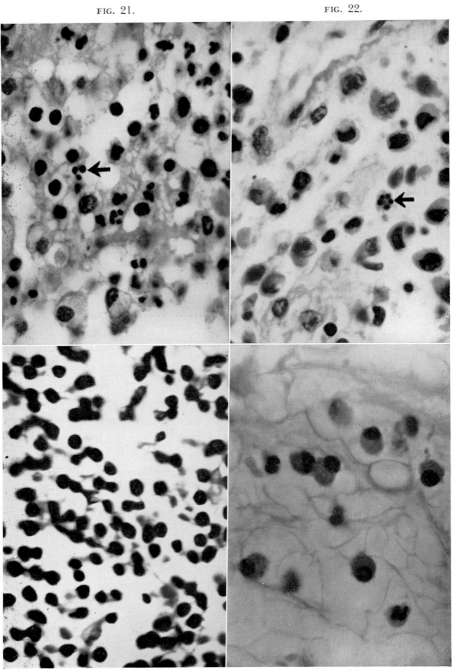

FIG. 23.   FIG. 24.

FIG. 21.   Neutrophils. ($\times$ 760.)
FIG. 22.   Eosinophils. ($\times$ 760.)
FIG. 23.   Lymphocytes. ($\times$ 760.)
FIG. 24.   Plasmacytes. ($\times$ 760.)

FIGURE 21.   This is an illustration of a suppurative exudate. The neutrophils are represented by the clusters of two to five small, round, black bodies. Each of these is a multilobed nucleus of a polymorphonuclear leukocyte. The nucleus of all cells contains large quantities of desoxyribose nucleic acid, the main constituent of chromatin. It takes the hematoxylin stain and in sections it is dark blue. The cytoplasm of most cells takes the pink eosin stain in various densities. In sections of tissue the cytoplasmic borders are not usually seen, the nuclei appearing in a more or less homogeneous background of cytoplasm. In exudates the cells are more widely separated so that cytoplasmic borders are usually apparent. In smears of exudate prepared with Wright's stain the various lobes of the nuclei of the neutrophils are seen to be connected by fine filaments of chromatin. In H and E sections these are rarely demonstrable. The more mature the neutrophil the greater the number of lobes in its nucleus. The arrow designates a typical neutrophil.

FIGURE 22.   The eosinophil is a type of granulocyte. The cytoplasm is filled with eosin-staining granules which are quite obvious in the section but do not appear in the black and white photograph. The nucleus of the eosinophil is apt to be immature and so may appear as a single body of irregular outline. The arrow designates a mature eosinophil. Most of the other cells in the illustration are immature eosinophils.

FIGURE 23.   The nucleus of the lymphocyte is round or ovoid. Its chromatin is usually heavily condensed so that it appears a solid dark blue or even black in the section. Sometimes the chromatin is irregularly broken, causing clear lines and spaces between the fragments. As the nucleus undergoes degenerative change it takes the hematoxylin less and less heavily and develops a washed-out appearance. The cytoplasm of the lymphocyte is sparse or completely undemonstrable in sectioned tissue. When seen it usually appears as a narrow demilune of a pale gray-blue about one side of the nucleus. All the cells in the illustration are lymphocytes.

FIGURE 24.   The nucleus of the plasmacyte is somewhat larger than that of the usual lymphocyte. It, too, is heavily chromatized but more apt to be broken. The fragments are sometimes arranged about the nuclear periphery beneath the nuclear membrane. This may give a clock-face or spokes-of-a-cartwheel appearance. The cytoplasm of the plasmacyte has a peculiar blue-rose color which is very characteristic. In most instances the nucleus is eccentrically placed, sometimes appearing halfway out of the cell and thus giving the cell a piriform outline. The cells in the illustration are typical plasmacytes.

FIG. 25.   FIG. 26.

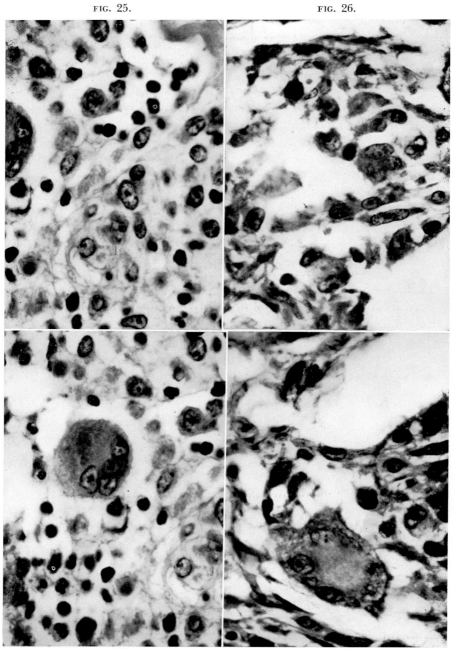

FIG. 27.   FIG. 28.

FIG. 25.   Macrophages. (× 760.)
FIG. 26.   Epithelioid cells. (× 760.)
FIG. 27.   Giant cell of inflammation. (× 760.)
FIG. 28.   Giant cell of granuloma. (× 760.)

FIGURE 25.   The large ovoid structures in this illustration are the nuclei of macrophages. Their magnification is the same as that of the exudative cells on the previous page. Note that they are much larger. Other names for the macrophage are histiocyte, clasmatocyte and mononuclear phagocyte. They are the largest of the mononucleated ameboid cells. Their cytoplasmic borders are demonstrable only if the cell is relatively isolated. The cytoplasm stains pale pink. The large nucleus is usually ovoid and frequently indented or reniform. The chromatin is usually finely divided and evenly dispersed. The nucleolus is often prominent. In this illustration there are also nuclei of lymphocytes and in the lower right corner a neutrophil.

FIGURE 26.   When macrophages (or fibroblasts) aggregate to form a granuloma they are called epithelioid cells. The nuclei are often elongated and lie side by side. Early pathologists saw these cells and because of their parallel arrangement compared them to the cells of an epithelial membrane. Realizing, however, that these were not true epithelial cells they devised the descriptive term epithelioid cells. The name has persisted and is applied whether or not the cells have a palisade arrangement. Toward the center of the lesion they may undergo necrosis; toward the periphery they may revert to collagenoblasts.

FIGURE 27.   This illustration shows a multinucleated giant cell of inflammation. The nuclei are identical with those of macrophages. The cytoplasm often contains phagocytized particles. This cell probably represents an agglomeration of macrophages or a group of macrophages whose cytoplasm has failed to divide.

FIGURE 28.   This picture shows a granuloma giant cell. It is a type of giant cell of inflammation and of the same order as the Langhans giant cell of tuberculosis. These cells are not the same as osteoclasts though they may sometimes resemble them. Another cell which must be differentiated is the megakaryocyte which is found in active marrow and produces blood platelets. The granuloma is a specific type of inflammatory reaction produced by certain agents: lipids; waxes and other foreign body materials; fungi; parasites; and some bacteria, such as the tubercle bacillus. Granulation tissue is a general reparative response to any tissue injury and should not be confused with granuloma. Granulomas are often encountered in granulation tissue.

FIG. 29.

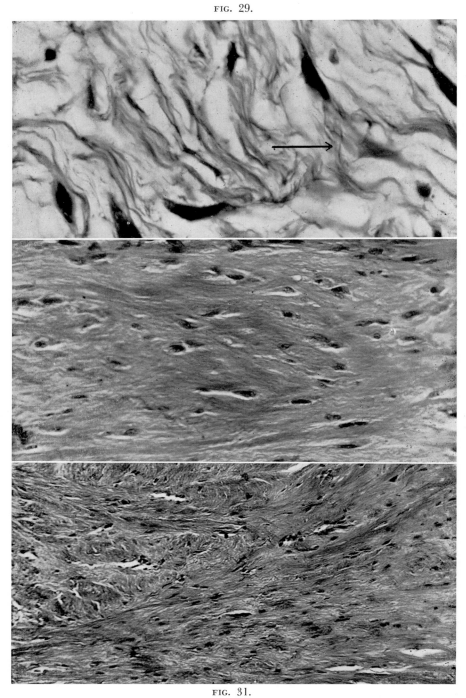

FIG. 31.

FIG. 29.   Very young collagenoblasts. (× 760.)
FIG. 30.   (middle). Young connective tissue. (× 265.)
FIG. 31.   Mature connective tissue. (× 132.)

The collagenoblast (fibroblast) is found throughout all tissues and areas of the body. It provides the collagenized connective tissue which supports all the functioning parts and binds these parts into a unit. The term collagenoblast is preferred, designating the particular cell which is involved in collagen formation. The term fibroblast is used to designate the forerunner of any of the three cells which form the three types of fibrous matrices, the collagenoblast forming collagen, the osteoblast forming osteoid and the chondroblast forming hyalin. The collagenoblast and the fibroblast are morphologically identical and actually may be the same cell. The osteoblast and chondroblast are shaped and identified by their related intercellular substance. The production of the various fibrous substances may be the result of a variety of stimuli acting upon the same cell.

FIGURE 29.   The illustration at high magnification reveals several young fibroblasts. They have passed out of the polyhedral into the fusiform stage. The nuclei are still plump but the ends are tapered. The cytoplasm-nucleus ratio is much smaller than in the polyhedral stage. At the ends of the cell the fibrils emerge and weave throughout the matrix. Most of the cells are bipolar but some are stellate. The arrow designates a stellate form which is deeper in the section than the others and, therefore, slightly out of focus.

FIGURE 30 represents an area of a section of collagenous connective tissue at medium magnification. The nuclei are thinner and more compact. The cytoplasm is no longer demonstrable. The network of fibrils is now filled in with collagen. The nuclei take the usual blue hematoxylin. The matrix takes the eosin lightly, assuming a pale pink to buff color. Collagen has much the same appearance in sections as osteoid but it is never lamellated, and of course there are no lacunae in which the osteocytes are entombed. Collagen stains green with Masson's trichrome, blue with Mallory's and brown with silver. The fibrils of the collagenoblasts stain black with silver stain.

FIGURE 31.   This is an area of nearly adult collagenous connective tissue at low magnification. The strands are woven together in such manner as to give great tensile strength. When completely mature the nuclei appear as hard black lines. The intercellular collagen may hyalinize, obliterating the fibrous character and giving the matrix a homogeneous, glassy appearance.

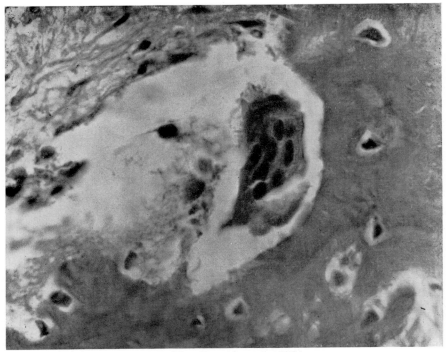

FIG. 32.   Osteoclast. (× 870.)

FIGURE 32.   The osteoclast is a huge cell containing from five to twenty nuclei in a single plane. The nuclei are usually dispersed throughout the cell but may be arranged about the periphery or clumped in the center. The magnification is high (× 870).

FIGURE 33.   A section of soft tissue illustrating a small artery and its accompanying vein. The artery has a thick wall. Usually the lumen measures slightly less than twice the thickness of its wall. The lumen is lined by a layer of endothelial cells and its supportive areolar tissue which together comprise the intima.

FIGURE 34.   This is also a section of soft tissue. The cross sections of two arteries are seen embedded in fat. The fat is composed of adult fat cells which in the section appear as large, round spaces surrounded by a delicate membrane. The spaces represent the area which was occupied by neutral fat which has been dissolved by the processing fluids. The nuclei of adult fat cells are small and they are pushed to the periphery by the intracytoplasmic fat. Unless the knife passes through the plane in which they lie they are not seen. Crossing the field from below to the right is a small nerve. Its fibrillar appearance is due to the fibrous supportive tissue. It has a characteristic wavy pattern. A cross section of this nerve can be seen in the upper right.

FIG. 33.

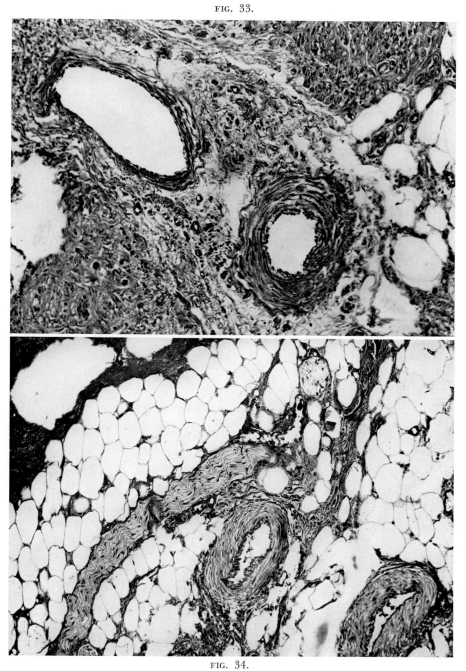

FIG. 34.

FIG. 33.   Artery and vein. ($\times$ 132.)
FIG. 34.   Artery, fat and nerve. ($\times$ 115.)

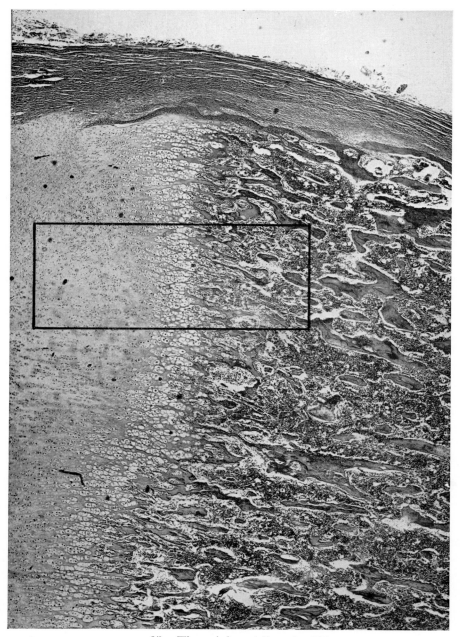

FIG. 35.   The epiphyseal line.   ($\times$ 12.)

FIGURE 35.   This is a very low magnification of a section taken through the epiphyseal line showing the enchondral plate on the left, the epiphyseal line through the center and the subepiphyseal metaphysis on the right. The perichondrium (over cartilage) and the periosteum (over bone) are at the top. The lined rectangle represents the area from which the four following illustrations were taken. Figure 36 comes from the extreme left of this rectangle, Figure 37 from the area of large, vacuolated, columnated chondrocytes, Figure 38 straddles the epiphyseal line and Figure 39 comes from the extreme right portion of the area.

FIGURE 36.   This picture is of an area deep within the enchondral plate. The osseous nucleus was to the left and the epiphyseal line to the right. The following three illustrations were taken consecutively from the same section by moving the slide to the left, thereby including fields progressively nearer the diaphysis. The right side of the field in each is nearest the diaphysis; thus if the four illustrations were placed end to end they would represent a nearly continuous progression from the depths of the enchondral plate through the epiphyseal line and into the metaphysis. In Figure 36 the cartilage cells are young, small and quite evenly dispersed through the hyalin matrix. The cytoplasm contains little or no glycogen.

FIGURE 37.   This area is several fields nearer the epiphyseal line. The chondroblasts are more mature. They are larger and the cytoplasm contains vacuoles from which glycogen was dissolved by the processing fluids. Note that by enlarging in a plane horizontal to the epiphyseal line which is to the right of this picture, the cells have become flattened and have achieved the effect of columnation. Between the columns of maturing chondroblasts remain pillars of hyalin.

FIGURE 38.   This section straddles the epiphyseal line; the epiphysis is to the left, the metaphysis to the right. The cartilage cells are now mature and greatly distended with glycogen. The metaphyseal granulation is breaking into the bases of the columns and the cells are being utilized in the process of mineralization. The pillars of mineralized hyalin now protrude into the metaphysis. Osteoblasts have separated from the mass of undifferentiated fibroblasts and are beginning to line up along these pillars and to lay down seams of osteoid.

FIGURE 39.   The mineralized hyalin pillars have been largely replaced by osteoid which, toward the left in the younger portion of the area, appears in narrow seams. The entire process is known as enchondral ossification.

FIG. 36.

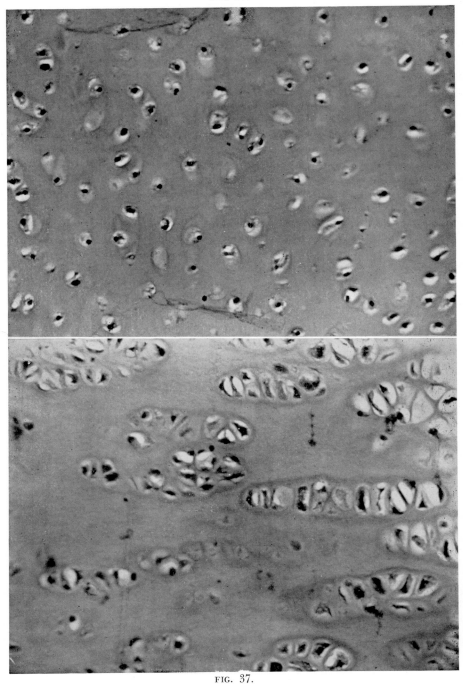

FIG. 37.

FIG. 36.   Chondroblasts of enchondral plate. ($\times$ 266.)
FIG. 37.   Columnation of chondroblasts. ($\times$ 266.)

FIG. 38.

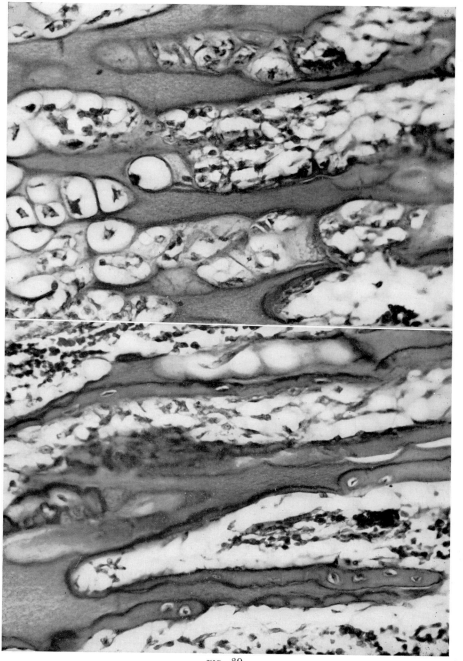

FIG. 39.

FIG. 38.   Epiphyseal line. (× 266.)
FIG. 39.   Subepiphyseal metaphysis. (× 266.)

FIG. 40.

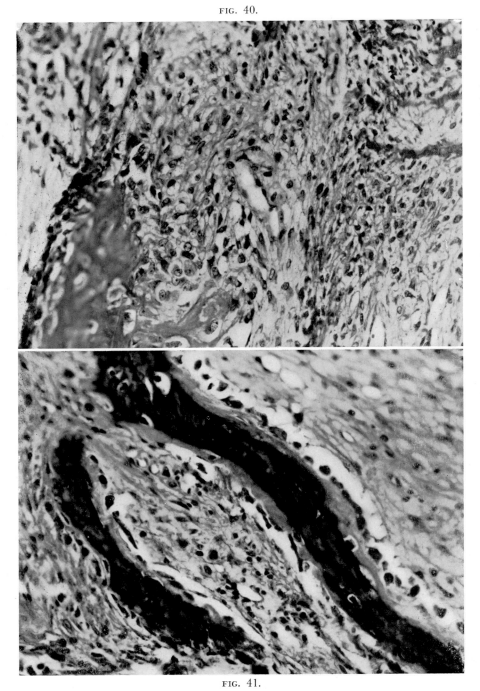

FIG. 41.

FIG. 40.   Fibroblasts migrating to form osteoblasts. ($\times$ 260.)
FIG. 41.   Osteoblasts laying down osteoid. ($\times$ 260.)

FIGURE 40.   Three types of cells emerge from the primitive fibro-blasts, the collagenoblasts illustrated in Figures 29, 30 and 31, the chondroblasts illustrated in Figures 36 and 37, and the osteoblasts. On the right side of the field in Figure 40 one finds an aggregate of round or ovoid nuclei of these fibroblasts. The cytoplasmic outlines, where visualized, are still polyhedral or round. As one progresses left across the field the nuclei become larger and the cell outline elongated. In the lower left portion of the field there is a mass of osteoid. As the undifferentiated cells approach this osteoid they become more rounded or cuboidal in shape. They line up along the margins of the osteoid and enter into the production of that substance. They are now known as osteoblasts. The mechanism of osteoid production is still unknown. Osteoid appears to be made up of certain polypeptides and amino acids from the blood stream which are acted upon by a substance, perhaps a mucopolysaccharide, secreted by the osteoblasts. It is inter-esting that when osteoblasts become neoplastic in nature they are apt to revert back to their undifferentiated elongated, fusiform or even spindled shape.

FIGURE 41.   This is a section taken from an area of actively forming bone. The osteoblasts are fully differentiated and are now seen as cuboidal cells arranged in rows along the surfaces of immature bone. The core of the latter has already mineralized and thus appears black in the illustration and dark blue in the section. Calcium salts take the hematoxylin stain. Between the row of osteoblasts and the core of mineralized bone one finds a layer, a "seam" of unmineralized osteoid. This stains a rather intense pink with eosin. Normal osteoid mineralizes very rapidly, probably within a matter of hours after it is formed. One can judge the rate at which ossification is proceeding by the amount and width of the osteoid seams. Under normal circum-stances one never sees unmineralized osteoid except in forming bone. When bone undergoes lysis the organic matrix (osteoid) apparently disintegrates, first releasing the mineral salts. Nothing is left to indicate where bone had been. When bone is demineralized in the laboratory the calcium salts are removed, leaving the organic matrix. We still do not know what artefacts are induced by this process.

FIG. 42.

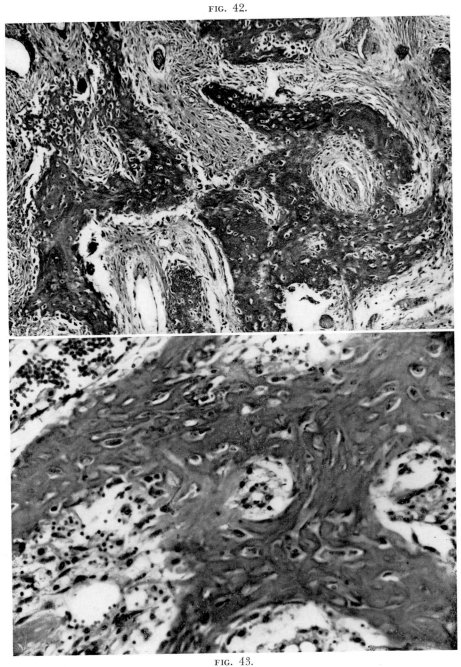

FIG. 43.

FIG. 42.   Primitive fiberbone. ($\times$ 115.)
FIG. 43.   Primitive fiberbone. ($\times$ 260.)

FIGURE 42.   As the mass of bone increases by the apposition of osteoid along its surfaces, some of the osteoblasts disappear and others are caught in the substance which forms around them. The osteoid then mineralizes and these cells become incorporated into the newly formed bone. They are now known as osteocytes and the spaces they occupy are called lacunae. They retain their fibrillar processes which emerge from the lacunae like spider legs and travel through the bone matrix in their minute channels, called canaliculi. These channels appear to constitute the apertures through which nutrients reach and sustain the cell within the lacuna. As the osteocyte matures, the nucleus shrinks and the chromatin condenses and consequently stains more darkly. The cytoplasm which in life fills the lacunar space does not withstand the process of demineralization and so is seen as an amorphous substance condensed around the nucleus. The space which results is an artefact.

FIGURE 43.   This picture illustrates at higher magnification a piece of recently formed fiberbone. Young fiberbone is easily distinguished from mature bone because the osteocytes are greater in number and larger. The fibers of the matrix are coarser. The bone may be laid down in layers but there is no organization of these layers into a lamellar pattern. Enchondral ossification, producing fiberbone, is responsible for the original shape of the bone. But fiberbone is weak and withstands stress badly. The process of conversion of fiberbone to stronger mature bone is a slow process and results in the modeling of bone to its final shape and in the pattern of cancellous bone in stress trajectories. To accomplish this the fiberbone undergoes a slow, progressive lysis and replacement. Osteoclasts are seen on those surfaces which are receding and osteoblasts on those which are being built up. Thus there is a gradual transition without weakening the area. The bone mass shifts in position as it changes its character.

FIG. 44.

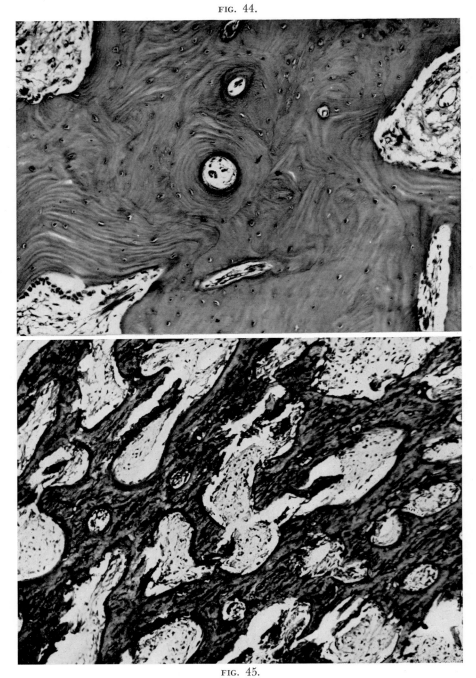

FIG. 45.

FIG. 44.   Mature bone, demineralized. (× 115.)
FIG. 45.   Mature bone, undemineralized. (× 130.)

FIGURE 44 represents an area of cortical bone from which the mineral salts have been removed in a bath of weak nitric acid. It takes the eosin stain because the salts are no longer present. The striations seen in the illustration represent lamellar bands. The fibrillar structure is much finer than that of fiberbone—too fine to appear at this magnification. Note that the osteocytes are fewer in number. In the center of the field there is a haversian system. This system of concentric lamellae is laid down about a haversian canal which appears in the center as a space. A haversian canal is shown at higher magnification in Figure 46. The cells are caught in flattened lacunae lying between the lamellae. When a haversian system is cut in cross section it is delineated from neighboring systems by a fine blue line along the surface of the outer lamella. This is known as a *cement line,* and probably represents a narrow crevice or space between the surface of the enclosed system and contiguous systems which have grown independently. There probably is no cement substance which binds the systems together. When osteoblasts lay down an osteoid seam on preexisting bone no cement line is seen, but when a system is completed and approximated by another system the line of contact appears through the microscope as a black line. The configuration of the lamellae and of the haversian systems is exceedingly important in judging new bone growth and in the diagnosis of several bone diseases. In Paget's disease the pattern is so completely changed that one can frequently make the diagnosis at a glance. Osteopetrosis is another example.

FIGURE 45 represents an area of cancellous bone which was sectioned without removal of the mineral salts. The bone now stains deep blue because of the presence of calcium. The irregular dark lines represent fractures produced by the passage of the knife. No cellular detail is retained in sections prepared in this fashion. The uninitiated, when looking at undemineralized normal bone, often call it necrotic because of its deep blue color and ragged edges. This mistake can never be made once the microscopist has compared the two types of preparations. There are numerous disturbances in the mineralization of bone. By removing the mineral salts so that the tissue can be sectioned we may efface the character of the disease we are trying to diagnose. For this reason sections of undemineralized bone are sometimes made with a special microtome. The procedure is technically difficult and not yet suited to routine diagnosis.

FIG. 46.

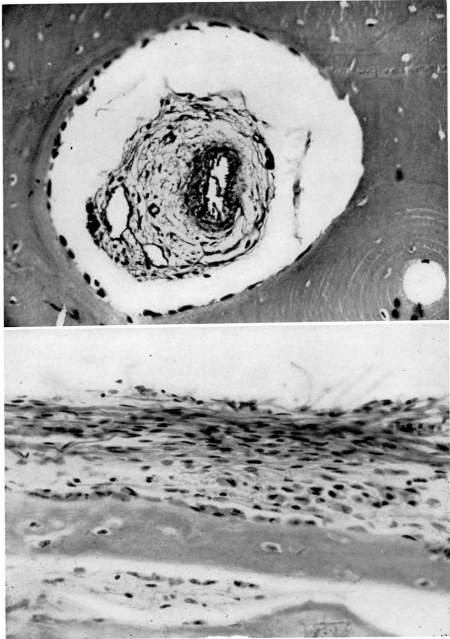

FIG. 47.

FIG. 46.   A haversian canal. ($\times$ 266.)
FIG. 47.   Young periosteum. ($\times$ 266.)

FIGURE 46.   This haversian canal contains an artery and two small veins. Nerve fibrils have been demonstrated in haversian canals by special technique. These structures are supported by loosely arranged collagenoblasts which form what is called areolar tissue. In preparation, this areolar tissue shrinks away from the rigid walls of the canal so that an artefactual space appears. This space is lined by a layer of cuboidal osteoblasts in this picture, suggesting that osteogenesis is still progressing. In the lower right corner there is another haversian canal the contents of which has dropped out of the section. It is surrounded by concentric lamellae to form a haversian system. Note that the lamellae about the larger canal are not concentric. Apparently the systems are built from without inward so that the same lamella may be involved in the outer structure of more than one system as illustrated in this picture. The haversian system cannot be considered as a unit except in relation to the vasculature pattern. Since the mature bone is laid down around the vessels, the canals run parallel to the trajectories of stress. Thus the lamellar pattern in any given area is the same as that of the same area in any other bone of the same type. In disease processes these patterns are disturbed and they change as stress trajectories are altered.

FIGURE 47 is a picture of a section taken through the cortex of the shaft of a fetal bone. It beautifully illustrates the components of periosteum. The periosteal membrane covers the upper (outer) surface of the portion of cortex seen in the lower portion of the field. Periosetum is composed of two layers which merge and are coextensive with each other. The outer half is made up of spindled collagenoblasts which are quite compactly arranged. A small amount of collagen appears between the cells. Collagenation increases with age. The inner half of the membrane is composed of elongated or fusiform cells which are much more loosely arranged. This layer is called the cambium. It is composed of cells which are in the process of differentiating into osteoblasts. A layer of more cuboidal osteoblasts can be seen approximated to the cortical surface. Bone is added by apposition in seams just as in enchondral ossification. The only difference is that here there is no intermediary stage of cartilage. The cambium has the ability to produce cartilage under abnormal circumstances. One frequently encounters casual reference to an endosteum, which is supposed to be a membrane like the periosteum applied to the inner surface of the cortex. The writer has examined many sections of cortex without finding any such membrane. In actively forming bone a single layer of osteoblasts may be seen but this can hardly be construed to compose a collagenic membrane.

FIG. 48.

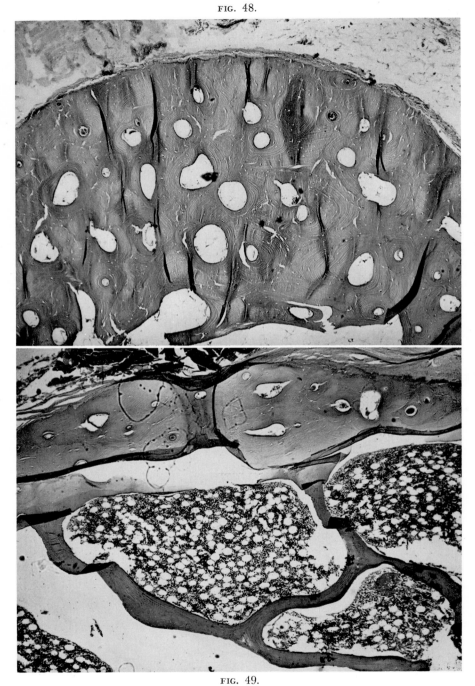

FIG. 49.

FIG. 48.   Section through diaphyseal cortex. ($\times$ 24.)
FIG. 49.   Section through metaphyseal cortex. ($\times$ 24.)

FIGURE 48. This picture shows an area from a cross section through the diaphysis of a phalanx of an adult. The full thickness of the cortex is represented. Over the upper surface one sees the periosteum. Note that there is no "endosteum" lining the inner surface. Since the section is through the shaft, the medullary cavity appears along the lower central margin of the picture. It is filled with fatty marrow. The vertical dark lines which mar the photograph are artefactual folds in the section. A patient technician can tease these out while they are floating on the surface of a water bath but this is rarely done in routine work. One has the opportunity of studying the pattern of the haversian systems in this illustration. Note that the canals and therefore the lamellar cylinders run parallel to the long axis of the bone. Note also that the canals are not always in the center of the systems and that some lamellae enter into the composition of more than one system. Some bones have an outer and an inner layer of lamellae which contain no haversian systems. The lamellae which constitute the cortical tissue between the systems always parallel those of one or more of the contiguous systems. This suggests that the haversian canals are actually not planned spaces but merely leftover areas where vessels are crowded by the growing bone. Studies of films made by roentgen micrography indicate that the lamellae nearest the canals are the least mineralized and probably the last to be infiltrated with calcium salts.

FIGURE 49. This illustration represents a section through a much thinner cortex at the level of the metaphysis. In the lower half of the field one finds the metaphyseal cancellous tissue. The "spicules" are in reality a continuous membrane of bone just as the partitions which surround the holes in a sea sponge constitute a continuous membrane. The cancellous bone is also continuous with the cortical bone. The spaces and lines in the illustration are artefactual splits and folds. In this bone the metaphysis still contains active marrow. The metaphysis is interposed between the articular plate and the medullary cavity. It braces and strengthens the thin metaphyseal cortex which surrounds it.

FIG. 50.

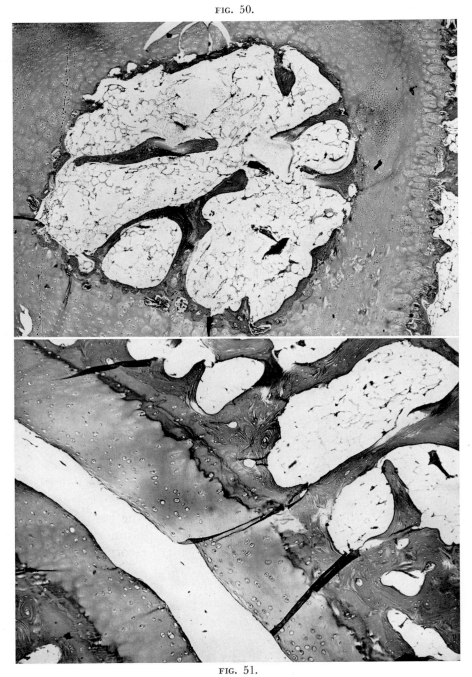

FIG. 51.

FIG. 50.   Osseous nucleus of the epiphysis. ($\times$ 16.)
FIG. 51.   Section across a joint. ($\times$ 16.)

FIGURE 50.   This picture shows a section through an immature epiphysis. The osseous nucleus occupies the central and greater portion of the field. To the right is the enchondral plate and the epiphyseal line along its right margin. To the left is the articular plate and the articular surface is further left, just out of the field. The time of the appearance of the osseous nucleus is specific for each epiphysis. Vessels reach the center of the epiphysis from the periphery (and sometimes through the center) of the enchondral plate. The fibroblasts lay down a nidus of bone. An epiphyseal line forms about the periphery of this nidus and, as the epiphysis ages, its chondroblasts in the vicinity of this line mature, a line of provisional calcification is established and enchondral ossification takes place just as it does on the meta-physeal side of the epiphyseal line. As the epiphyseal chondroblasts are used up the osseous nucleus expands to take their place. A thin spherical shell of bone is formed which surrounds a ball of cancellous tissue. Gradually the sphere becomes lens-shaped, its convex surfaces facing the articular plate on one side and the enchondral plate on the other, thus dividing the epiphysis into two parts. As it progresses the ossification line is halted on the articular plate side and an arch of bone seals off the cartilage, thus preserving the articular plate at a constant thickness. On the opposite side of the lens-shaped nucleus chondro-blasts are added as the cartilage cells of the enchondral plate are dis-sipated. Thus enchondral ossification is allowed to proceed until the cylindrical bone has reached its full stature. At another specified time, the chondroblasts cease to proliferate and those of the enchondral plate are used up as the epiphyseal line advances. Eventually the cancellous bone of the metaphysis meets the shell of the nucleus, the enchondral plate is spent and no cartilage intervenes between the two bone masses. At this point growth of the cylindrical bone at this end is completed. Conversion of the fiberbone into adult bone proceeds so that the two bone masses become continuous. Until this time the vasculature of the epiphysis and that of the metaphysis are almost distinct, but now vessels from the more vascular metaphyseal area penetrate the epiphysis and the blood supply becomes continuous and more adequate. Now the only way the bone can increase in length is by reactivation of chondroblasts at the cartilage-bone line of contiguity beneath the articular plate. This may happen in acromegaly in which there is excessive secretion of somatotropic hormone.

FIGURE 51 illustrates two apposed articular plates in the lower left half of the field. The bone arches are complete beneath the plates. The joint space crosses the lower left field.

FIG. 52.

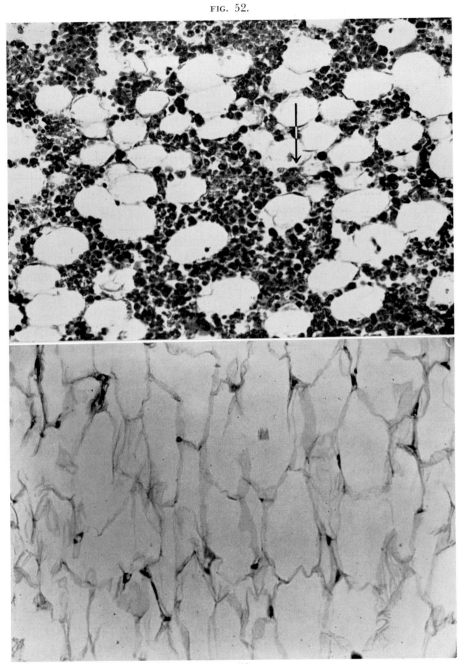

FIG. 53.

FIG. 52. Active bone marrow. ($\times$ 275.)
FIG. 53. Fatty bone marrow. ($\times$ 275.)

FIGURE 52.   This is a photograph of a section made through cancellous tissue containing active or hematopoietic bone marrow. No bone "spicules" are included in the field. The microscopist must learn to distinguish hematopoietic marrow from inflammatory exudate and it is not always easy since many of the same cells are involved. The novice is apt to interpret a section such as that illustrated here as chronic osteomyelitis. The difficulty is not eased by the demineralizing process which blurs the detail of all viable cells in the section. One of the most helpful features is the regular disbursement of large round or oval spaces which represent the fat cells. These always appear in normal marrow and are rarely seen in exudate. Also the variety of cell types is usually greater in marrow than in exudates. Normal marrow contains all the cells of the myelogenous series including normoblasts and erythrocytes. One cannot do an analytic count of these cells in demineralized sections because the demineralizing agent destroys the nuclear detail which is necessary for such a count. One can get a fair idea of the cellular constituents, however, in a thinly cut, well stained section. In the illustration one can make out the large, dark nuclei of the young myelogenous forms and the clusters of smaller bodies which represent the nuclei of granulocytes. With the advantage of color in the sections one can distinguish the yellow-pink color of the hemoglobin in erythrocytes. The arrow in the illustration points to a megakaryocyte, a large cell with a multilobulated nucleus which is responsible for the formation of blood platelets. It is rarely mistaken for an osteoclast. Just below the megakaryocyte there is a mature fat cell which has been sectioned through the plane of the nucleus. The latter is seen as a line of chromatin at the extreme periphery of the cell. It represents the nucleus which has been flattened to a plate and pushed to one side by the large globule of fat which now distends the cytoplasmic membrane. The fat, of course, has been dissolved out by the processing fluids. It may be demonstrated by doing a frozen section and staining with certain dyes such as Scharlach R which have an affinity for neutral fat.

FIGURE 53.   This picture illustrates the fatty marrow which fills the medullary cavity. Only the cytoplasmic membranes and here and there a flattened nucleus can be seen. This type of marrow is the normal component of the medullary area but in emergency states it may revert back to hematopoietic marrow, illustrating the versatility of the mesenchymal derivatives.

FIG. 54.

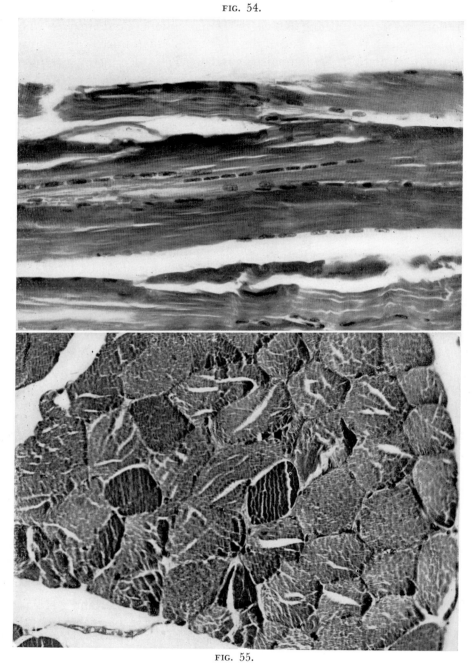

FIG. 55.

FIG. 54.   Longitudinal section of skeletal muscle. ($\times$ 275.)
FIG. 55.   Cross section of skeletal muscle. ($\times$ 275.)

FIGURE 54. This is a picture of a rather highly magnified longitudinal section of skeletal or voluntary muscle. Running horizontally through the major portion of the field there is a muscle bundle. Each bundle is made up of a group of parallel muscle fibers. Each fiber is a syncytium covered by a cytoplasmic membrane, the sarcolemma, which surrounds a bundle of parallel fibrils, the sarcoplasm, and a number of nuclei which are always located eccentrically beneath the sarcolemma. The sarcoplasm stains a deep rose-pink with eosin. The fibrils are cross-banded and these striations should be seen in a reasonably good preparation if the muscle is healthy. Diseased muscle first shows a blurring or loss of its striations. Next the nuclei swell and the chromatin becomes fragmented. Finally the muscle fiber fractures at various levels and may disappear. The products of degeneration elicit an inflammatory reaction and exudative cells may infiltrate into the area. The space occupied by the fibril is taken by fat cells and fibroblasts. Some fibers may atrophy and shrink to a fraction of their normal diameter. The remaining healthy fibers called on to do the work of the whole may hypertrophy to several times the normal diameter. Skeletal muscle is a highly differentiated structure and when injured it attempts to regenerate with but little success. The nuclei divide to produce excessive numbers in long chains but the sarcoplasm is unable to produce new fibrils. One can judge the extent of injury of a muscle field by noting the variation in fiber diameter, the number of nuclei in relation to the amount of sarcoplasm, the inflammatory reaction and the extent of fat and fibrous replacement. It should be remembered, however, that a muscle may reveal severe damage in one area and a short distance away it may appear perfectly healthy. Thus muscle biopsies are notably inaccurate in estimating the extent of disease of the entire structure.

FIGURE 55 represents a cross section of muscle photographed at the same magnification as the longitudinal section. The ends of the fibrils are seen, surrounded by the sarcoplasm. Here and there an eccentric nucleus is found in the plane of section. The fibrils which stain darkly in the illustration show what appears to be a condensation of their sarcoplasm. Unfortunately, this is an artefact seen in most muscle sections. These dark-staining fibers must not be interpreted as evidence of disease unless one is very sure of the technique.

FIG. 56.

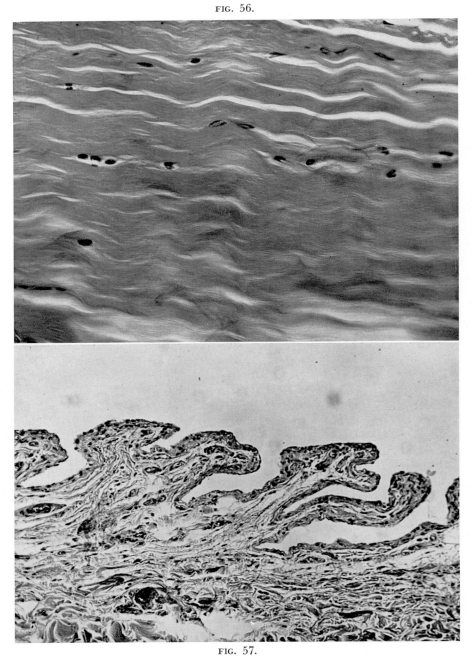

FIG. 57.

FIG. 56. Longitudinal section of tendon. (× 275.)
FIG. 57. Synovial joint lining. (× 125.)

FIGURE 56. Tendons, ligaments and fascia are types of collagenous fibrous connective tissue. They are produced by collagenoblasts which lay down a dense matrix of collagen fibrils so arranged as to achieve a maximum of tensile strength. Tendons are composed of parallel bundles of parallel fibrils. Many fewer cells are caught in this matrix than in ordinary collagen, osteoid or bone, so that the structure is relatively acellular. This material takes the eosin stain and depending upon numerous local factors it may appear pale pink or deep red. When sectioned the fibrils usually assume a wavy pattern such as that seen in the illustration.

FIGURE 57. Synovial membrane lines joint cavities, bursae and tendon sheaths. It consists of a layer (usually single) of cells whose centrally placed nucleus is thicker than the flattened cytoplasm. Thus the membrane in cross section has a cobblestone appearance. Supporting this membrane is a thin layer of fibroblastic cells with a small amount of intercellular collagen. The membrane does not cover weight-bearing surfaces of the articular cartilage. Where the joint capsule is folded the membrane takes a villous configuration. The core of each villous process carries numerous large thin-walled vessels to supply the membrane with an abundance of blood. The joint is lubricated with synovial fluid, a viscous substance composed predominantly of hyaluronate. This fluid is probably secreted largely by the synovial cells. When injured by trauma, infection or impairment of blood supply or when there is alteration of metabolic activity, possibly by change in permeability of the ground substance, the synovial cells may respond by proliferation to form a membrane of several cells' thickness. Exudative inflammatory cells infiltrate the underlying supportive tissue and may penetrate out to the surface where they are caught in the meshwork of fibrin which often forms a covering membrane.

6

Radiology of
the Skeletal System

Skeletal structures are uniquely suited to radiographic examination. The technical aspects are relatively simple, the facilities are readily available and the results tend to be definitive since bone, because of its physical characteristics, casts a distinct image that is in sharp contrast with the surrounding soft tissues. Of even greater importance, however, is the fact that bone is living tissue, less permanent than the soft tissues attached to it, and so reflects alterations in anatomy and physiology of either a local or systemic nature. It is the recognition and interpretation of these alterations that is significant. To a degree, the radiograph of a diseased bone often substitutes for the gross pathologic specimen. The radiologist, however, is denied knowledge of the nature of the abnormal tissue which is present, for pus, blood and neoplastic tissue cast identical shadows. The examination, therefore, is not an end in itself but is rather a part of the whole that must be evaluated in light of all of the known clinical and laboratory data.

The value of radiographic study depends upon an understanding of anatomy, physiology, pathology and the physical principles of radiography. This understanding permits an interpretation of the findings coupled with a realization of the limitations of the method. Overemphasis and failure to realize the limitations are as much to be avoided as is neglect of the method, resulting from a lack of knowledge of its value. The sections of this book dealing with the radiographic manifestations of orthopedic diseases will attempt to correlate the radiographic appearance with the altered morphology wherever possible. For detailed radiographic description, competent texts and appropriate references are readily available. In many sections, descriptions of the gross pathology are applicable to the radiographic manifestations.

In order to interpret a radiograph and to realize its limitations as well as its value, some understanding of the principles of physics as related to radiography is necessary. Why does bone cast a sharp, opaque and contrasting image? Why do soft tissues, pus and blood cast non-contrasting shadows which do not permit differentiation of these structures? X-rays are electromagnetic in nature. By virtue of their wave-length, which approximates 1 Å, they are distinct from other radiations constituting the electromagnetic spectrum. A radiograph results from the differential absorption of the primary x-ray beam as it passes through the tissues to strike the sensitive emulsion of the photographic film. Bone absorbs a significant amount of x-rays as compared with the soft tissues; as a result, few of the rays which strike bone pass through to the film, which after processing is therefore clear or white. Air does not absorb significant amounts of x-rays, so that the emulsion is more affected and after processing the film is black. The soft tissues are intermediate as to absorption. The final image is modified by scattered radiation, geometric factors and by the character of the photographic film, of the processing solutions and of the techniques employed in processing the film.

Absorption of x-rays depends upon the atomic number of the irradiated material and on the wave-length of the radiation employed. An increase in either results in increased absorption. The wave-length of the radiation bears a definite relation to the voltage applied to the x-ray tube and is thus important from the technical standpoint in obtaining radiographs of satisfactory quality. The organic constituents of the body comprising hydrogen, carbon, nitrogen and oxygen have low atomic numbers and the chemical compounds formed by these elements absorb only small amounts of radiation. The inorganic constituents, calcium and phosphorus, have significantly higher atomic numbers, and tissues containing these elements absorb significant amounts of x-rays in contrast with the soft tissues. Differences as to density also affect absorption but to a lesser extent. Alterations in the mineral content of bone may be appreciated and under the most favorable circumstances fat may be seen in contrast with muscle. Shades of black and white (or radiolucency and opacity) may thus be distinguished, dependent upon the elements which are present and to a certain extent upon the density of the tissues which are exposed. Gas, air and at times fat are radiolucent, in contrast with soft tissue and body fluids which are intermediate as to lucency. These in turn are in contrast with bone and other structures containing calcium salts, which are opaque.

As x-rays pass through matter some of the rays are absorbed, some are scattered by collisions with atoms and some pass through unchanged. Scattered x-rays fog the ultimate image by exposing portions of the film not affected by the primary beam. This may be controlled by the use of cones and grids. The former limit the beam and the latter absorb the scattered radiation before it strikes the film. From the geometric standpoint, an x-ray beam is divergent, so that there is an optimum distance from the tube to the film and from the part to be examined to the film. The closer the part to the film and the further the tube from the film, the less magnification and the less distortion. Needless to say, the speed of exposure must be such as to prevent motion being manifest on the radiograph. Processing techniques and the type of film employed in departments of radiology are usually well standardized and will not be considered.

Thus the foundation of radiology is physical. Radiology is not a science of signs but represents the application of physics to anatomy, physiology and pathology. Descriptions of the radiographic appearance of diseased bone are replete with such phrases as "sunburst appearance," "ground-glass appearance of the shaft," "pencil-line cortices" and many others. These signs are only descriptive and are not specific for any disease. They do have a basis in fact, however, and an understanding of the mechanisms responsible for these manifestations is mandatory to the understanding of the disease in question. For example, a long bone of a patient with scurvy may be described as having "pencil-line cortices" and a "ground-glass-like" shaft. Such descriptions refer to osteoporosis in which, because of a lack of organic matrix coupled with continued resorption of bone, the trabeculae become thin and sparse and the cortices become thin. The fine trabeculae absorb less x-rays than do normal ones and thus produce less contrast with the soft tissues of the marrow.

These facts do not lessen the importance of experience. One who sees many bone lesions may recognize alterations that fall into a pattern which he has come to associate with a particular disease. Such experience only serves to strengthen the objective evidence at hand.

In like manner, one must remember that joint spaces are potential spaces and not gross areas of intermediate density as seen by x-ray. The apparent space is in fact cartilage which has the density of soft tissue and which contrasts sharply with subchondral bone. This understanding is essential to the study of joints and particularly to the study of growing bone. The epiphyseal center is a center of bone located within a large mass of cartilage, i.e., the epiphysis. Therefore in diseases involving primarily the joint, cartilaginous destruction must precede destruction of subchondral bone and cartilaginous destruction is manifest by narrowing of the distance between the ossified ends of participating bones.

From the anatomic standpoint, one must recognize the existence of normal variations. Prominent nutrient foramina are often confused with fracture lines, and irregularities in bone configuration may be confused with periosteal new bone formation. Such variations are usually symmetrical and examination of the "opposite side" for comparison will make their significance evident. Bizarre configurations of the bones and joints may be seen as a result of faulty projection or positioning; reexamination is always indicated when the radiographic appearance of a structure does not correlate with anatomic or pathologic information.

The correlation of physiology and radiology is best illustrated by the changes observed in a growing cylindrical bone. The growing ends of a bone will reflect the earliest and most severe changes of metabolic bone disease. The rate of growth of a long bone differs at its proximal and its distal ends, and it is the faster growing of the ends that will present the most apparent alterations. It is for this reason that the wrist and knee are examined when rickets or scurvy is suspected, not because of convenience or for other arbitrary reasons. It is important to note that the epiphyseal center is opaque, not the epiphysis. The zone of provisional calcification, which abuts on the metaphysis, is quite dense and represents the area in which calcium salts are deposited in the cartilaginous intercellular matrix between degenerated cartilage cells. As the blood vessels and osteoblast invade this zone of degenerated cartilage cells, osteoid is deposited on the surface of the exposed cartilaginous matrix. The metaphysis is that area in which osteoid is being laid down and bone is being formed. With a deficiency of mineral salts, as in rickets, the zone of provisional calcification is the first to be affected and thus disappears early in the course of the disease. When organic matrix is deficient, as in scurvy, new bone is not formed and a radiolucent area is evident adjacent to the zone of provisional calcification, the so-called scorbutic zone. Under normal circumstances the trabecular pattern and the thickness of the cortex are dependent in large part on stress and strain; in bowing of a bone, for example, thickening of the cortex and of the trabeculae along the weight-bearing line will be evident.

The soft tissues must not be neglected during the study of bones. They often reflect disease of the underlying bone even when osseous alterations are not apparent. In osteomyelitis, inflammatory exudate in the soft tissues adjacent to the involved bone may distort radio-

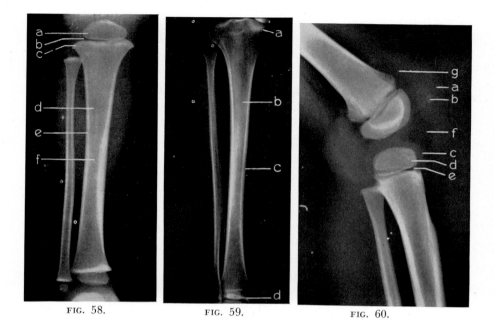

FIG. 58.   FIG. 59.   FIG. 60.

FIG. 58.   Male age 2 years. Radiograph of the tibia and fibula. a, Epiphyseal center; b, epiphyseal line; c, zone of provisional calcification; d, nutrient canal; e, cortex; f, medullary canal.

FIG. 59.   Male age 31 years. Radiograph of the tibia and fibula. a, Residual of epiphyseal line; b, medullary canal; c, cortex; d, subchondral bone at ankle joint. Compare with Figure 58. The epiphyseal centers enlarge and assume a definite configuration as growth occurs. Note the change in the appearance of the ankle joint that occurs when final growth is attained. The amount of epiphyseal cartilage is appreciated.

FIG. 60.   Male age 5 years. Lateral radiograph of the knee. a, Soft tissue shadow of patellar cartilage in contrast with suprapatellar and infrapatellar fat pads (f-g); b, center of ossification for patella; c, proximal tibial epiphyseal cartilage evident because of contrast with infrapatellar fat pad; d, epiphyseal center; e, epiphyseal line. The distal femoral epiphysis and the proximal tibial epiphysis are evident anteriorly. The joint space is appreciated as a "potential" space, not a real one.

lucent muscle planes to indicate the presence of an abnormality before there is evidence of bone destruction. Effusion into a joint may widen the normal radiolucent zone and at times may be associated with dislocation of the participating bones. Fat around the capsule of a joint will often outline the limits of the capsule and reflect its distention by fluid or neoplastic tissue.

The first aim of radiographic study is to find evidence of disease and to note its exact location and extent. Objective analysis of the abnormality on the basis of anatomy, physiology and physics then follows. Finally, the radiographic information is correlated with clinical and laboratory data. The following outline is an attempt at such organized thinking.

I. Normal
II. Abnormal
    A. Benign
               generalized
               localized
        (1) congenital malformation
        (2) infectious
        (3) traumatic
        (4) metabolic
        (5) neoplastic
        (6) adaptive (stress and strain)
    B. Malignant
        (1) primary in bone
        (2) primary in tissues contiguous to bone
        (3) metastatic

Radiographic interpretation is then on a firm basis and the limitation of the method and its worth are evaluated logically and speculation kept at a minimum.

REFERENCE

1. Glasser, Otto, Quimby, E. H., Taylor, L. S., and Weatherwax, J. L.: Physical Foundations of Radiology, 2nd Ed. Paul B. Hoeber, Inc., New York, 1952.

Disturbances in Skeletal

Development

Congenital Developmental Disturbances

ACHONDROPLASIA

Achondroplasia is a hereditary, congenital, familial disturbance in epiphyseal chondroblastic growth and maturation causing inhibition of enchondral bone formation which results in a peculiar type of dwarfism. Some ossification centers appear to be affected more than others, particularly those of the base of the skull and at the ends of long bones. Intramembranous bone formation is normal except as it is secondarily affected by disturbances in length growth. The condition is sometimes called chondrodystrophia fetalis or achondroplastic dwarfism.

The cause of the inadequate cartilage development is entirely unknown. It was long thought to be a disorder of endocrine function, and when certain types of dwarfism were found to be related to pituitary insufficiency, achondroplasia was placed in this group. Failure to find a disturbed function of the pituitary, the thyroid or any other ductless gland has necessitated a reclassification of the condition as a germ plasm defect. This classification may not be entirely healthy because it tends to close the issue and discourage further investigation. Since the condition is hereditary it is doubtless caused by abnormal genetic components, but no one has shown, as improbable as it may seem on mention, that the failure of cartilage growth and maturation is not due to a lack of response to vitamin A. If some such cause could be identified, the course of the abnormality might be altered just as the prognosis of erythroblastosis fetalis has been bettered, even though its cause is genetic.

There is evidence of the existence of achondroplastic dwarfs as far back as antiquity. Because the condition is not necessarily incompatible with vigorous health and a long life, this peculiar body conformation has always excited a considerable amount of curious interest. Since his mentality is usually not affected, the achondroplastic is faced with the same problems of earning his livelihood as are those of normal physique. Even in ancient times he shrewdly evaluated his assets and turned to the field of entertainment, becoming the clown and jester of those who could afford to keep him. Today one will find a considerable proportion of the world's achondroplastics following their traditional occupation. They are frequently referred to as "circus dwarfs."

Achondroplasia is the commonest type of dwarfism. Were it not that over half of these persons die of a severe form of their malformation in utero and during the first few months of infancy, or during a difficult parturition because of the narrow pelvic outlet of their achondroplastic mothers, the number of cases would be greatly increased because the condition is a simple Mendelian dominant and fertility is not affected.

Achondroplasia exists in all degrees of advancement. It may be so severe that it is diagnosed in utero and the patient does not survive fetal life. In its usual form the cases are diagnostically obvious as they walk down the street (Fig. 61). But there are lesser degrees of involvement in which the stature may be almost normal and only a roentgenographic skeletal survey will demonstrate the stigmata of the condition.

The average achondroplastic attains a height of about 50 inches. His head is apt to be enlarged, though it appears relatively bigger than it is because of his inadequate stature. There is some degree of hydrocephalus in most cases, caused by deficient brain space in the posterior fossa. The hydrocephalus is usually of the communicating type and is rarely severe enough to inhibit mental growth. The failure to provide sufficient space for the brain is due to lack of growth along the intersphenoid and spheno-occipital synchondroses. The four principal epiphyseal ossification centers of the base of the skull normally close in early adult life. In the achondroplastic they may ossify in utero or infancy. This accounts for the prominent brachycephaly, the decreased diameter of the foramen magnum and the saddling of the nose. The brain is obliged to grow upward and forward owing to the short base, resulting in a characteristic bulging of the forehead and bossing of the frontal bones. The relatively normal growth of the mandible, which enlarges by both enchondral and intramembranous bone formation, makes it look relatively large, resulting in prognathism. These facial features are so constant that most achondroplastics have the appearance of belonging to the same family.

Since only enchondral bone growth is affected, there is less inhibition of trunk growth than of that of the extremities. The vertebral column may achieve normal length resulting in the characteristic disproportion of the stem and the arms and legs. However, vertebral development is usually not normal. The body may be formed in the shape of a wedge and thus be crowded backward to cause angulation. This may happen anywhere along the column, but is most common between the twelfth dorsal and third lumbar vertebrae. Lordosis is usual, resulting in a horizontal tipping of the sacrum. This produces a characteristic prominence of the buttocks. Kyphosis is apt to develop in the thoracic and cervical areas. Sometimes a gibbus is produced. Since there is inadequate growth of the pedicles there is barely sufficient space for the cord and cauda equina without angulation. Distortion and abnormal pressures cause rupture of the intervertebral discs. Pressure upon the cord and nerve roots, particularly in the lower spine, is the most common complication in the adult achondro-

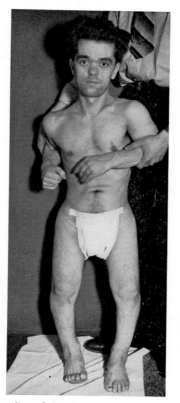

FIG. 61.   Achondroplasia. An adult chondroplastic revealing dwarfism, large head, wide face, saddle nose, prognathism, short extremities and bowed legs.

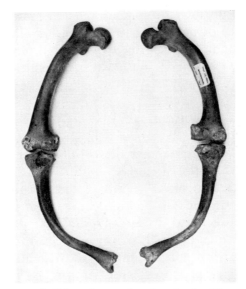

FIG. 62.   The femora and tibias of an achondroplastic. They are short, thick and heavy. The ends are flared. The shafts are bowed.

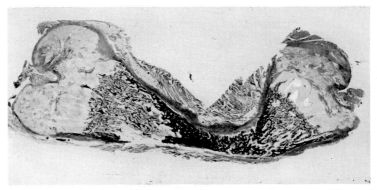

FIG. 63.   Achondroplasia. Longitudinal section of a long bone. The ends of the bone are widened in relation to the diameter of the mid-shaft. This gives the x-ray appearance of "trumpeting" which is highly characteristic of this condition.

plastic.[1] This often results in paraplegia and disturbance of bladder function.

The ribs frequently fail to grow to normal length, producing a flattened and narrow chest. All of the long bones are widened at the ends and thus the rib cage may show a prominence of the costochondral junctions.

The long cylindrical bones of the extremities, depending entirely upon enchondral growth for their length, are the most dramatically altered. The finger tips reach only to the hip joint instead of the mid-thigh region and the patient has a duck-legged appearance. The legs are frequently bowed (Fig. 62). The fingers are stubby. The trumpeting of the bone ends may cause enlargement of the joint region (Fig. 63).

Achondroplasia may be accompanied by other congenital malformations. These are particularly apt to occur in the skin and sometimes in the heart. A rare variation of the condition is a combination of achondroplasia, ectodermal dysplasia (skin, hair and teeth),[2] polydactyly and Roger's disease (cardiac septal defect). This has been called Ellis-van Creveld syndrome.

ROENTGENOGRAPHIC MANIFESTATIONS

As a reflection of a disturbance in enchondral bone formation, the roentgenographic manifestations of achondroplasia are most marked in the long bones. The base of the skull is short and the deformity of the pelvis characteristic. In the severe and often fatal form of the disease the ribs are markedly shortened so that the volume of the thorax is reduced. Alterations in the vertebrae are present in most cases but the length of the spine usually approximates normal. The vertebrae may appear as thin discs surrounded by abundant cartilage or there may be only minimal loss in stature, compensated in part by intervertebral disc spaces that are normal or slightly increased in width. The short thick pedicles and laminae cause a narrow and shallow spinal canal. Myelography will demonstrate the deformity of the spinal canal and often, in the adult, rupture of intervertebral discs. Marked lumbar lordosis is present and the sacrum is angled sharply posteriorly.

The long bones, because of disturbed enchondral osteogenesis, are short and their ends flared. The zone of provisional calcification and epiphyseal center are usually smooth in outline, but in the hyperplastic type may be quite irregular. The epiphyseal center may be partially enclosed by marginal overgrowth of the end of the shaft. Periosteal osteogenesis is normal so that the diameter of the bones is normal. Bowing is common, as is cortical thickening at the sites where muscles attach.

The ilia are broad and short. A broad, flat pelvis is a common finding in association with large acetabula with horizontal roofs.

The lack of growth of the bones at the base of the skull results in a short base (Fig. 65). The cranial vault is often increased in size and the frontal regions tend to bulge. In the child, the synchondrosis between the occipital and sphenoid bones closes quite early in life.

Radiographic manifestations of achondroplasia vary as do the clinical manifestations. The classic achondroplastic dwarf shows short cylindrical bones, in relation to the length of the trunk. Severe deform-

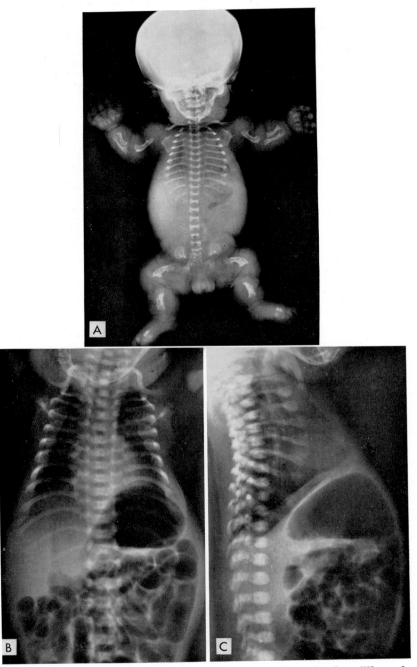

FIG. 64.   Achondroplasia—severe forms. *A* is the radiograph of a stillborn fetus. Marked skeletal deformity is evident. Anterior-posterior (*B*) and lateral (*C*) radiographs of an infant with extreme deformity of the ribs. Respiratory distress was marked. Note the bell-shaped trunk.

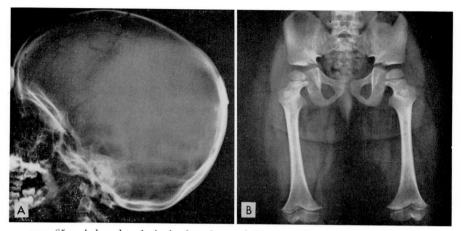

FIG. 65. Achondroplasia in female aged 5 years. The base of the skull (*A*) is short and the spheno-occipital synchondrosis is closed. Frontal bulging is evident and contributes to the depressed bridge of the nose noted clinically. The deformity of the pelvis and femora (*B*) is typical.

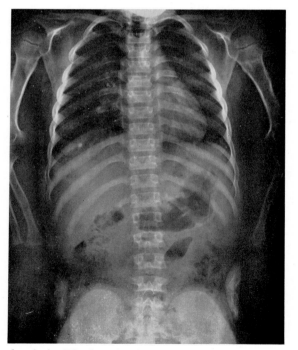

FIG. 66. Achondroplasia. The length of the upper extremities may be compared to the length of the trunk. There is little deformity of the spine and ribs.

ity is incompatible with life, and all of the skeletal structures will show marked alteration. In others, the radiographic features may be almost entirely lacking.

MICROSCOPY

The changes apparent on microscopic examination are best seen in sections made through the epiphyseal plate of a long bone during the growing period (Fig. 67). The epiphyseal plate is not as thick as normal, but it has a greater circumference to cover the flared end of the diaphysis. This increase in width is probably due to subchondral appositional growth. The decreased thickness appears to be the result of inadequate interstitial chondroblastic division. Not only is there a paucity of chondroblasts but those formed fail to mature properly. They do not acquire their enzymatic and glycogen content as normal cells do and they fail to form definite columns. Thus, the surrounding cylinders of hyalin are not produced, resulting in a failure to produce a normal continuous line of provisory calcification. Without adequate bars of calcified hyalin, the scaffolding of the lattice fails to form (Fig. 68). Some bits of mineralized hyalin protrude into the metaphysis and about these there is normal osteoid production, suggesting

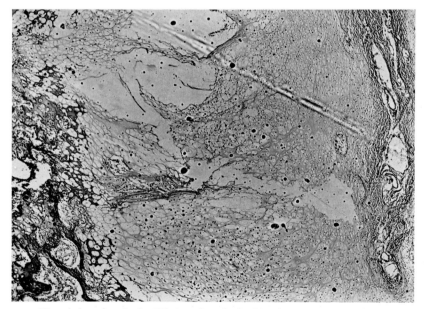

FIG. 67.   Achondroplasia. The enchondral plate is seen on the right, the "epiphyseal line" and metaphysis along the left margin. The plate is thin; columnation is extremely irregular if it occurs at all. No scaffolding is formed and there is an incomplete line of provisional calcification. (× 30.)

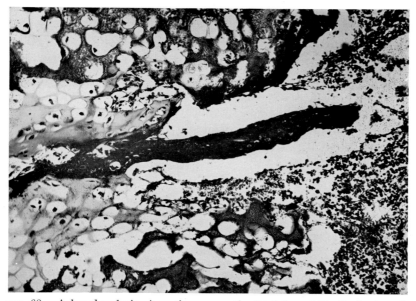

FIG. 68. Achondroplasia. A section across the "epiphyseal line" of a long bone. The metaphysis is on the right. There is a failure of orientation and maturation of the chondroblasts which throws all subsequent events in this region into confusion. (× 180.)

that the fault is not in osteoblastic activity. But the scaffolding is so irregular and sparse that little osteoid can be laid down in a systematic fashion. Intramembranous, periosteal bone formation appears not to be affected. Compacta is produced and the cortices appear wider and sturdier than normal because of the shortness of the diaphysis. The production of a heavy cylinder of compacta with deficient supporting spongiosa may be the cause of the flaring with stress on the epiphysis. The thin epiphysis and its lack of support by an adequate spongiosa result in sagging, so that the diaphysis appears to partially surround the epiphysis and the epiphyseal line is curved and irregular.

PROGNOSIS

If the achondroplastic survives the trauma of childbirth he stands a good chance of living well into adult life. During late middle age he is apt to be plagued by symptoms caused by pressure upon the cord and the spinal nerves. Thus backache, sciatica, paresthesias and even paraplegia may develop. A herniated disc may add to these difficulties. If he marries a normal spouse he has a 50 per cent chance of fathering a normal offspring. If he marries another achondroplastic, he may be fairly sure of helping to perpetuate his kind.

MORQUIO'S DISEASE

This condition has been called chondro-osteodystrophy or eccentro-chondro-osteodystrophy. The eponym "Morquio's" is retained here only because it is the one most widely used.

The condition is a hereditary disease often occuring in multiple siblings and causing dwarfism, kyphosis and severe disability. It was incompletely described several times in the years from 1913 to 1928 but it was in Morquio's report[4] in 1929 that it was first completely set forth as an entity. In a series of three reports he eventually described four cases in a single family.

Morquio's is a rare disease. At this writing there are a few less than one hundred cases reported in the world literature. It is usually considered to be a disease of childhood, the signs most often appearing between the sixth and eighteenth months. It occurs in both sexes with about equal incidence. Its hereditary nature is now thoroughly established since approximately 50 per cent reveal this characteristic and the majority of these show sibling relationship. It is recessive. The condition has occurred in mother and offsprings more than once. There is more than a suggestion that consanguinity plays a role since it appeared five times in forty-one families, an incidence of 12 per cent and about sixty times more frequently than might be expected in an average cross section population.[5]

A variety of accompanying malformations have been reported, one of the commonest being dolichocephaly. When the latter occurs there may be mental impairment.

In only a few cases has there been a suggestion of the disease at the time of birth. In almost all, the first symptoms appear at about the time weight-bearing begins by sitting or standing. Since there are no reports of prenatal x-ray studies it is impossible to say whether or not skeletal changes occur in utero. If it could be shown that the disturbance does not begin until after birth one might conjecture, as the cause, a deficiency of some substance which was supplied by the mother until placental separation.

The first sign noted is usually a dorsilumbar kyphosis (Fig. 69), and as an attempt at weight-bearing continues, a galaxy of skeletal distortions appear. The neck is short so that the head appears to be thrust forward and jammed down into the thorax. The sternum is prominent with a horizontal displacement. The chest is increased in the anteroposterior dimension. The head is normal in size though it appears large because of the lag in growth of the rest of the body, this lag being progressively more apparent as the more caudad parts are approached. Thus, the legs appear less well developed than the

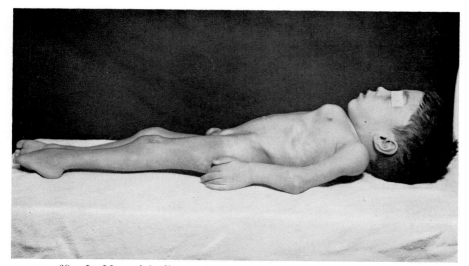

FIG. 69. In Morquio's disease the caudad portions of the body are poorly developed. The head is relatively large, the neck short. The plastron is bulged forward. The legs are undeveloped. (From Shriners' Hospital.)

trunk and the trunk less so than the arms. The joints are widened. The wrists and ankles and sometimes larger joints are abnormally mobile owing to muscle and tendon laxity, but extension at the elbows, hips and knees may be incomplete because of an elongated olecranon and epiphyseal distortion. As the patient ages the characteristic stance with kyphotic back and partially flexed hips, knees and elbows develops. The hands are short and trident with thick fingers and ulnar deviation. The feet are short, wide, flat and everted at the ankles. The deciduous teeth are usually well formed but the permanent teeth are distorted both as to position and shape. Since most of the decidual tooth buds develop in utero and the permanent buds after birth, this selectivity in tooth development further suggests that the cause of the disease is postnatal in influence.

ROENTGENOGRAPHIC MANIFESTATIONS

The roentgenographic manifestations of Morquio's disease reflect abnormal conversion of cartilage to bone. Alteration in the size and contour of the vertebral bodies is constant and distinctive. The long bones are affected in most instances, and while the degree of deformity varies, it is the growing ends of the long bones that show abnormality. There is no disturbance in the density or the architecture of the diaphyses in most instances except when deformity progresses to the degree that disuse osteoporosis results.

The vertebral bodies are flat (universal vertebra plana) with

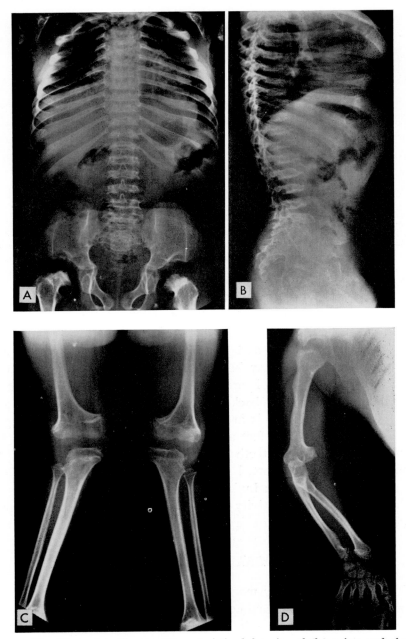

FIG. 70.   Morquio's disease. Characteristic deformity of the spine and chest is evident (*A* and *B*). The acetabula are deep and irregular. The proximal femoral epiphyseal center is poorly formed, and the neck of the femur is short and bent. The bones of the lower extremities are of normal length (*C*); those of the upper extremity are shorter than normal (*D*). Flat, irregular and wide epiphyseal centers are evident. Knock-knee deformity is present (*C*).

rough, irregular contours and an anterior central projection or tongue. The intervertebral disc spaces are narrower than is normal. Kyphosis is common and may be aggravated by posterior displacement or wedging of one or more vertebra. A small sacrum is common. An increase in the anterior-posterior diameter of the chest occurs as a result of kyphosis. The ribs tend to be broad and deformed at both their anterior and posterior ends.

The cylindrical bones may be normal in length. In some instances they are short and it is usually the bones of the upper extremities that manifest this alteration. The growing ends of the long bones are broad with irregular zones of provisional calcification and irregularly ossified, flattened epiphyseal centers. The proximal femur may show marked deformity, and subluxations at the hip are not uncommon. The acetabula tend to be deep and irregular in contour and the ilia to flare laterally.

A decrease in muscle mass may be evident about the lower extremities. Knock-knee deformity is extremely common as a result of the relaxation of muscles and tendons about the knees.

MICROSCOPY

The opportunity of obtaining material for microscopic study has been extremely limited and consequently conclusive descriptions cannot as yet be given. Opie and Harrison[6] described a case under the title of "hypertrophic chondrodystrophy" which now appears to be Morquio's disease. They gave a detailed description of the microscopic features of the head of the femur. They reported an abortive and disordered maturation of the epiphyseal chondroblasts with failure to produce an oriented, calcified hyalin scaffolding. There was sealing off of the epiphyseal plate with an irregular vault of bone and islands of cartilage within the metaphysis. The writer found much the same picture in two cases with repeated biopsies at intervals in one of them (Fig. 71). The improper chondroblastic maturation, some chondroblasts collecting glycogen in the depths of the epiphyseal plate and others none at all, resulted in a distorted hyalin bar production and irregularities in the epiphyseal line. The line of provisional calcification was broken and distorted and here and there the hyalin matrix showed focal areas of degeneration. The result was a helter-skelter production of primary spongiosa. Lamellated cortex formation appeared to be relatively normal.

Because bone deformity appears on weight-bearing one might conjecture that there is an inability to convert primitive fiberbone to adult bone. The skeleton, remaining soft, is unprepared for the stress of

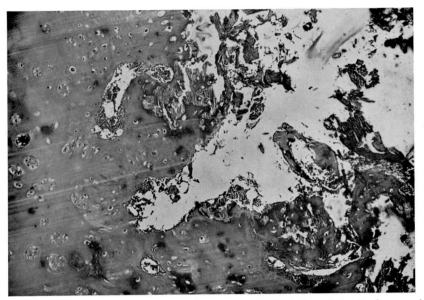

FIG. 71.   Morquio's disease. A section across the "epiphyseal line" of a growing bone showing a completely chaotic arrangement of the chondrocytes, provisional line of calcification and hyalin scaffolding. The epiphysis is on the left. Note the irregular maturation of the cartilage cells and wandering line which represents the junction of the epiphysis and metaphysis. ($\times$ 40.)

normal weight-bearing. A single biopsy specimen removed from the shin of a nine year old patient with Morquio's disease revealed fiber-bone where adult bone normally should have been. One must not draw conclusions from such limited material and it is fortunate for the pathologist that the diagnosis does not depend upon the micro-scopic appearance.

DIFFERENTIAL DIAGNOSIS

Hurler's disease (gargoylism) is the condition most frequently confused with Morquio's. The radiologic aspects are so similar that numerous cases of the former have been reported in series under the title of the latter. Though the two conditions may closely resemble each other, both clinically and radiologically, at present they appear to be quite distinct entities. Mental deficiency may be seen in both, but when found in Morquio's disease it is probably an accompanying condition and not a part of the process sui generis. Clouding of the corneae probably does not occur in Morquio's. In the latter, the liver edge may descend below the costal margin, but this is because of liver displacement rather than enlargement. The spleen and lymph nodes are not enlarged. If a biopsy of the liver, spleen or lymph nodes

is done and globules of an alien substance found within the cell cytoplasm, the condition is probably lipochondrodystrophy. The leukocytes of the peripheral blood should be stained with Wright's stain
and searched for coarse, dark, violet granules. This finding, according
to a recent report, is diagnostic of Hurler's disease.

PROGNOSIS

The progress of Morquio's disease usually slows as the patient
ages. Some cases seem to be arrested with puberty though a few continue through adolescence and even into adult life. Formes frustes
have been described on radiologic evidence alone but this is hazardous
business since the radiologic findings in Morquio's disease are not
pathognomonic. Whether or not the disease is arrested, the skeletal
distortion is usually so marked that woeful crippling is inevitable.
Once the progress has come to a halt the patient may live as long as
his deformities are compatible with existence.

OSTEOGENESIS IMPERFECTA

Osteogenesis imperfecta has been called osteitis fragilitans,
fragilitas ossium congenita, osteopsathyrosis idiopathica and brittle
bones. It is a hereditary, often congenital and familial disease which
is manifested by an inability to produce the adequate and normal
intercellular substances of certain mesenchymal derivatives, particularly osteoblasts and fibroblasts, in various body areas. The result is a
young patient with a fragile skeleton, thin skin and sclerae, poor teeth,
a tendency to macular bleeding and hypermotility of joints.

There are two forms of the disease. Osteogenesis imperfecta congenita is noted at birth and it has obviously developed in utero. It is
often fatal. Osteogenesis imperfecta tarda starts its course some time in
childhood. It may produce symptoms of only one or two system disturbances and its effects are much less severe than those of the congenital form.

The disease is quite rare, but because of its unique symptomatology it has been recognized as an entity for nearly two hundred years.
Its peculiar and dramatic expression has resulted in the reporting of
over two thousand cases and even in the older literature the diagnoses
appear to be quite accurate.

Several writers have concerned themselves with the hereditary
features of this disease. It apparently occurs as a spontaneous muta-
tion and once established in the hereditary apparatus it persists as a
dominant. Thus, it may appear in a single member of a family and

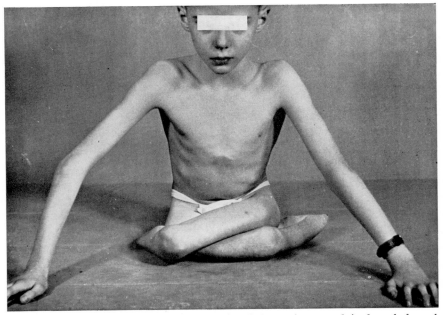

FIG. 72. In osteogenesis imperfecta the skeleton is normal in length but the cortices are deficient in thickness and strength. The extremities are long and gracile. The fragile bones of the lower extremity often show multiple fractures because they are subjected to stress. (From Shriners' Hospital.)

his offspring are apt to inherit the disease while those of his siblings show no trait. Since the congenital form is severe and affects children before reproductivity, the affected branch soon dies out.

The outstanding characteristic in the full-blown disease is the skeletal fragility and proclivity for fracture on slight trauma. Thus, the case which develops in utero may not survive the rigors of parturition. Some doggedly tenacious writers have recorded thousands of fractures in a single case. If the patient survives the neonatal period or if the disease begins later in childhood, he is haunted for the remainder of his life by the specter of fracture on minor trauma. If the fractures are numerous and the deformity profound (Fig. 72) he may literally grow smaller instead of larger as overriding and bending cause loss in stature.

Though the bone is inadequately formed to resist normal stress, the fractures heal, often within a normal time. Callus formation may be frugal or it may be exuberant, but the bone that is formed is of the same poor quality as that it replaces. Ordinary activity may cause partial fractures which eventually may result in bending. Manifestations are usually more obvious in the lower extremities, probably because these are more vulnerable to trauma; invalidism is therefore a common sequence of the disease.

Those who have had the opportunity of observing considerable numbers of patients with osteogenesis imperfecta[7] state that bone growth is abnormal apart from the fractures and subsequent deformities. The cylindrical bones of the extremities are apt to be long and gracile and skeletal muscles poorly developed. The skull is reported to be misshapen with protrusion of the frontal and parietal regions and a deeply overhanging occiput.

Though pathologic fractures are the most trying features of the condition, the inability to produce normal components of intercellular matrix is manifested elsewhere. The blue sclerotics are probably of this order. The sclerae may range from a blue-white tint to a deep sky blue color. Some observers insist that the shade is not constant and that it may vary from time to time within the same patient. Others have described a "Saturn's ring" of white about the cornea. The color is apparently due to the intraocular pigment which is visible through the sclera. Some writers have reported sclerae of subnormal thickness; others contend that the thickness is normal, but that the substance is translucent. The abnormality does not affect vision.

The teeth are often poor because of malformation of the dentin.[8] Both deciduous and permanent teeth are affected. When the teeth alone are involved, the condition has been called "dentinogenesis imperfecta" or "hereditary opalescent dentin." They are usually discolored bluish gray to a yellowish brown and they often have an opalescent appearance. The enamel, being a product of cells of ectodermal rather than mesenchymal derivation, is normal, but since it rests upon a foundation of poor dentin it chips and the teeth may be lost by the age of thirty. Roentgenograms show short roots and sometimes obliterated pulp canals.

Deafness is frequently mentioned as a characteristic feature of osteogenesis imperfecta tarda during adult life. Some authors believe that this is the result of pressure upon the eighth nerves as they emerge from the cranial vault, but others state that its onset is like that of otosclerosis and is due to abnormal proliferations of cartilage which become calcified and result in sclerosis of the petrous portion of the temporal bone.

The hypermotility of the joints, especially at the wrists and ankles, has been frequently noted. It may be due to a disturbance in the production of the collagen components of tendons and ligaments.

Follis[9] has noted a peculiar appearance of the skin on microscopic examination. By special staining technique he has demonstrated the presence of an immature collagen of the corium and suggests that there is an inability to transform fetal collagen into the mature adult form.

A tendency for macular hemorrhage into the tissues has been noted. The Rumpel-Leede test may be positive. This again may be the result of an inability to produce a normal intercellular cement substance; thus capillary permeability is altered.

There is still controversy concerning whether there is normal scar formation in patients with osteogenesis imperfecta. Scot and Stiris[7] investigated this question and concluded that though healing occurs, and often within a normal time, the resulting scar is broader than normal and the collagen of poor quality.

ROENTGENOGRAPHIC MANIFESTATIONS

Osteogenesis imperfecta affects the entire skeleton. Roentgenographic manifestations vary according to the severity of the disease, but in general the bones are osteoporotic and often show evidence of old or recent fractures. The osteoporosis reflects inadequate osteoblastic activity. The trabeculae are fine and sparse and the cortex thin. Because cartilaginous maturation proceeds normally, the cylindrical bones are of normal length. Their diameter, however, tends to be

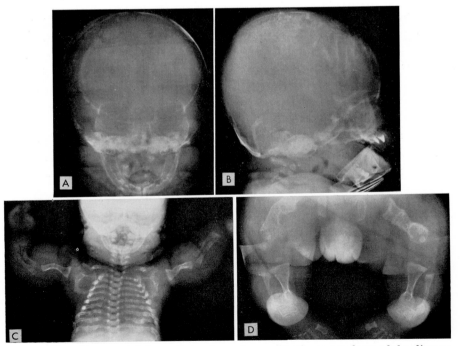

FIG. 73.   Osteogenesis imperfecta. A newborn with the severe form of the disease. In *A* and *B* note the inadequate mineralization of the cranial bones, the wide sutures and multiple centers of ossification. Multiple fracture of the extremities and rib cage are evident in *C* and *D*. The cortices are thin and the spongiosa is markedly deficient.

smaller than normal as a consequence of disturbed periosteal osteo-genesis. The ends of cylindrical bones appear wide when compared to their shafts, and because the trabeculae are sparse the zone of pro-visional calcification may appear more opaque than normal.

Bones of intramembranous origin are affected, and in the severe, early form of the disease the radiographic appearance of the skull may be striking. Multiple centers of ossification, less opaque than normal, are evident, and as these slowly enlarge the cranial bones exhibit a mosaic pattern. Chipping and crumbling of the teeth may result in radiographic abnormality akin to caries.

Fractures and deformity are an integral part of the radiographic appearance. Deformity, the result of muscle pull, may be evident. Compression fractures of the vertebrae are not uncommon and are manifest by a decrease in the stature of the vertebral bodies. In the less severe forms of the disease, frequent fractures may be the dominant feature with little recognizable abnormality of the cortex and spongiosa.

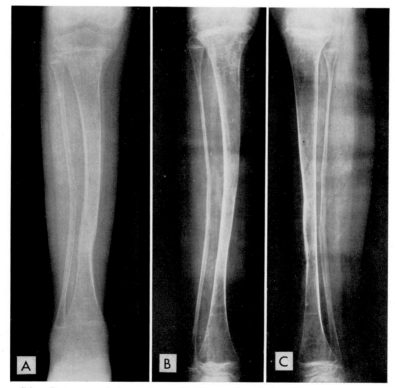

FIG. 74. Osteogenesis imperfecta. Radiographs of the tibia and fibula of a child exposed at the age of 5 years (A) and 7 years (B and C). Longitudinal growth is evident over the two-year interval but note the change that occurred in the diameter of the bones, particularly the fibula. The cortex is narrow and trabeculae sparse. Healing of the fracture of the shaft of the tibia (A) occurred, but with deformity.

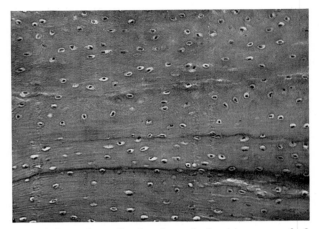

FIG. 75.   Osteogenesis imperfecta. Section through the thin cortex of a long bone. The bone is immature in type with lack of lamellation and haversian systems. ($\times$ 200.)

MICROSCOPY

Demineralized sections of bone in osteogenesis imperfecta reveal a disturbance in both enchondral and intramembranous bone formation. The cartilaginous epiphyses are normal and the secondary ossification centers appear on schedule. Chondroblastic proliferation is present and orderly and maturation with columnation and glycogen imbibition appear to be undisturbed. Mineral salts are deposited in the line of provisional calcification and a hyalin lattice is formed. Here, enchondral growth appears to stop. Osteoblasts fail to emerge in proper numbers from the undifferentiated cell mass and consequently the fingers of calcified hyalin remain naked or inadequately covered, since a paucity of osteoid is laid down. Very few osteoclasts appear, whether because there is no use for them or because of an inability to form them is unknown. Thus, the spongiosa is exceedingly scant. It consists of a few thin and often fractured spicules of primitive bone in a relatively large marrow space. Follis[10] and Weber[11] independently reported wide seams of an unknown substance which takes a deep blue stain with hematoxylin surrounding the fragments of mineralized hyalin lattice.

Osteoid formation by the periosteal osteoblasts is equally deficient. Some primitive fiberbone is laid down, but there is no transition to adult bone and therefore no lamellation and no haversian system formation. The result is a deficient cortex and one which lacks continuity. The bone that is formed remains in the coarsely fibered state and never becomes arranged in the lines of normal stress. (Fig. 75) There is apparently no fault in mineralization since the osteoid becomes mineralized promptly and adequately.

The above descriptions were made from sections of bone in cases of fatal osteogenesis imperfecta congenita. All degrees of bone production are seen in cases of osteogenesis imperfecta tarda but the spongiosa almost always appears scant and the compacta inadequate.

Sections of the skin in the fatal congenital form were stained by Follis[9] using the periodic acid–Schiff and silver techniques. He interpreted the persistent metachromasia and argentophilia as evidence that the collagen of the corium was immature.

Some interesting studies have been done by Engfeldt et al.[12] utilizing microradiography, x-ray diffraction and polarized light techniques. These methods demonstrate irregular mineralization of osteoid which appears to be on the basis of a disturbance in osteoid production rather than in the mineralization itself. The osteoid is of a peculiar fetal character, coarsely fibered and arranged without regard to vasculature. There is consequently no lamellation and no haversian system formation. There is little or no attempt at replacement by secondary or mature osteoid. The defect appears to lie either in an inability of the osteoblasts to differentiate from the multipotent cell mass or in some deficiency which prevents them from providing the normal constituents necessary for osteoid formation. Since presumably there is no inadequacy in the nutrients supplied to the cell, the fault would appear to lie within the cell itself which is either refractory to normal stimuli or lacking in a normal enzyme equipment.

It is of great interest that in osteogenesis imperfecta there is a dissociation of chondroblastic and osteoblastic activity. Cartilage appears to develop normally and is affected only because of the abnormal mechanical stresses which result from inadequate bone formation. The only other condition in which this dissociation is so clearly apparent is scurvy. In ascorbic acid deficiency, there is normal chondroblastic activity but the osteoblasts fail to develop normal components of phosphatase and cytoplasmic ribose nucleic acid and there is a comparable failure of osteoid and collagen production.

Osteogenesis imperfecta now appears to be a systemic inability to produce normal and adequate osteoid and collagen. This inability is registered in the skeleton, the teeth, the sclerae, the joints, the skin and the blood vessels. Some of these areas are likewise affected in scurvy. However, no one would seriously propose that osteogenesis imperfecta is due to a tissue refractoriness to vitamin C since the two diseases are so different symptomatically.

PROGNOSIS

The patient with severe osteogenesis imperfecta in childhood is almost certain to develop disabling skeletal deformity if indeed he survives to adulthood. At the time of cessation of normal skeletal growth the severity of the condition may subside but the fabric re-mains shoddy and the patient must continue to avoid trauma of all degrees. The abatement of symptoms at adulthood has led some to consider endocrine dysfunction as a possible cause. There are no facts to substantiate this hypothesis. It appears that the condition is a dis-turbance in skeleton formation and is, therefore, most manifest at the time skeletal bone is being produced. As the rate of growth diminishes, the manifestations of the disease become less obvious and if the victim survives to maturity he may learn to live with his affliction.

OSTEOPETROSIS

Osteopetrosis, also known as Albers-Schönberg disease, osteo-sclerosis, osteosclerosis fragilis, marble bones and chalk bones, is a rare hereditary, congenital and familial abnormality in bone growth, the disturbed mechanism of which appears to be a failure or inhibi-tion of resorption of calcified hyalin and primitive bone. Since there is little or no inhibition in the formation of cartilage and primitive bone, growth continues but, lacking resorption, the cores of calcified cartilage and their sheaths of unlamellated osteoid persist, interfering with the formation of adult bone which normally replaces it and crowding the areas where resorption should produce the medullary cavity.

Recognizable cases of osteopetrosis have been described since the middle of the eighteenth century under a variety of names but Albers-Schönberg was the first to report a roentgenographic description of the condition in 1907 and it has since borne his name. Karshner[13] intro-duced the term osteopetrosis in 1926 and since that time numerous papers have appeared ascribing an amusing variety of alterations in physiology to account for the clinical and morphologic findings of the disease.

The terms osteopetrosis and marble bones were suggested because of the density to x-ray and a few descriptions of the bones as harder than normal. Other reports state that a drill sinks into the bone as though it were chalk and call attention to the high incidence of patho-logic fractures. These features have inspired the terms chalk bones and osteopetrosis fragilis. It is true that transverse fractures do occur, indicating that the affected bones are brittle rather than soft. It is also true that in a few instances the bone is eburnated causing the drill to smoke as penetration is attempted, but in most instances the bone is hard but actually of a chalky consistency.

Some writers have contended that the disturbance is due to an excessive deposition of normal calcium salts. It is true that, for any measured volume of bone, the mineral content is greater than that of normal bone, but if the normal spaces of the latter are taken into consideration the quantitative relation of mineral to organic matrix of osteopetrotic bone remains about that of the normal. Others have contended that the type of mineral in osteopetrosis is abnormal and compare these bones to those seen in cases of fluorine, strontium and phosphorus toxicity. Chemical analysis of the salts extracted from osteopetrotic bone has not corroborated this hypothesis. Some have thought that the crystalline architecture was altered by an abnormal quantitative variation in the normal constituents. The results of several analyses are conflicting and the facts are not as yet clear, but it is probable that at least in some cases of osteopetrosis chemical make-up of the bone salts is the same as that of normal bone.

Because of failure to find a cause for the condition in the mineral content it was suggested that the disturbance was due to an abnormal proliferation of bone by the endosteum. Actually, in the sense of a periosteum-like membrane lining the medullary cavity, an endosteum does not exist and in osteopetrosis bone does not grow into the medullary cavity from the inner surface of the cortex. Cortical bone remains from its embryonal inception so that a normal medullary cavity is never formed. It has been stated that only enchondral bone is affected because, grossly, the metaphyseal areas are the most dramatically altered, but actually all bone, both enchondral and intramembranous, is involved. A comparison of large sections of infant and adult osteopetrotic bone with the normal of comparable ages bears out this statement.

A careful reading of the admirable paper by Zawisch[14] is infinitely helpful in understanding the process that results in the changes which characterize osteopetrosis. It must be stated that the exact mechanisms of the disease are not known. The most that can be said is that there appears to be a failure or an inhibition of the resorption processes so that primitive chondro-osteoid persists and interferes with its replacement by normal mature bone.

Osteopetrosis is a rare condition, there being less than two hundred cases reported in the literature. It has been diagnosed by roentgenograms of the fetus in utero. In most fatal cases death is due to anemia during the second year. The average case is diagnosed some time during adolescence, attention being directed to the condition by fracture, anemia, failing vision or osteomyelitis of the jaw. Rarely, cases are diagnosed in adult life and at least one instance is recorded in advanced senility. Like most of the congenital diseases of the skeleton, the earlier the manifestations occur, the worse the prognosis is apt to be. The severest type, often placed in a special group, dies in utero or, if these patients survive the fetal period, they usually succumb before their second birthday. Those who live through childhood may develop difficulties at any time thereafter with a progressive anemia.

Occasionally one finds a focal area of sclerosis in a single bone of an adult and biopsy shows the characteristic microscopy of osteopetrosis. Whether these are bona fide instances of solitary, focal osteopetrosis or a variety of some other sclerosing disease is not certain. The incidence of the generalized type suggests that it is inherited as a simple Mendelian recessive. Some have suggested that the more florid type behaves as a Mendelian dominant. There is a higher incidence of consanguinity in the parents than in the average population.

In the cases of osteopetrosis which manifest themselves early the skull bones are usually quite drastically involved. Since the major cartilaginous growth centers are within the base it is this area which is most extensively involved. The failure in modeling which characterizes the disease results in the formation of a massive base with improper and inadequate formation of the various fossae. There may be inadequate room for the growth of the pituitary with disturbed function of that gland. Inadequate space for the circulation of the cerebrospinal fluid about the hemispheres results in hydrocephalus in many cases. This may be severe enough to cause widening of the sutures and delayed closure of the fontanels. Consequently, the head may be enlarged. In the same manner, there is apt to be incomplete formation of the foramina so that there is inadequate room for the passage of the cerebral nerves. Atrophy of the optic nerves causes failing vision and this may be accompanied by nystagmus and occular palsy. Many of the juvenile cases progress to complete blindness. Deafness and facial palsies are also common. The teeth are apt to be late in erupting and severe caries develops early. Caries is followed by infection with eventual osteomyelitis and necrosis of the mandible. These difficulties are attributed to the inadequate bony channels for nutrient circulation.

The vertebrae are usually severely involved and there may be impingement on the spinal nerves as well. Cylindrical bones develop a highly characteristic conformation. At times, the shaft is widened throughout its entire length, but more often the middle third of the diaphysis is of about normal width. The ends of the diaphysis develop a peculiar bulbous clubbing which extends to the epiphyseal line. This is due to the failure in absorption of both the calcified hyalin islands and the young bone which is laid down about them. Normally this first product in the formation of bone, osteochondroid, undergoes a slow lysis and replacement with adult, lamellated bone in stress trajectories. Since absorption of the osteochondroid does not occur, modeling cannot take place and the bone elongates, maintaining the diameter of the metaphysis. This elongated "metaphysis" is the hall-mark of osteopetrosis, but if a careful examination is made the bone of the shaft laid down by the cambium will be seen to be involved also.

Fractures are common in osteopetrosis. They are often character-istically transverse. These have puzzled investigators who have assumed that, because the bones are more massive and opaque, they should be stronger. It has been suggested that the crystalline lattice in osteo-petrosis is abnormal and, therefore, lacking in strength. The little investigation that has been done in this field has not substantiated this view. When one examines osteopetrotic bone under the micro-scope, the reason for its tendency to fracture becomes obvious. Nor-mally, a fine lamellated bone is laid down in lines which are arranged so as to most effectively resist stress. In osteopetrosis, finely lamellated bone is not formed nor is there organization of the unresolved osteo-chondroid in trajectory lines. Consequently, though the bone is hard to the touch since it contains large quantities of calcium salts, the alignment and reenforcement is defective and it breaks like chalk, transverse to the long axis.[15] Fractures heal producing a callus which has the same abnormal features as the original bone.

Normal growth is impeded. The skeleton is apt to be moderately stunted. Ossification centers appear and close on schedule except where there is secondary interference by fracture, abnormal pressures or dis-use atrophy.

A myelophthisic anemia is apt to be a most troublesome compli-cation and is frequently the cause of death. In the advanced case one can find no gross evidence of hematopoietic marrow since the spongiosa and the medullary cavity are replaced by porous bony tissue. The spleen and, in children, the lymph nodes and liver attempt to com-pensate for this lack by myeloid metaplasia. The enlargement of these organs constitutes a part of the clinical expression of osteopetrosis.

ROENTGENOGRAPHIC MANIFESTATIONS

Radiographically, osteopetrosis is manifest by striking opacity of the bones and obliteration of the normal architecture. In many areas the cortex and spongiosa are of the same density, and in the growing long bone the zone of provisional calcification will be indistinguish-able from the adjacent spongiosa. The entire skeleton is affected.

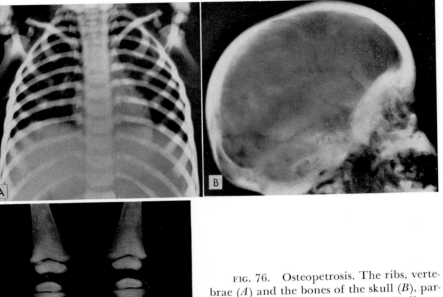

FIG. 76.   Osteopetrosis. The ribs, vertebrae (A) and the bones of the skull (B), particularly those at the base of the skull, are
thick and uniformly opaque. Widening of
the distal femora (C) is apparent and the
medullary canal is almost obliterated in the
diaphysis of the tibias. Striations in the
diaphyses of the long bones are evident. The
epiphyseal centers are involved.

The bones at the base of the skull tend to show the most marked
change but all of the cranial bones may be involved. The mastoid
air cells and paranasal sinuses may never develop and distortion of
the cranial fossae and foramina may be evident.

The ends of the long cylindrical bones are widened as a manifestation of failure of modeling. This widening is most marked where
bone growth is rapid; particularly do the distal femora show this
alteration (Fig. 77). Obliteration of the medullary canal, totally or in
part, is a manifestation of failure of normal resorptive processes.
Radiolucent striations, vertical or horizontal, in the distal diaphyses
of long bones are common. A radiolucent outline of a bone within a
bone may be evident.

The roentgenographic manifestations then are a reflection of the
persistence of primitive chondro-osteoid and inhibition of normal

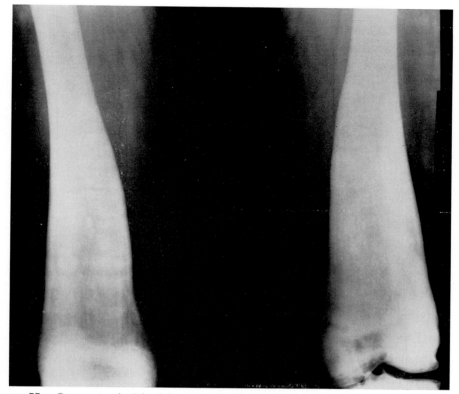

FIG. 77.   Osteopetrosis. Distal femora of a 61 year old white male. The inhibition of
normal modeling and the uniform opacity of the bones are evident.

resorptive processes. The radiolucent striations in the bones probably
represent remissions of the process with transient formation of more
normal bone trabeculae.

MICROSCOPY

The morbid microscopy of osteopetrosis can be best appreciated
by examination of sections made through the epiphyseal plate and
metaphysis of a growing bone. It will be seen that chondroblasts
multiply quite adequately and follow the normal pattern of maturation. Columnation is poor with crowding at the frontier of provisory
calcification. It is impossible to be sure whether this irregularity is due
to the essential mechanisms of the disease or whether it is secondary
to the more obvious changes which take place within the metaphysis.
A lattice of mineralized hyalin bars is formed and normal appearing
primitive osteoid is laid down in wide seams about them. This combination of cartilaginous nucleus with a perimeter of osteoid may be

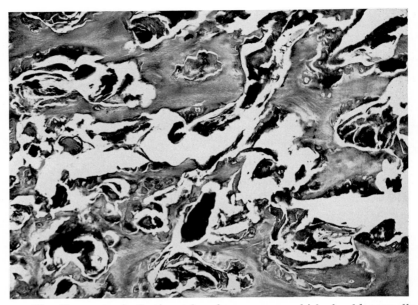

FIG. 78.   Osteopetrosis. Section taken from an area which should normally be cancellous tissue. The bone is laid down about nidi of densely calcified cartilage producing a helter-skelter arrangement without spicule formation.

designated as osteochondroid. Under normal circumstances the cartilage portion gradually fades away as the epiphyseal frontier advances beyond it, but in osteopetrosis it persists. Osteoid continues to pile up about these cartilaginous islands, occupying the space which is normally devoted to the vascular granulation. The latter is gradually squeezed out of existence so that there is little remaining to penetrate the feet of the cartilage cell columns distally. This may account for the crowding that occurs in this area. Since the osteochondroid persists, new, lamellated osteoid cannot replace it and so the metaphysis gradually increases in length as the bone grows, forming the distal enlargement of the "clubbed diaphysis." The failure of lysis of the osteochondroid also results in an obliteration of the space normally occupied by the medullary "cavity," which is filled with fat, and the areas at either end where the spongiosa and hematopoietic marrow should be. The metaphyseal cortices which are normally formed by a combination of the outermost spicules of spongiosa covered with a layer of cambium bone are made up of the same type of primitive bone as that found deeper in the metaphysis. The alternating horizontal bands of opacity and translucency which are seen in roentgenograms crossing the clubbed areas of long bones are caused by layered strata of almost solid osteochondroid and more normal appearing bone. One gets the impression from examining these areas that the more normal bands represent periods when the disease process is arrested and the resolution of osteochondroid proceeds normally. Nearer the center of the diaphysis bands of the same type may be seen running longitudinally, signifying the same activity sequence in the bone that is laid down by the periosteum.

Sections through the diaphysis proximal to the clubbed ends also reveal the presence of cartilage and primitive osteoid. It is unknown whether such sections have represented fortuitous examples of post-fracture callus, remnants of the originally formed metaphyseal cortex or an example of cambium cartilaginous metaplasia.

When one examines a section of osteopetrotic bone, it is difficult to make out any normal, organized bone structure. Irregular patches of hyalin containing scattered chondrocytes are embedded in a ragged matrix of coarse fibered bone. The latter is put together in a coarse mosaic which has a resemblance to that of Paget's disease except that the fragments are larger and their shape conforms to the cartilage islands which they surround (Fig. 78). The cement lines are wide and prominent. In the opaque bands there are no forms which even remotely resemble a normal spicule. The translucent bands are made up of connecting trabeculae largely without cartilage remnants and composed in part by adult bone. The haversian spaces are wide and contain loose aggregates of spindled and stellate fibrous cells. Islands of hematopoietic marrow appear here and there.

It is obvious that the regions which normally support cell-forming marrow are deficient. The anemia may be ascribed to this deficiency. In the opinion of some the condition is the result of the multipotent mesenchyme which should normally differentiate into the various components of bone, cartilage, fibrous and marrow tissue. From examination of the sections, one gets the impression that all the skeletal elements could be normally formed if only the products of the first stage could be cleared away to give them space. The myeloid metaplasia in the spleen and lymph nodes appears to support this impression.

PROGNOSIS

The symptoms and ultimately the course of osteopetrosis depend largely upon the severity of the involvement and the age at onset. If the patient survives early childhood, he has a fair chance of attaining adulthood. The longer he lives the less likely he is to die of his disease though sarcoma has been reported as a late complication.

MISCELLANEOUS SCLEROSING DISTURBANCES

There are several rare conditions, all of them probably congenital, which are characterized by streaks, patches, nodules or points of abnormal density on the roentgenograms. Among these should be included melorheostosis, progressive diaphyseal dysplasia (Engelmann), hereditary multiple diaphyseal sclerosis (Ribbing), osteopathia striata (Voorhoeve), osteopoikilosis (spotted bones) and chondrodystrophia fetalis calcificans (stippled epiphyses). Most of them are without symptoms and are consequently discovered only when x-ray examination is done for an accompanying condition. In most of them the material is so scant that inadequate microscopic material is available for conclusive descriptions. It appears at present that all are abnormal condensations of normal bone tissue and they have been described as variants of osteopetrosis. This would appear to be fallacious since in the latter the bone is not normal. One is tempted to classify all these conditions together because of their many similarities, but with our present state of knowledge it is probably better to consider them separate entities until sufficient data are collected to group them according to the disturbed physiology which accounts for their appearance.

MELORHEOSTOSIS

This is a rare condition in which there are curious linear longitudinal thickenings of the shafts of long bones. These irregular streaks of thick bone protrude both internally into the medullary tissues and externally beneath the periosteum. Since they appear to start proximally and progress distally along the entire length of the shaft and epiphysis, involving the bones of an extremity consecutively, the roentgenograms have the characteristic appearance of a molten substance flowing down one side of the bones of a member. It has been repeatedly likened to melted wax flowing down the side of a lighted candle.

Leri and Joanny were the first to describe this condition in 1922. They suggested the name "melorheostosis" which means flowing member. Since that time something less than fifty cases have been reported.

The disease has usually been diagnosed in patients between the ages of five and twenty years, but in several instances there has been evidence of onset in infancy. It appears, therefore, that the malformation is congenital in origin. No hereditary features have been reported.

The presenting symptom of melorheostosis is most often pain.[16] This pain may be severe but difficult of localization since an entire bone or several bones may be involved. More than three quarters of the reported cases have involved the bones of but a single extremity, monomelic. Usually the side of the pelvis or shoulder girdle corresponding to the involved member is affected. Involvement of one side of the mandible and maxilla has been reported. If the condition is marked and begins early the epiphysis may close prematurely, causing shortening of the extremity. The hyperostosis may extend in the soft tissues across the joint to cause interference with motion and even ankylosis. The outward protrusion may press upon nerves to cause sensory disturbance or upon the vasculature of the part with consequent edema. At least two cases have been reported in which a thickening and induration of the skin over the bony lesion has resulted

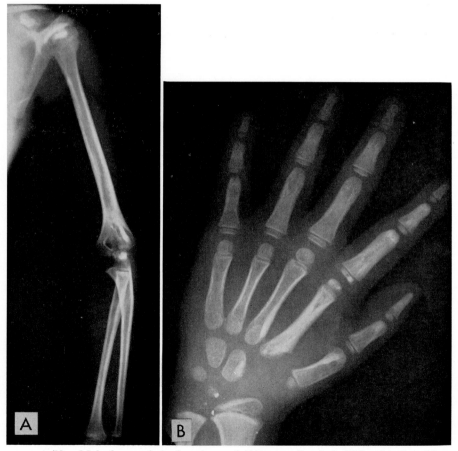

FIG. 79.   Melorheostosis in female aged 4½ years. Cortical thickening is evident in the humerus and radius (A). The wavy, dense cortex encroaches on the medullary canal and is most marked in the distal diaphysis of the radius. B is a radiograph of the hand and wrist on the same side as A. Phalangeal, carpal and metacarpal involvement is present as well as involvement of secondary epiphyseal centers (proximal humerus, capitellum and proximal phalanx of second digit).

in a diagnosis of scleroderma.[17] The diagnosis is usually made on the appearance of the roentgenograms.

MICROSCOPY

Complete studies of the skeleton in melorheostosis have not been reported. Only a few biopsy descriptions are available. The substance of the bone is apparently normal but the mass in the regions involved is increased. There appears to be a condensation of bone at the expense of the haversian and interspicular spaces.

The nature of the disturbance in physiology which accounts for the excessive production of bone in this peculiar pattern is entirely unknown. Numerous theories have been offered, but none of them seems sufficiently plausible to be worthy of listing.

PROGNOSIS

The malformations may advance throughout the years of skeletal growth and cease progression at the age of maturation of the bone involved. Since the bony lesions, once developed, do not regress, the patient must be resigned to his malformations unless they can be altered by surgery. Pain from the lesion itself is troublesome only during the developmental stage.

PROGRESSIVE DIAPHYSEAL DYSPLASIA
(Engelmann)

This condition was described by Engelmann in 1929. Since that time an additional thirteen cases have been reported, the largest series being four.[18] The skeletal lesions consist of a cortical thickening of the midshaft area principally in long bones, which progresses toward the epiphyses, both proximally and distally. The medullary area is encroached upon and there is appositional bone formation beneath the periosteum. The shaft may become fusiform in shape. Usually the entire circumference of the cortex is involved.

Most of the cases have been noted first in early childhood, but one report describes the characteristic bone changes in an infant, so there is some evidence to suggest that the condition is congenital. To date there is little evidence of a hereditary factor, though the infant mentioned was the son of a father who had been reported as having hereditary multiple diaphyseal sclerosis.

The large bones of the extremities are the ones usually affected but in a few cases flat bones, including those of the skull, have shown the characteristic thickenings. The small bones of the hands and feet are usually spared.

Progressive diaphyseal dysplasia differs from other congenital sclerosing disturbances in that it is coupled with a curious neuro-muscular dystrophy and general wasting. The nature of the former is quite unknown though it results in a peculiar, stifflegged, waddling gait with a wide base. The tendon reflexes may be hyperactive and easy fatigue has been the chief complaint in several instances. The undernourished status may respond to strict dietary measures but recurs if dietary supervision becomes lax. The skeletal lesions have not given rise to symptoms and are noted only when roentgenograms are made.

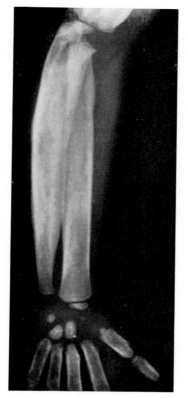

FIG. 80.   Progressive diaphyseal dysplasia. The radiograph of the forearm shows fusiform enlargement of the bones occasioned by new bone formation, endosteal and periosteal. The medullary canal is irregularly narrowed. Sharp demarcation of the process at the distal diaphyses is evident and the metaphyses and epiphyses are spared. Elongation of involved bones is common. (Courtesy of E. B. D. Neuhauser, M.D., Children's Medical Center, Boston, Mass.)

MICROSCOPY

Biopsy descriptions are given in two reports. Heavy masses of compact bone without other distinguishing features are noted. In one case the biopsy was repeated after an interval of several years and it was stated that resorption of bone along the inner cortical surface was combined with apposition along the outer. If such is the case, then the roentgenograms should reveal diaphyseal expansion with medullary widening rather than cortical thickening with medullary narrowing. It must be admitted that insufficient material has become available for conclusive opinions. These cases have not been followed sufficiently long to make prognostication possible.

HEREDITARY MULTIPLE DIAPHYSEAL SCLEROSIS
(Ribbing)

A few cases of this condition have been reported[19] as separate entities though the child of one patient was reported as having progressive diaphyseal dysplasia (Engelmann's disease). Ribbing first described the condition[20] in four siblings.

The bone lesions are much like those of Engelmann's disease, i.e., there is cortical thickening of a portion of the shaft of one or more long bones. This thickening is largely due to new bone formation along the outer surface of the cortex, but there may be some medullary narrowing. The tibia and femur are most commonly involved. Sometimes the distribution is symmetrical. These lesions may be symptomless and without evidence of accompanying disease or they may give rise to a "boring type" of bone pain.

The condition as described may be different from Engelmann's disease in that there is a high familial incidence and the neuromuscular disability and wasting have not been reported as accompanying conditions.

MICROSCOPY

The very scant amount of material which has become available has shown only an increase in bone mass at the expense of the haversian spaces. The bone is otherwise normal in appearance.

OSTEOPATHIA STRIATA
(Voorhoeve)

Voorhoeve described this condition as a distinct radiologic entity in 1924. The abnormality is characterized by multiple condensations

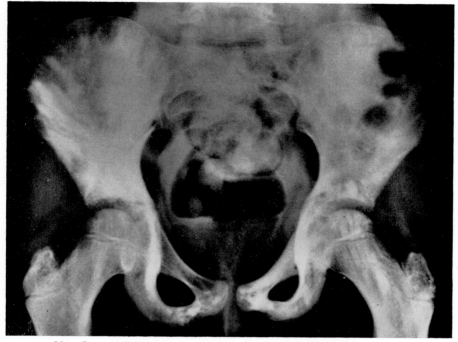

FIG. 81.   Osteopathia striata. Condensation of cancellous bone is manifest by opaque streaks in the ilia (particularly the right ilium) and in the proximal femora. (Courtesy of E. B. D. Neuhauser, M.D., Children's Medical Center, Boston, Mass.)

of cancellous bone tissue which begin at the epiphyseal line and extend into the diaphysis. In the ilium, the striae form a sunburst about the acetabulum and fan out toward the iliac crest. Any or all of the long bones may be involved and the end of greatest growth is said to be more obviously involved. The condition differs from osteopetrosis, melorheostosis, progressive diaphyseal dysplasia (Engelmann) and hereditary multiple diaphyseal sclerosis (Ribbing) in that cancellous bone and only cancellous bone is affected. However, the condition has been described in association with osteopetrosis in other bones[21] and in one instance in the same bone. The lesions are without symptoms and are discovered only on radiologic examination. At least one case showed accompanying punctate opacities in the epiphysis and another an elevated serum alkaline phosphatase.

OSTEOPOIKILOSIS
(Osteopathia Condensans Disseminata)

Spotted bones was described by Stiede in 1905. Since that time over a hundred cases have been reported. Since the condition is with·

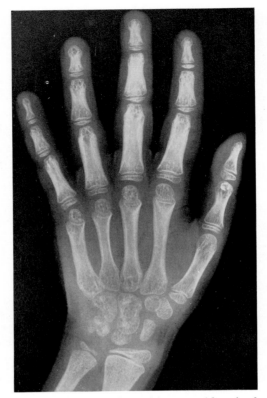

FIG. 82.   Osteopoikilosis. Spheroid opacities are evident in the carpal ossification centers as well as in the epiphyseal centers of the metacarpals. (Courtesy of E. B. D. Neuhauser, M.D., Children's Medical Center, Boston, Mass.)

out symptoms these cases have been discovered by roentgenologic examination for coincidental disease. The abnormality is characterized by numerous spheroid or lenticular nodules of condensed bone occurring in the spongiosa of the metaphysis or epiphyseal osseous nucleus. Schmorl published a description of the microscopic appearance in 1931. These well delineated opacities have been described in almost every bone, but they are most commonly encountered in the small bones of the hands and feet,[22] at the ends of the large bones of the extremities or in the pelvic bones about the acetabulum. They are rarely found in the skull.

The condition is apparently congenital since it has been diagnosed in a fetus and again in a newborn. It is familial and hereditary. One report describes the lesions in eight siblings.

It may be accompanied by hereditary, multiple exostoses, by a tendency to form keloids, and more than one case has been associated with dermatofibrosis lenticularis disseminata.[23]

MICROSCOPY

Several biopsy and a few autopsy studies have been done. The nodules are found within the cancellous tissue, sometimes with a peripheral attachment to the inner surface of the cortex. They are not cortical ingrowths. They may be round, lens shaped or elongated, composed of lamellated bone. They merge with the surrounding spongiosa; i.e., the spicules of cancellous tissue appear to blend into their substance but their mass has a greater density so that they can be dissected quite easily. Sections show them to have haversian spaces in about the same proportion as dense, cortical bone.

PROGNOSIS

Osteopoikilotic nodules may be present at birth or they may appear and increase in number during the growing period. In some cases they have been periodically checked over a period of years and they are said to grow larger or diminish in size and may even fade away completely.

CHONDRODYSTROPHIA FETALIS CALCIFICANS
(Stippled Epiphyses)

This is an exceedingly rare condition in which multiple punctate opacities appear in the unossified epiphyseal cartilage, usually at birth. The infants are frequently stillborn, and microscopic sections show great irregularity in vascularization of the epiphysis and chondroblastic maturation. Areas of ectopic ossification and hyalin mineral deposition are responsible for the stippled appearance on the roentgenogram.

MISCELLANEOUS DEVELOPMENTAL DEFORMITIES

In certain instances the formation of bone tissue is normal, but the bones fail to grow to proper size and shape. The resulting congenital anomalies are grouped under the heading of miscellaneous developmental deformities. Included here are brief accounts of arachnodactyly (Marfan's syndrome), acrocephalosyndactylism (Apert) and cleidocranial dysostosis (mutational dysostosis).

ARACHNODACTYLY
(Marfan's Syndrome)

Archnodactyly is a rare, hereditary, congenital growth disturbance of the muculoskeletal, cardiovascular and ocular systems. It was first

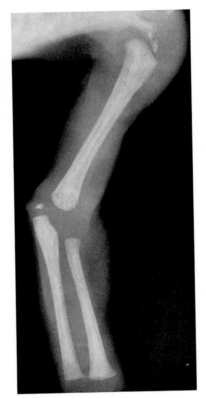

FIG. 83.   Chondrodystrophia fetalis calcifans. Opaque, punctate stippling of the epiphyseal cartilage at the shoulder and elbow may be seen. Stippling of vertebra cartilage was present. The cylindrical bones were of normal length. In some instances, normal enchondral bone growth is inhibited, as is seen in achondroplasia. (Courtesy of E. B. D. Neuhauser, M.D., Children's Medical Center, Boston, Mass.)

described by Marfan in 1896 and named "arachnodactyly" by Achard in 1902. The name was inspired by the appearance of the hands and feet because the digits are abnormally long and slender, suggesting the appendages of a spider. Whittaker and Sheehan[24] suggest that because the peculiar deformities of the hands and feet constitute only part of the syndrome and, indeed, may be lacking, the name "Marfan's syndrome" be retained as the term of choice.

There are numerous reports of this syndrome in both the foreign and American literature and any active orthopedic, cardiovascular or ophthalmologic service is apt to encounter at least one of these patients with one or more of its manifestations from time to time.

There is a strong heredity factor in the incidence of Marfan's syndrome. If the genealogy is carefully searched, perhaps 50 per cent of patients will reveal at least some of the stigmata among their progenitors.

All of the cylindrical bones are abnormally long and slender, thus producing the conformation of the hands and feet which has suggested the name of the condition. The patient is tall, the adult usually attaining a height of over six feet. The extremities are long and gracile. The arch of the palate is unusually high and there may be a double row of teeth. The latter are often unusually long and poorly spaced. There is apt to be dolichocephaly. The thorax may be funneled. The muscles are poorly developed and show poor tone. Hypotonicity of muscles, tendons and ligaments results in hypermobility of the joints.

Numerous congenital anomalies have been reported in the heart, including patent foramen ovale, mitral stenosis, aortic insufficiency and dilatation of the aortic arch. Myocardial strain frequently leads to endocarditis just as in other cardiac anomalies which interfere with normal function. The most common and important cardiovascular complication is aneurysm formation. The aneurysms are usually of the dissecting type and often terminate the life of the patient in the early adult period.

Poor vision is a common accompaniment of this condition. It is usually due to dislocation of the lens.

Sections of bone have shown no departure from the normal microscopy. It appears that Marfan's syndrome is a disturbance in skeletal growth rather than in the formation of cartilage and osteoid tissue.

ROENTGENOGRAPHIC MANIFESTATIONS

The roentgenographic manifestations of arachnodactyly are secondary in importance to the clinical findings. The cylindrical bones are longer than is normal but there is no abnormality of bone density or architecture.

ACROCEPHALOSYNDACTYLISM
(Apert)

This is an uncommon, congenital disturbance in the growth of bone and soft tissue affecting principally the head, the hands and the feet. As the name suggests, the head is elongated and peaked, and the hands and feet show various degrees of syndactylism.

The name "acrocephalosyndactylism" was suggested by Apert in 1906 though several cases had been reported before his paper appeared. The condition is now frequently called "Apert's syndrome."

The most complete review was published by Park and Powers[25] in 1920. A recent review[26] states that there are at least forty-nine published cases to date.

The condition is congenital since numerous cases have been described in the newborn. There have been no published data to indicate that Apert's syndrome is hereditary though both syndactylism and scaphocephaly (usually a part of the syndrome) commonly show a hereditary incidence. It may be that those with severe cases do not reach the age of reproductivity or are unable to bear children, thus concealing a heredity factor. There are no data on this phase of the subject.

The peculiar appearance of these patients is such that one might mistake them for members of the same family. It has been stated that the finer facial characteristics and traits of expression are masked by the changes so that there is a species resemblance.

The head is vertically elongated and peaked, the highest point varying between the anterior and posterior fontanels. The dome slopes sharply on both sides (Fig. 84). The face is usually considerably widened. The head is shortened in the anteroposterior diameter. The planes of the face and the back of the skull, which is often flush with the neck, are flattened and remarkably parallel. The calvarium appears to have increased in volume chiefly by growth above the level of the face.

The cause of this curious malformation of the head, according to Park and Powers who go with considerable length into the existing theories of mechanism and offer some of their own, is a premature synostosis of the cranial bones due to inadequacies on the part of the non-ossifying mesenchymal tissue to separate the various ossification centers. The synostoses result in inadequate expansion in certain directions and increased intracranial pressure caused by the enlarging brain. The latter undergoes convolutional atrophy. Impaired mental development is reported in a few cases. In some instances an internal hydrocephalus has developed, its cause and association not understood.

The increased intracranial pressure is the cause of the disturbance in vision which is one of the outstanding symptoms of the condition. The eyes are displaced forward so that their transverse axes diverge and slant downward. There is often strabismus. The contents of the orbit are pushed forward so that the eyes bulge prominently and may develop staphylomas. In severe cases they have been completely displaced. Progressive impairment of vision is the usual result. Fusion defects of the maxilla and mandible occur, particularly notable in the posterior palate, which may be narrow and high-vaulted. There is often interference with the normal development of the teeth. The mandible

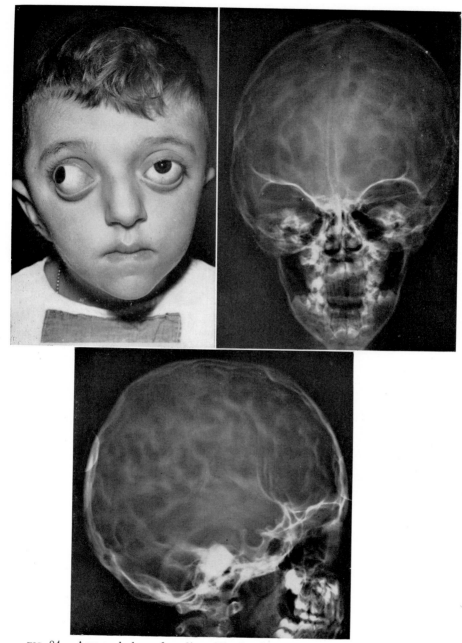

FIG. 84. Acrocephalosyndactylism. The head is elongated and peaked with slop-ing sides; it is shortened in the anteroposterior diameter with parallel planes of the face and back of the skull. The eyes are displaced forward with divergence of their axes. (Courtesy of Dr. Michael Scott.)

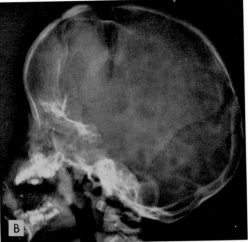

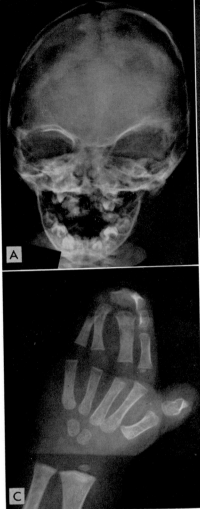

FIG. 85. Acrocephalosyndactylism in male aged 19 months. There is marked deformity of the skull secondary to premature closure of the coronal sutures (*A* and *B*). The patient was operated upon at the age of 6 months and the craniectomy defects are evident. The anterior fossa is small, the sphenoid bone abnormally formed. Hypoplasia of the maxilla is apparent. The orbits are shallow. Syndactylism (*C*) is present in the hands, and the bones of the feet showed similar abnormality.

has been reported to be prognathic in some cases and recessive in others.

The excessively high forehead, often with a prominent horizontal, supraciliary groove, the peaked head flattened posteriorly, the wide-spaced bulging eyes, flat face and short nose constitute the characteristic facies of the acro-scapho-brachycephalic portion of the condition.

Syndactylism is another prominent feature of this malformation. It may be complete or partial. There may be synostoses between metacarpals and between metatarsals. There are often synostoses between the phalanges of different digits and there may be failure of joint formation between the various units of the same digit.

The syndactylism is apparently due to the same disturbance in growth which causes the malformations of the head bones, a failure of the non-osteogenic mesenchymal tissue to isolate the various ossification centers. It is of interest that in both instances the defects are the result of the failure of a process which normally occurs toward the end of the sequence of events which result in the formation of the skeleton.

Sections of the involved bone, when examined with the aid of the microscope, show only normal bone tissue. The condition is apparently a disturbance in skeleton formation, not in bone tissue production. It appears to be, as Park and Powers insist, the result of a germ plasm defect. The literature is lacking in long term follow-up data. It is known that some of the cases have become progressively worse throughout childhood, but it is not clear what course the disease takes after cessation of skeletal growth.

CLEIDOCRANIAL DYSOSTOSIS

Cleidocranial dysostosis is a developmental disturbance of the skeleton in which a wide variation of deformities occurs involving numerous bones. There is almost always involvement of the skull bones or the clavicles or both.

The first report of such a case (quoted from Soule[27]) was that of Cutter in 1870. Marie and Sainton recognized the condition as an entity, supplied the name of cleidocranial dysostosis and reported two cases in 1897. Since that time approximately 350 cases have been described in the literature. The most complete recent survey is that of Soule[27] who added six additional cases.

A familial incidence was recorded in approximately two thirds of the reported cases and the condition was found in as many as five successive generations. The trait is passed on by either the mother or father who manifests the deformities. The condition is congenital. Well documented sporadic cases have been noted.

Rhinehart suggested that since either, or in rare cases both, the clavicular or/and the cranial deformities may be lacking, the term "cleidocranial dysostosis" should be abandoned and replaced by "mutational dysostosis." This suggestion was supported by Soule.

The condition appears to be a germ plasm defect in skeletal development. The substance of bone is normally formed, but the conformation is faulty. Both enchondral and intramembranous bone formation are affected and the disturbance starts very early in embryonal life.

There is a marked brachycephaly with widening of the interparietal diameter above. The skull thus appears excessively broad. The foramen magnum is larger than normal and slants forward and downward; the mandible is prognathous. The maxilla appears underdeveloped as do the other bones which compose the face. The malar, lacrimal and nasal bones may be deficient or absent. The palate is narrow, sometimes cleft, and the arch is high. The paranasal sinuses are small. The frontal and parietal bones are prominently bossed. The principal sutures are greatly delayed in closing, giving a "hot cross bun" appearance to the head. The metopic suture may persist throughout life. Wormian bones commonly develop from secondary centers within the suture membranes.

Since the clavicle is produced from three separate centers, the ends by enchondral growth and the center intramembranous, great variation occurs in its development. In a small percentage of cases it is absent entirely. Only the sternal third may be present, or the acromial third, or the two ends without the middle, or all three portions without uniting. The scapula is small and often winged. These abnormalities allow great mobility of the shoulders. One or both sides may be involved. In the latter instance the patient may be able to approximate the shoulders until the tips of the acromial processes touch beneath his chin.

The large bones of the arm are less frequently involved but occasionally the radius fails to attain proper length, causing abduction at the wrist. Extra epiphyses may appear in the metacarpals and phalanges and the second metacarpal is excessively long.

The pelvic bones appear underdeveloped with contraction and asymmetry of the pelvic canal. Fusion at the symphysis pubis may fail to occur. The sacrum and coccyx are often poorly formed, the latter sometimes absent. The neck of the femur may be deformed to cause coxa vara. Abnormalities in the bones of the feet may be similar to those of the hands.

Poorly developed vertebrae with fusion defects of the spinous processes and laminae may cause lordosis, scoliosis or kyphosis.

There is marked disturbance in formation of the teeth. The deciduous teeth are usually normal though often delayed in eruption. Shedding of the deciduous teeth is usually delayed or does not occur so that eruption and growth of the permanent teeth are markedly impaired. Caries and premature periodontitis are excessive. Dentigerous cysts may develop.

The literature contains no account of morbid microscopy so we must assume that the cellular and intercellular components of the deformed bones are normal.

The disturbance in dentition or difficulties in gait due to femoral

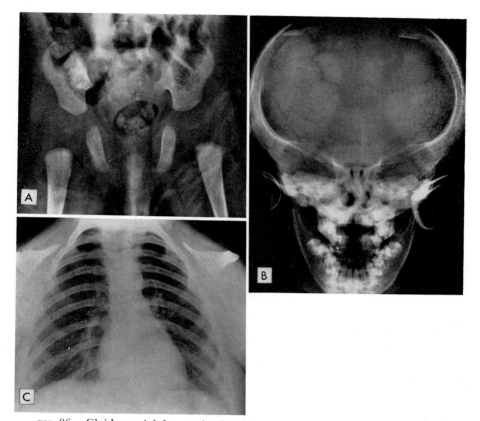

FIG. 86. Cleidocranial dysostosis. *A* and *B* are radiographs of the pelvis and skull of a male age 6 months. The pubic bones are underveloped; only a small portion of the body of each is evident. The epiphyseal center for the heads of the femora is tiny. The radiograph of the skull (*B*) shows widely patent sutures and fontanels, numerous centers of ossification in the cranial bones and an increase in the biparietal diameter. The facial bones are small. This child had no clavicles and the radiograph of his mother's chest (*C*) reveals absence of clavicles.

neck deformity are the commonest causes of complaint. The failure of proper development of the clavicles causes little or no disability.

REFERENCES

ACHONDROPLASIA

1. Spillane, J. D.: J. Neurol., Neurosurg. & Psychiat., *15*:246; 1952.
2. Keizer, P. R., and Schilder, J. H.: Am. J. Dis. Child., *82*:341; 1951.
3. Epstein, J. A., and Malis, L. I.: Neurology, *5*:875; 1955.

MORQUIO'S DISEASE

4. Morquio, L.: Arch. de med. d. enf., *32*:129, 1929.
5. Whiteside, J. D., and Cholmeley, J. A.: Arch. Dis. Childh., *27*:487; 1952.
6. Opie, E. L., and Harrison, N.: J. Med. Research, *31*:277; 1917.

OSTEOGENESIS IMPERFECTA

7. Scot, D., and Stiris, G.: Acta med. Scand., *145:*237; 1953.
8. Bergman, G., and Engfeldt, B.: Acta path. et microbiol. Scand., *35:*537; 1954.
9. Follis, R. H.: J. Pediat., *41:*713; 1952.
10. Follis, R. H.: Bull. Johns Hopkins Hosp., *93:*225; 1953.
11. Weber, M.: Arch. Path., *9:*984; 1930.
12. Engfeldt, B., Engstrom, A., and Zellerstrom, R.: J. Bone & Joint Surg., *36B:*654; 1954.

OSTEOPETROSIS

13. Karshner, R. G.: Am. J. Roentgenol., *16:*405; 1926.
14. Zawisch, C.: Arch. Path., *43:*55; 1947.
15. Pines, B., and Lederer, M.: Am. J. Path., *23:*755; 1947.

MISCELLANEOUS SCLEROSING DISTURBANCES

16. Franklin, E. L., and Matheson, I.: Melorheostosis. Brit. J. Radiol., *15:*185; 1942.
17. Dillehunt, R. B., and Chuinard, E. G.: Melorheostosis Leri. J. Bone & Joint Surg., *18:*991; 1936.
18. Neuhauser, E. B. D., Schwachman, H., Wittenborg, M., and Cohen, J.: Progressive diaphyseal dysplasia. Radiology, *51:*11; 1948.
19. Paul, L. W.: Hereditary multiple diaphyseal sclerosis. Radiology, *60:*412; 1953.
20. Ribbing, S.: Hereditary multiple diaphyseal sclerosis. Acta radiol., *31:*522; 1949.
21. Hurt, R. L.: Osteopathia striata—Voorhoeve's disease. J. Bone & Joint Surg., *35B:*89; 1953.
22. Hinsen, A.: Familial osteopoikilosis. Am. J. Surg., *45:*566; 1939.
23. Martincic, N.: Osteopoikilosis. Brit. J. Radiol., *25:*612; 1952.

MISCELLANEOUS DEVELOPMENTAL DEFORMITIES

24. Whittaker, S. R. F., and Sheehan, J. D.: Dissecting aortic aneurysm in Marfan's syndrome. Lancet, *16:*791; 1954.
25. Park, E. A., and Powers, G. F.: Acrocephaly and scaphocephaly with symmetrically distributed malformations of the extremities. Am. J. Dis. Child., *20:*235; 1920.
26. Kahn, A., and Fulmer, J.: Acrocephalocyndactylism. New England J. Med., *252:*379; 1955.
27. Soule, A. B.: Mutational dysostosis. J. Bone & Joint Surg., *28:*81; 1946.
28. Yakovac, W. C.: Calcareous chondropathies in the newborn infant. Arch. Path., *57:*62; 1954.

8

Developmental Disturbances of Childhood

ENCHONDROMATOSIS

There were numerous reports of disturbances in enchondral bone formation between 1900 and 1937. It is regrettable that in several papers a variety of entities is grouped under one of several headings, so that it is quite impossible on analyzing certain series to be sure exactly which entities are being reported. The term "dyschondroplasia" has been used by Mahorner[1] to include enchondromatosis, hereditary multiple exostoses, stippled epiphyses and osteopoikilosis, and the same term has been used to report separate series of enchondromatosis and of hereditary multiple exostoses. Apparently Ollier,[2] in reporting four cases of "dyschondroplasia" in 1899, confused the last two conditions but it was he who pointed out the metaphyseal radiolucency which today characterizes enchondromatosis. Since his report the terms "Ollier's disease" and "dyschondroplasia" have been used more or less interchangeably and recently the more exact name of "enchondromatosis" has been largely substituted for both. Since Ollier emphasized the unilaterality of the condition, some writers use the name "Ollier's disease" to designate those cases in which the lesions are entirely or predominantly in one side of the skeleton. In 1881, Maffucci reported an association of enchondromatosis and multiple cavernous hemangiomas and this rare combination has since been known as "Maffucci's disease."

There is fairly general agreement today that enchondromatosis and hereditary multiple exostoses represent two quite separate entities, and with the available modern means of diagnosis they should never again be confused.

Enchondromatosis is essentially the hamartomatous proliferation of cartilage cells within the metaphysis of several bones, causing thinning of the overlying cortices and distortion of length growth. It was formerly thought to be hereditary in nature but if, on close scrutiny of the reports, one discards the cases which are probably not true enchondromatosis, the hereditary and familial features of the disease are lacking. It is also difficult to ascertain with certainty whether or not the condition is congenital. Examination of the reports of bona fide cases failed to reveal unequivocal x-ray evidence of the disease at birth.

The first manifestations of enchondromatosis are usually noted in early childhood. In the more florid instances an obvious impairment of length growth becomes apparent, usually unequal growth of the lower extremities, but in more occult cases the presenting symptom may be pathologic fractures in adolescence or even adult life. Pain is rare unless fracture has occurred or unless there is reactivation in later life with a spurt in growth. This often signifies malignant alteration.

The lesions apparently represent a perversion of enchondral growth and, therefore, are usually confined to cylindrical bones. Occasionally focal masses of cartilage may be found in sites other than the metaphyses, especially in the ribs, combined with the typical metaphyseal lesions of enchondromatosis. A single cartilaginous mass may occasionally be found in a flat bone and this may or may not represent a solitary manifestation of the disease. The bones of the hands and feet are most frequently involved (Fig. 87). Because some cases are limited to these areas there has been a tendency to consider this a special group. At present it appears that this curious localization is but a partial manifestation of the disease as a whole. In those cases with extensive long bone involvement there is almost always at least some evidence of the lesions in the small bones if they are carefully examined. The most vigorous growths are usually seen at the end of greatest activity in the long bones of the extremities.

There can be little doubt that the disturbance seen in enchondromatosis is due to an abnormal proliferation of cartilage cells which arise either from embryologic rests within the metaphysis or from epiphyseal chondroblasts which fail to mature properly and, therefore, migrate into the metaphysis or, more likely, are overtaken by the advancing epiphyseal line and are left stranded there. The latter appears to the writer to be the more logical explanation since normal growth may be disturbed, possibly as a result of improper chondroblastic maturation. Retaining their proliferative potency these cells produce masses of useless, disorganized cartilage cells. As such they mimic neoplastic chondromatous growth so closely that the differentiation cannot be made on microscopic examination. The fact that they are not true neoplasms is evident in that they obey, to some extent, the normal growth laws and after a certain period cease to proliferate. Usually this point in time is about that of the normal cessation of growth of the bone involved.

If during childhood and adolescence the growth is florid, the overlying cortex may be "expanded" producing the "trumpeting" that is characteristically seen. The cortex may be weakened to the point of pathologic fracture. Aggregates of viable cartilage cells protruding through the thin shell of metaphyseal cortex may be pinched off and continue to grow, producing extracortical masses of cartilage. These have been mistaken for exostoses but except for their position they are in no way similar. The lesions of hereditary multiple exostoses or the solitary osteochondroma is actually an example of enchondral bone formation, normal in every respect except for the direction of growth. The cartilage cells of enchondromatosis never fulfill their normal destiny of provoking bone formation.

Eventually, epiphyseal orientation may be regained and normal

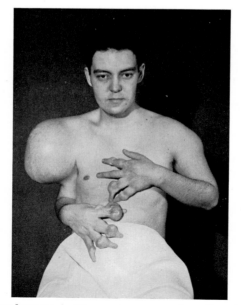

FIG. 87.   Enchondromatosis. The most common site of involvement, the bones of the hands, is here dramatically illustrated. In the large cylindrical bones the enchondroma is more apt to become malignant.

enchondral bone growth may then proceed beyond the island of cartilage cells. Thus, the abnormal cartilage mass appears to drift into the diaphysis, though in reality the advancing epiphyseal line merely leaves it behind. In large long bones the cartilage masses are always found in the end third or quarter of the bone. In the small bones of the hands and feet they may replace the entire length of the medullary tissues. In some instances the growth is an irregularly lobulated conformation and the roentgenogram has a correspondingly mottled appearance. In other cases there appears to be a semblance of orientation in as much as the cells proliferate in a linear pattern producing longitudinal strands of translucency which separate the more opaque bands of normal spongiosa.

ROENTGENOGRAPHIC MANIFESTATIONS

The roentgenographic manifestations of enchondromatosis reflect a hamartomatous proliferation of cartilage cells within the metaphysis of one or more long bones. Because cartilage has the density of soft tissues, the masses of cartilage contrast sharply with the adjacent bone. The involved bone is often shorter than normal and the distal shaft is replaced by a large mass of cartilage in which streaks and spots of opacification (calcification) are evident. Widening of the end of the bone is common as a result of failure of tubulation or modeling. The epiphyses are spared.

At times, the only manifestation may be the presence of radio-

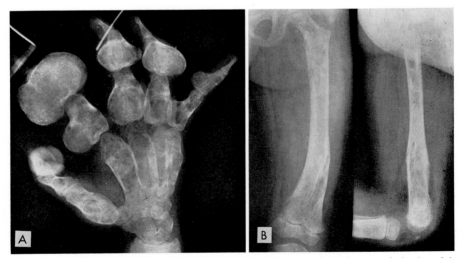

FIG. 88.   Enchondromatosis. Extensive involvement of the bones of the hand is illustrated by *A*. The lesions have expanded the cortex to a marked degree but a thin shell of bone covers the proliferating cartilage. In *B*, radiolucent streaks are evident in the distal diaphysis of the femur. Deformity of the bone is evident.

lucent, longitudinal streaks extending into the shaft from the metaphysis. The cortex is thinned over the proliferating cartilage and may in fact be perforated so that there are external projections of the cartilaginous mass. In the small bones of the hands and feet the entire bone is often involved with resultant thinning and expansion of the cortex. Pathologic fractures may occur as a consequence of the cortical thinning and weakness.

MICROSCOPY

When one sections the curetted material from a lesion of enchondromatosis (Fig. 89) one finds masses of cartilage cells in a hyalin matrix. These cells range from small chondroblasts to relatively mature, large vacuolated chondrocytes but their pattern is quite disorderly. Areas of "myxomatous degeneration" are common and may dominate the picture. This is probably less a matter of degeneration than an inability to produce normal hyalin with the physical and staining properties of that seen in the epiphysis. The cells are usually irregularly grouped (Fig. 90) and it is not always easy for the microscopist to be sure that he is not dealing with chondrosarcoma. The nuances of microscopic differentiation will be dealt with in the chapter concerning chondrosarcoma. On microscopic examination alone the lesions of enchondromatosis and those of solitary enchondroma or even ecchondroma cannot be separated.

As the lesions age they almost always become infiltrated with amorphous calcium salts. That there is a failure of crystal lattice formation is shown by the lack of rigidity of the calcified areas. The

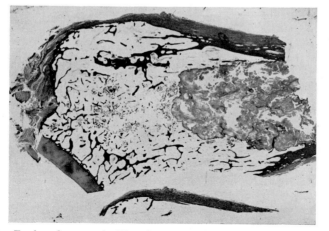

FIG. 89. Enchondromatosis. Very low magnification of the end of a cylindrical bone with an enchondroma deep in the metaphysis. Note that its borders are distinct and that there is no tendency to infiltrate like a true neoplasm. ($\times$ 4.)

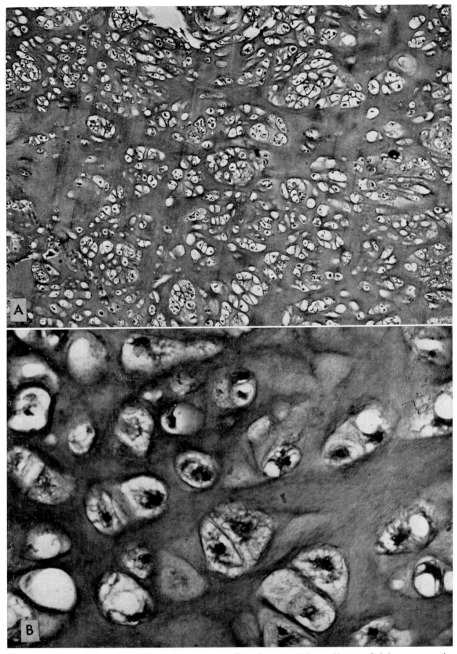

FIG. 90.   *A,* Section taken from an enchondroma. The cells are fairly mature in type but their arrangement is quite disorganized. The cells are also more thickly dispersed than those of normal hyalin cartilage. (× 40.) *B,* Higher magnification of an area from Fig. *A.* The cells are relatively small and there is but one nucleus to a cell and one cell to a lacuna. (× 400.)

salts are laid down in irregular patches, striations and points which produce the characteristic roentgenograms of these lesions.

PROGNOSIS

Concerning the fate of the patient with enchondromatosis there is almost no factual data on which one may base a valid opinion. It is certain that lesions of enchondromatosis have been discovered in advanced years without evidence of true neoplastic change. It is just as certain that neoplastic growth is the event that leads to the discovery of many of the cases in adult life. Some writers have attempted on the basis of limited series to express the prognosis in percentage figures, the figures of malignant change ranging from 5 per cent upward. To the writer and at the moment this seems unwarranted; the matter had best be left with the statement that the patient with enchondromatosis stands a greater chance of developing a malignant cartilaginous tumor than the average. Therefore, all known lesions should be periodically surveyed and any reactivation of growth in adult life should be regarded as malignant neoplasm until proven otherwise.

HEREDITARY MULTIPLE EXOSTOSES

As the name implies, this is a condition in which multiple bony excrescences grow out from the cortical surfaces, forming tubular extensions roughly transverse to the long axis of the bone involved. This skeletal deformity was known to Virchow, but little was written about it until Ehrenfried reviewed the literature and reported twelve cases in 1917. He suggested the term "hereditary deforming chondro-dysplasia." Keith (1920) called it "diaphyseal aclasis," a name which is still preferred by the British. Jaffe[3] proposed the term "hereditary multiple exostoses," which because it is descriptive and simple is the one most widely used today. It is also reported under the titles "cartilaginous exostoses" and "hereditary osteochondromatosis." The latter is eminently descriptive, but should not be used because the same name has been used for a condition characterized by the production of spheroid masses of cartilage within a joint and in the periarticular tissues.

The condition is familial and there is a prominent hereditary incidence in the histories of nearly 75 per cent of the cases. The trait is usually passed to his children by the father but there are several well documented cases in which the mother only was afflicted. Several children in one family are not uncommonly involved and the condition has been traced through five consecutive generations. Males are affected almost three times as often as females.

These bony outgrowths are usually discovered some time during childhood or adolescence. None has been reported present at birth. The exostoses themselves are usually symptomless but they may cause pressure upon tendons which must slide over them and thus bursae are formed which may become inflamed. At times they may compress vessels and interfere with blood supply or cause pain by pressure on nerves. Accompanying the exostoses there is frequently incomplete length growth of the radius and fibula. These bones are thus shorter than their paired ulna and tibia, with a resultant characteristic curving at the elbow and knee.

Hereditary multiple exostoses most frequently appear on the long bones of the extremities, but the flat bones of the pelvis, the scapula, the ribs and the vertebrae are sometimes involved. Since these exostoses are disturbances in the enchondral growth of bone they are never found in areas resulting from intramembranous formation, though they have been reported arising from portions of skull bones in the vicinity of a cartilaginous ossification center. The small bones of the hands and feet are sometimes affected. In long bones the exostoses usually appear at the end of greatest growth, at the knee when they involve the femur or tibia and at the shoulder and wrist when they arise from humerus or ulna.

These lesions probably always begin their growth at the extreme end of the shaft in the vicinity of the periphery of the epiphyseal line. As the latter advances they are left upon the cortical surface and a progressively widening breach separates them from their point of origin. At the same time there is a failure of modeling of the involved metaphysis so that it remains wider than normal. The exostoses, the broad metaphyses and the short radii and fibulae compose a triad of characteristic features of the disease (Fig. 91). One can roughly judge the date of onset of the disturbance by the distance of the exostosis from the epiphyseal line and the length of the widened area.

The exostoses are usually bilateral and frequently symmetrical though at times one side is predominantly involved. Several may grow from one metaphyseal area. They are usually flattened transversely, often appearing as a short, tall ridge in the long axis of the host bone. They are capped by a layer of hyalin cartilage. This cap frequently extends well down over the pedicle, sometimes approaching the normal cortex. The base is often wider than the apex so that the growths may be triangular or fin-shaped. They almost always lean in a direction away from the nearest epiphysis and toward the center of the diaphysis. Rarely the pedicle is slender and the distal end bulbous.

The cartilaginous surface usually reveals numerous lobular irregularities.

The structure is essentially a cylinder of cortical bone surrounding a core of cancellous tissue and covered with a layer of cartilage which acts as an epiphyseal plate. The cancellous bone is coextensive with that of the host bone and frequently supports hematopoietic marrow. The cartilaginous portion is comparable to the epiphysis of a long bone except that it has no osseous nucleus. It acts as both an epiphyseal and an articular plate. The bony portion is covered with an extension of periosteum from the normal cortex and the cap is covered with perichondrium.

Exostoses are morphologically identical to the solitary lesion which is known as osteochondroma.

The cause of the disturbance which results in hereditary multiple exostoses is unknown. The hereditary incidence, the failure of metaphyseal modeling and the impaired growth of the radius and fibula suggest an inherent germ plasm defect. Virchow suggested that a piece of the active epiphyseal plate was pinched off and set up independent growth in a direction transverse to the normal long axis. Others have found islands of cartilage cells in the deep layers of the periosteum and have suggested that they are embryonal cell rests or areas of

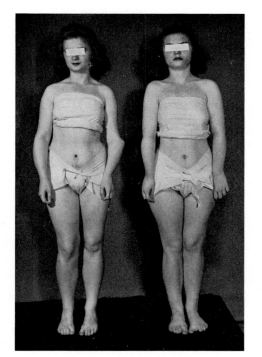

FIG. 91.   Hereditary multiple exostoses. Two sisters show the typical deformity of the elbow and knee. (From Shriners' Hospital.)

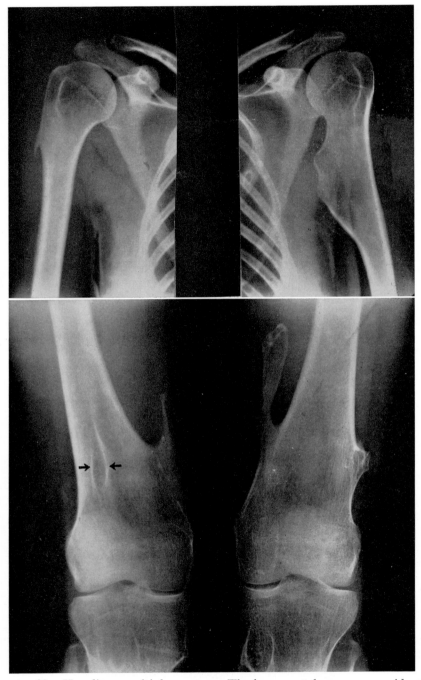

FIG. 92.   Hereditary multiple exostoses. The bony protuberances are evident at the ends of the bones. The end of the diaphysis and the metaphyseal area are broad as a consequence of failure of tubulation. The cartilaginous cap on several of the exostoses is irregularly opacified. When seen end-on, the site of origin of the exostosis is visible by virtue of its cortex which casts a dense round or oval shadow (arrows).

metaplasia which may be activated to produce the exostoses. Keith found instances in which the periosteum did not completely reach the epiphyseal line and thought that, lacking the restraining influence which he felt the periosteum exerted on the epiphyseal cartilage, the latter was allowed exuberant growth. Jansen[4] believed that the deformity was the result of an impairment in osteolysis during modeling. Failure of resolution left the wide metaphysis and a fragment of the periphery of the epiphysis which continued to proliferate and form an epiphyseal line at right angles to the normal. In the light of present knowledge one will probably agree with Jaffe that the process probably represents a combination of the various hypotheses offered.

MICROSCOPY

Sections taken through the bone of the pedicle show it to be of the cortical type with normal lamellation and haversian systems. The trabeculae of the cancellous tissue appear normal in all respects. The marrow may be fatty or actively hematopoietic. The appearance of the covering cartilaginous plate varies with the age of the lesion and the stage of its growth. In the depths of the cartilage near the exterior surface the cartilage cells are young, small and evenly dispersed. As the line of junction with cancellous bone, the "epiphyseal line," is approached the chondroblasts are seen to mature. They enlarge, the cytoplasm becomes vacuolated, they flatten transversely and arrange themselves in recognizable though often irregular columns (Fig. 93).

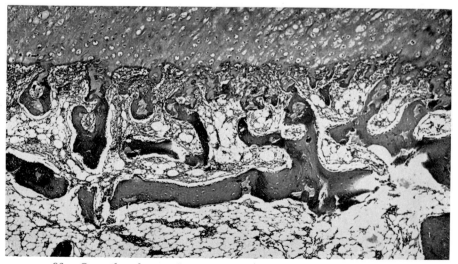

FIG. 93.   Osteochondroma. Low magnification of a section taken through the cartilage cap and adjacent pedicle. The lesion mimics the epiphysis and metaphysis of the growing bone from which it arises. ($\times$ 27.)

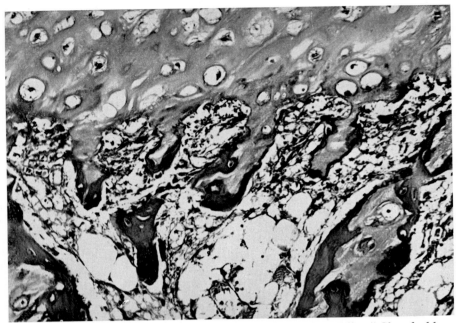

FIG. 94.   Osteochondroma. Section through the "epiphyseal line." Chondroblasts mature, form a line of provisional calcification and a hyalin scaffolding for osteoid apposition. (× 290.)

The intervening acellular hyalin becomes infiltrated with bone salts to form a provisional line of calcification. The "epiphyseal line" is usually quite irregular but vascularized tongues of fibrous tissue break into the bases of the cell columns just as in normal enchondral bone formation, and a hyalin lattice is formed. The projecting bars are usually widely separated and run in various directions but seams of osteoid are laid down on their surfaces and bone trabeculae are thus formed (Fig. 94). As the lesion matures the cartilage columns peter out and an arch of bone seals off the cartilage from the bony portion. When the subchondral trabeculae fail to show cores of hyalin one can be sure that the growth period is approaching its end.

PROGNOSIS

The growth of the exostosis apparently begins in childhood and continues until the nearest epiphyseal center ossifies, i.e., its growth period is the same as that of its host bone. Occasionally one will find evidence of activity well into adult life but it is usually impossible to determine whether this is independent growth or whether there is still activity in the normal epiphysis. Reactivation should always be regarded with suspicion. A diagnosis of malignant change must be presumed until ruled out.

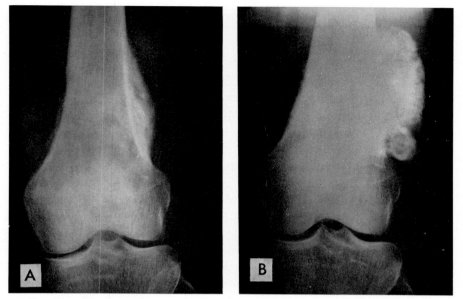

FIG. 95.   Hereditary multiple exostoses. A reactivated exostosis was surgically removed
(*A*). A few months later an osteosarcoma (*B*) was found growing at the site.

Malignant neoplastic change is encountered frequently enough
in hereditary multiple exostoses to make periodic examination mandatory. It is impossible to establish an accurate figure but most authors
agree that this unfortunate complication occurs in about 5 per cent
(Fig. 95). Trauma, particularly if it causes fracture, should most certainly be watched by x-ray examination.

The tumors usually arise from the cartilaginous cap and are therefore chondrosarcomas. In this case the growth is relatively slow and
metastasis is apt to be late. In some cases osteosarcoma has developed
from an exostosis. It may be expected to run the usual course with a
fatal termination within eighteen months.

FIBROUS DYSPLASIA

Fibrous dysplasia of bone is a disturbance in postnatal intramedullary bone maintenance. Normal bone undergoing physiologic
lysis is replaced by an abnormal proliferation of fibrous tissue. The
process is therefore slow, frequently requiring years to cause cortical
weakening and produce clinical lesions. The proliferation may eventually extend beyond normal boundaries, thus causing distortion and
"expansion." Since the inability to produce normal bone involves only
the intramedullary tissues and never cambium bone formation, the
lesions are always covered with a shell, however thin, of adult cortical
bone.

This condition was first recognized as an entity probably no earlier than 1922 when Weil (quoted from Schlumberger[5]) first reported it in the German literature. Since fibrous dysplasia is a fairly common disease, one wonders how cases were classified prior to this date. Solitary lesions were almost certainly confused with unicameral cyst, ossifying fibroma, non-osteogenic fibroma and subperiosteal cortical defect. At least some cases of multicentric but unilateral involvement were, from the authors' personal knowledge, diagnosed as Ollier's enchondromatosis. Cases with extensive skeletal lesions were categorized as hyperparathyroidism (osteitis fibrosa cystica), neurofibromatosis and, in the older age group, Paget's disease.

Freund and Moffert[6] reviewed the condition in 1936 under the title "fibrous osteo-dystrophy" and in the following year McCune and Bruch[7] recognized the entity and used the term "osteodystrophia fibrosa." In 1937, Albright[8] and co-workers reported five cases of bone involvement with disturbance of endocrine function and pigmented patches in the skin using the name "osteitis fibrosa disseminata." They noted its similarities to parathyroid adenoma (osteitis fibrosa cystica) and neurofibromatosis but considered it a separate entity. Since this paper the condition has frequently been referred to as "Albright's syndrome." It should be remembered, however, that these writers were concerned as much with the endocrine disturbance as with the bone lesions and, therefore, this eponym should not be used in considering most of the cases, i.e., those with bone involvement only.

In 1938, Lichtenstein[9] reported eight cases with detailed studies of the lesions in bone. He proposed the name "fibrous dysplasia" or "polyostotic fibrous dysplasia" when multiple bones were involved. Since then this has been the name of preference. Lichtenstein and Jaffe[10] added 15 more cases in 1942 and a considerable number have been reported since. Schlumberger[5] was able to collect 67 cases of monostotic fibrous dysplasia from his survey of the army material. He expressed the opinion that ossifying fibroma and non-osteogenic fibroma were variants of this condition. Thannhauser[11] thought that it was a skeletal manifestation of neurofibromatosis.

Sufficient material has been collected to show undeniably that fibrous dysplasia is an entity, though it resembles neurofibromatosis, since both are germ plasm defects involving fibroblastic proliferation and maturation and there is some, though not great, overlap in incidence. The microscopy of typical lesions of ossifying fibroma and non-osteogenic fibroma appears to be sufficiently unique to separate them from fibrous dysplasia but in atypical sections the distinction may be difficult or impossible.

Fibrous dysplasia may appear as a solitary lesion or there may be more than one lesion in a single bone. Sometimes several bones of a single extremity may be involved (monomelic) or only the bones of one side may be affected. In severe cases the lesions may be scattered throughout the skeleton.

When one divides the cases into minimal, moderate and severe, the complications of involvement of extraskeletal systems are found to fall into a pattern. Solitary lesions are rarely accompanied by endocrine disturbance, skin patches or irregularities of skeletal growth (monomelic hypertrophy), while severe cases usually show one or more of these complications.

Clinical evidence of the bone lesions usually becomes manifest in late childhood though a few severe cases have shown evidence of beginning in infancy. It is not uncommon to discover solitary lesions in the third decade and at times even much later, but the bulk of evidence suggests that most if not all areas of involvement begin during the growing period. All types of bones are affected though there is some slight predilection for the large bones of the extremities. Though any part of the latter may be the site of origin, fibrous dysplasia is apt to begin in the metaphysis and progress toward the mid-diaphysis. Both cancellous and cortical bone are affected. As mature bone undergoes physiologic lysis it is replaced by solid masses of proliferating fibrous cells. The process suggests an inability to maintain bone in certain focal areas but it must be admitted that as it progresses it may extend beyond the normal cortical limitations. The original mass usually extends peripherally in projecting lobulations so that the affected area is scalloped and highly irregular in outline. The cortex is eroded from within while the periosteum attempts to compensate by laying down a thin shell of normal bone on the outer surface. Cylindrical bones become expanded and large elevations appear on the surface of flat bones.

The cortex may be so weakened that pathologic fracture occurs and this may be the presenting symptom of the disease. The second most common complaint is the deformity which occurs, particularly when bones of the head are involved. These may involve the orbit, to cause exopthalmos, the maxilla or the mandible (Fig. 96). Pain is usually not an outstanding feature until infractions and deformity make weight-bearing difficult.

When the area is approached surgically it is seen that normal bone has been replaced by irregular masses of pale tissue streaked with brown and red where there has been hemorrhage (Fig. 97). This material is usually gritty and has been likened to putty containing granules of sand. On slight magnification the particles are seen to be irregular, spicular masses of bone lying in the fibrous matrix. Small

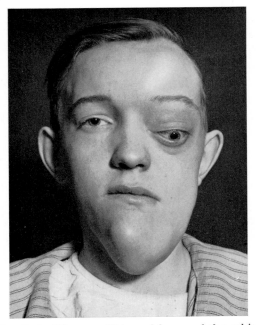

FIG. 96.   Fibrous dysplasia. The mandible and bones of the orbit are common sites
of involvement.

masses of cartilage are often found, and though these never constitute
the predominant element of the entire lesion they may be large enough
to confuse the issue in biopsy diagnosis. Small irregular regions of
fluid have been reported. These are areas of cystic degeneration rather
than true cysts and they are never a prominent part of the picture.
The "cysts" reported in roentgenograms are areas of relative translucency resulting from the replacement of bone by fibrous tissue. The
only true cysts of bone are found in "solitary cyst" though the cystic
degeneration of parathyroid adenoma (osteitis fibrosa cystica) may
be difficult to differentiate.

The pigmented, non-elevated skin patches occur in perhaps a
third of the cases of fibrous dysplasia, usually the more extensive.
They usually occur on the trunk, have a geographic outline and vary
from a few millimeters in diameter to the size of one's palm or larger.
They have a café-au-lait or chestnut color. The epidermis and underlying corium are normal in texture and consistency.

Endocrine dysfunction is almost restricted to females though a
few cases of hyperthyroidism have been seen in males. Again, the bone
involvement is usually severe. The usual complaint is precocious
menstruation which occurs in something less than one fifth of the
cases. The menarche appears early (it has been reported at three
years) and the menses are usually irregular in amount and periodicity
with a tendency to become regular at the normal age of puberty.

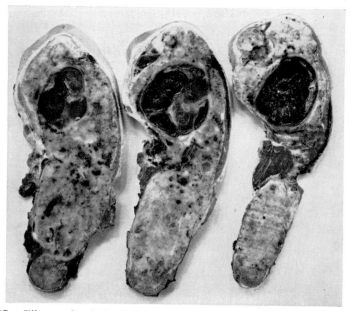

FIG. 97.   Fibrous dysplasia. It became necessary to remove the left arm because of multiple arteriovenous fistulae. Multiple anomalies are seen in many cases of fibrous dysplasia. In the lower portion of the specimen one finds the gritty, gray material that characterizes the condition.

Hyperthyroidism is also seen in patients with fibrous dysplasia in a higher incidence than in the normal population. Precocious skeletal growth has been reported in a few cases. There may be abnormally rapid growth during childhood but premature closure of the epiphyseal centers is apt to occur so that ultimate growth may fall short of average stature.

The precocious menstruation, which is presumably on the basis of premature ovarian stimulation, the hyperthyroidism and the early rapid growth and epiphyseal ossification all suggest the possibility that these disturbances may be the polyglandular effects of a dysfunctioning pituitary. Support is given this hypothesis by the fact that the base of the skull is frequently involved in fibrous dysplasia and this involvement may affect the pituitary space or the floor of the third ventricle above it. There has been insufficient investigation either to prove or disprove this theory. Against it is the occasional accompaniment of anomalies in other systems which could hardly be of endocrine origin. Such are reported in rather wide variation.[12]

ROENTGENOGRAPHIC MANIFESTATIONS

The lesions of fibrous dysplasia may not be radiolucent, but rather may be somewhat opaque because of the irregular, microscopic masses

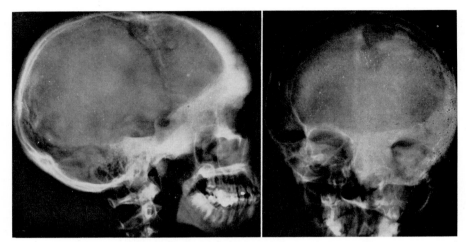

FIG. 98. Fibrous dysplasia. The bones at the base of the skull are opaque and markedly thickened. The paranasal sinuses, except for the right maxillary sinus, are obliterated and the left orbit is distorted. The patient is 17 years of age.

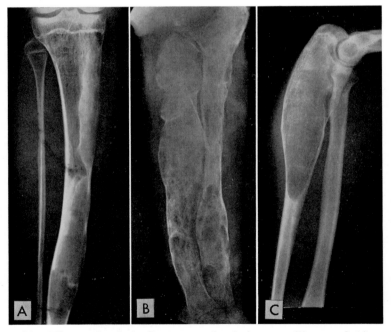

FIG. 99. Fibrous dysplasia. Representative lesions are illustrated (A) and (C). The semi-opacity of the lesions is evident as well as widening of the diaphysis and thinning of the cortices. Marked involvement with distortion of bone architecture is apparent in (B), the radiograph of a forearm of a young adult.

of bone which exist within the fibrous matrix. The individual lesion is not sharply outlined and in the advanced lesion the involved areas are lobular and scalloped in outline. The lesions which erode and expand the cortex are nevertheless covered by a layer of bone, since periosteal bone formation is normal. Abundant periosteal new bone is seen when pathologic fracture occurs through a lesion. The lesions are most frequently located in the proximal bones and decrease in severity and extent distally.

Deformity of the long bones in the form of bending and, in the severe disease, telescoping is not uncommon because of the fibrous nature of the lesion.

The manifestations of the disease as it involves the bones of the cranial vault are similar to those elsewhere. However, when the base of the frontal bone, the sphenoid, ethmoid and maxillary bones are involved, the results differ. Here there is marked thickening and opacity of the bones with obliteration of the paranasal sinuses and a decrease in the capacity of the orbits.

MICROSCOPY

Sections taken at random through a lesion of fibrous dysplasia should show a matrix of fibrous tissue in which are embedded sparsely scattered spicules of bone. The character of both the matrix and bone is important in reaching a decision on the basis of microscopy and the appearance depends greatly upon the age of the lesion. In the mature process the matrix is usually quite dense, the cells—fibrocytes—are well-spindled, the nuclei elongated and densely chromatic. There are considerable amounts of intercellular collagen. The cellular pattern is that of organized fibrous connective tissue seen elsewhere in the body. There is a paucity of vessels though the tissue cannot be described as being avascular (Fig. 100). Small aggregates of hemosiderin are common though hemorrhage is never a very important feature. In the vicinity of extravasated blood or old blood pigment there may be collections of giant cells. Usually these are sparse and they may be hard to find though at times these collections are large enough to suggest giant cell tumor or brown tumor of parathyroid adenoma. These cells are usually moderate in size and contain from three to twenty nuclei, generally grouped in the central portion of the cell. The giant cells appear to be formed by a merging of the individual matrix cells. Here and there one may find small numbers of pale xanthoid cells, their cytoplasm filled with lipid granules. Typical osteoclasts are found but are never very abundant.

The bone may appear quite normal in the older lesions but

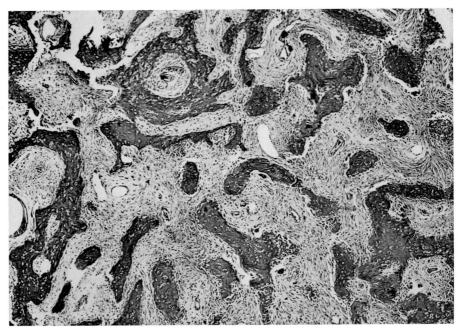

FIG. 100.   Fibrous dysplasia. A section to illustrate the spicules of fiberbone inter-spersed in a field of fairly mature collagenous tissue. This lesion is well established and probably no longer progressive. ($\times$ 40.)

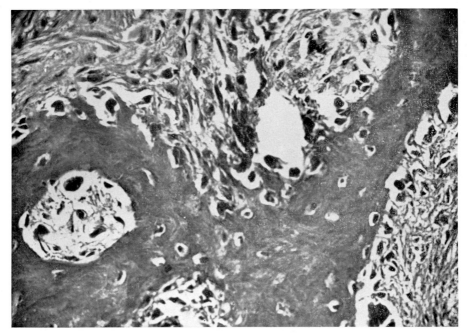

FIG. 101.   Fibrous dysplasia. Section of a bone spicule in a fibrous matrix. Along the upper margin there appears to be osteoblastic osteogenesis. ($\times$ 375.)

usually it is of the primitive type, coarse-fibered and contains numerous large lacunae with young cells. Mineralization is apt to be uneven. Sometimes the edges of the spicule are quite rough. Many of the spicules will show their convex surfaces to be covered with a layer of cells which are indistinguishable from normal osteoblasts (Fig. 101). Frequently a seam of pink-staining osteoid separates them from the mineralized portion of the spicule.

In younger lesions the matrix is composed of more loosely arranged fibroblasts. The cells are less spindled, their nuclei are larger and younger and there is less collagen. In these sections fibro-osseous metaplasia is usually prominent. At times the spicules appear to be no more than fibrous condensations (Fig. 102) with obvious transition of their cells into those of the surrounding matrix. Fibrous metaplasia is probably an important feature of the process but it quite certainly is not pathognomonic when present nor does its absence rule out the diagnosis. Actually, fibro-osseous metaplasia may be a difficult thing to recognize and one might reasonably ask the question "Just what is fibro-osseous metaplasia?"

We know that in normal osteogenesis cells emerge from the undifferentiated "fibrous" mass, line up about bars of calcified hyalin and engage in the laying down of an osteoid seam. It is only when the seam emerges that we recognize them as osteoblasts. Before then they cannot be distinguished, by any staining method yet devised, from

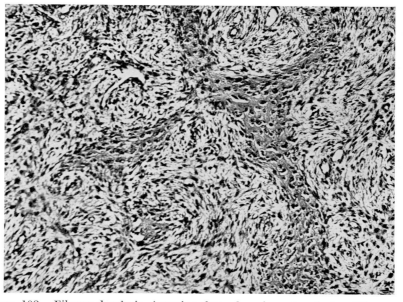

FIG. 102.   Fibrous dysplasia. A section through an immature lesion. Fibro-osseous metaplasia is quite obvious. The "bone spicule" is vaguely seen in a field of young collagenous tissue. (× 180.)

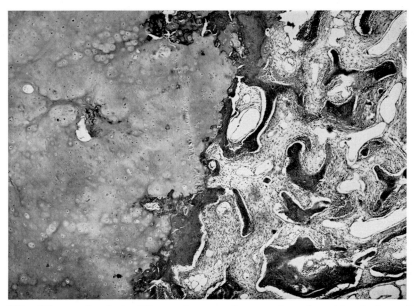

Fig. 103.   Fibrous dysplasia. The section reveals a portion of an island of cartilage on the left and fibrous dysplasia on the right. ($\times$ 35.)

collagenoblasts or, for that matter, from primitive chondroblasts. It is the intercellular environment that makes the distinction between these three types of cells. We speak of the periosteum as fibrous, yet physiologically there is osteoblastic metaplasia and the production of normal cortical bone. It is confusing to insist that the metaplasia in fibrous dysplasia is abnormal though admittedly the metaplastic transition is quite obvious. Actually, it is the character of the bone product and its relation to the matrix which is abnormal in fibrous dysplasia.

The islands of cartilage (Fig. 103) which are found in this condition have the same microscopic appearance as the cartilage of enchondromatosis and it is probable that they arise in the same manner, by a failure of normal differentiation of the cells of the primitive cell mass. One might hypothesize that the dysfunction in fibrous metaplasia is only one step further along the normal maturation path than that of enchondromatosis.

PROGNOSIS

If the lesions of fibrous dysplasia begin in early childhood, are multiple and progress throughout adolescence, skeletal deformity is apt to be advanced and crippling may be severe. If the lesion is solitary and first noted during adolescence, the patient may escape with scarcely a scar. One may expect the progress of the disease to slow or become completely arrested at the time of skeletal maturation. It is difficult to explain the lesions which make themselves known during adult life. Perhaps they began during the growth period, but why have they become activated? None of these is apt to produce serious skeletal damage, and it is possible that they have not become reactivated but that circumstances of aging such as osteoporosis or changes in stress trajectories point up a lesion which otherwise might have been carried unknown throughout life.

NEUROFIBROMATOSIS

Neurofibromatosis or von Recklinghausen's disease is a hereditary, often congenital and sometimes familial disturbance in the supportive tissue of the nervous system, both central and peripheral. It usually involves the skin, it may involve the skeleton, and disturbances in other systems such as the endocrine and gastrointestinal tract have been reported.

Ewing states that Kölliker was the first to describe the condition in 1860. In 1882, von Recklinghausen associated the lesions with the nervous system and the disease has since borne his name, though this sometimes leads to confusion since the same eponym is applied to parathyroid adenoma. Verocay (1910) suggested that the masses of proliferating cells arose from the Schwann syncytium rather than the fibrocytes of the nerve sheath. The work of Masson (1926) supported this contention since the nevus cells of the skin are also involved and both as well as the glial supportive cells are derived from the neuro-ectoderm. Stout and Murray have long contended that the neurilem-moma (sometimes spelled neurilemoma), a solitary, benign, encapsulated tumor of nerves, occasionally encountered in neuro-fibromatosis, is Schwannian in origin. They base their opinion on the morphology of cells grown in tissue culture. One might question the validity of such dogmatism and ask how the cells originally selected to establish the criteria were indubitably known to come from the Schwann sheath, since morphology becomes even less trustworthy than usual when the cell environment is changed as radically as is necessary for culture work. However, the matter is highly academic and hardly worth the polemics it has provoked.

Neurofibromatosis, as the name implies, involves principally the nervous system. Masses of spindled cells arise from either the Schwann or fibrous supportive cells or both, along the course of peripheral nerves, in branches of the autonomic nervous system and in the meninges. These masses are pale and moderately firm. They may involve a short segment or extend along the greater portion of the full length, sometimes continuing proximally to involve the substance of the cord. They greatly increase the diameter of the nerve trunk and often cause a tortuosity of its course—plexiform neurofibroma. Pain is not usual but at times it results from pressure on the contiguous nerve fibers. The meningiomas are not unusual as such. In a small percentage, glial "tumors" occur within the brain, often involving the floor of the third ventricle.[13] It is debatable whether these proliferations of the supportive cells of neurons are truly neoplastic or simply the product of an unrestrained, hamartomatous growth. The nerve enlargements, often called "neurofibromas," may occur along the cranial or spinal nerve roots (acoustic neuromas and spinal neurofibromas) and here cause bone changes by erosion. The endocrine disturbances which have been reported may result from pressure upon the hypophysis by enlargement at the chiasm.

The skin is almost always affected, not only by the neurofibromas, and less often neurilemmomas, but also because its supportive tissue, its nevus cells and appendages are involved.

Proliferations of melanoblasts may be limited to geographic brown patches within the skin, café-au-lait spots measuring from a few millimeters to several centimeters in diameter, or true benign dermal and compound nevi and even malignant melanomas may develop. The café-au-lait spots or chestnut patches are the commonest skin manifestation of neurofibromatosis. They are also seen sometimes in pseudarthrosis and fibrous dysplasia.

At the dermal nerve endings there are apt to occur poorly delineated proliferations of spindled cells within the corium which elevate the epidermal surface. Sometimes the epidermal melanin is heavier in these areas and they may support a thick growth of hair. Some of these elevations may become pedunculated. They may occur singly, in patches or literally cover the skin by the hundreds. These lesions are sometimes called fibroma molluscum (Fig. 104). They are not true fibromas since they are not encapsulated. Large areas of skin may become diffusely thickened and redundant so that it hangs in coarse, heavy folds, a condition called elephantiasis. Occasionally there are patches of hypertrophied sebaceous glands (Pringle) and there may be lipomas.

Lesions in the skeleton include bone erosion by the neurofibromas, scolioses, pseudarthrosis, abnormalities in size and areas of demineralization which have been called cysts on the basis of roentgenographic examination. The cause and the nature of the scolioses are unrecorded. The vertebrae are often found to be wedged. In pseudarthrosis a segment of diaphysis is known to undergo softening by deossification and replacement by masses of spindled cells similar to those found in the skin. It is probable that the vertebral lesion is analogous to pseudarthrosis in the extremities. The curvatures occur most commonly in the lumbar areas, the angulation is often sharp and as the lesion progresses paraplegia may occur.

Though pseudarthrosis is a relatively common complication it occurs apart from neurofibromatosis and so will be treated in a separate section (p. 161).

Skeletal enlargement or focal gigantism is perhaps the most bizarre and fascinating aspect of von Recklinghausen's disease. The hypertrophy may involve a single bone, the bones of a part such as a single digit or those of the entire extremity. The bones are usually normal in shape. The associated muscles and joints are proportionately enlarged. The involved part is usually in the distribution or segment of an affected nerve.

It would appear in surveying the many facets of this kaleidoscopic disease that the fault lies deeply buried within the germ plasm of one or more germ layers. The neuroectoderm is almost certainly involved judging from the incidence of lesions in the entire nervous system and also its related neuroepithelially derived supportive tissue, melanoblasts and related skin. It has been suggested[14] that the disturbance in the nerve impulse conduction channels results in altered nutritional supplies and growth potentials. Though at present this is

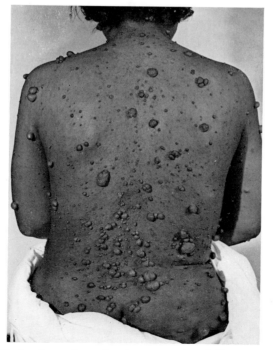

FIG. 104.   Back of a patient showing examples of fibroma molluscum.

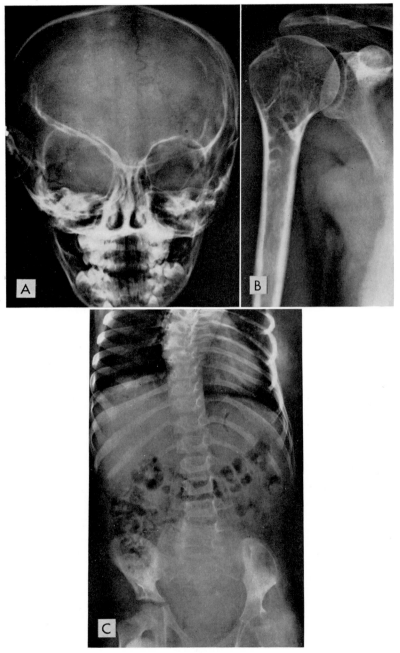

FIG. 105.   Neurofibromatosis. Involvement of the right orbit is illustrated (*A*). The orbit is enlarged and the orbital fissure is enlarged; exophthalmos was present. Small, radiolucent cyst-like areas with opaque margins are evident in *B*, the radiograph of the humerus. In *C*, a large mass of the density of soft tissue fills the pelvis (neurofibroma). Scoliosis and deformity of the pelvis and left femur are present.

nothing more than an unsubstantiated hypothesis, the distribution and character of the extraneural lesions lend some credence to it.

MICROSCOPY

Sections made through an area of bone softening reveal poorly delineated masses of spindled cells resembling rather mature fibrocytes (Fig. 108B). In some areas there is a tendency for trabeculation and palisading but the major portion of the mass shows no attempt at organization. Considerable amounts of collagen are readily demonstrable with special stains. In some areas there is a rather abortive attempt at fibro-osseous and fibrocartilaginous metaplasia. These sections suggest an inability to maintain and replace normal bone. Instead, fibrous connective tissue is produced and overproduced with some attempt at bone and cartilage metaplasia.

The lesions of the nervous system (Fig. 106) show a variety of pictures. The neurofibromas are made up of masses of spindled cells which with ordinary staining methods look much like those of the bone lesions. The occasional neurilemmoma may contain Verocay bodies, aggregates of palisaded nuclei (Fig. 107 *A*), and when this pattern predominates they are classified as Antoni Type A. When whorls, trabeculation and Verocay bodies are lacking and the tissue appears myxomatous with areas of cystic degeneration, the lesion is said to be of the Antoni Type B (Fig. 107 *B*). A variety of gliomas,

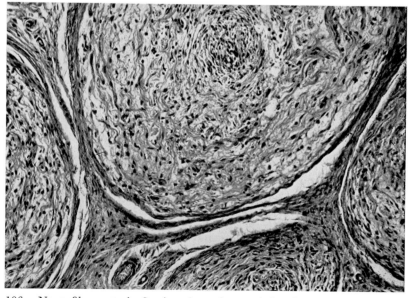

FIG. 106. Neurofibromatosis. Section through a peripheral nerve showing immense thickening due to proliferation of collagenoblasts of the supportive tissue.

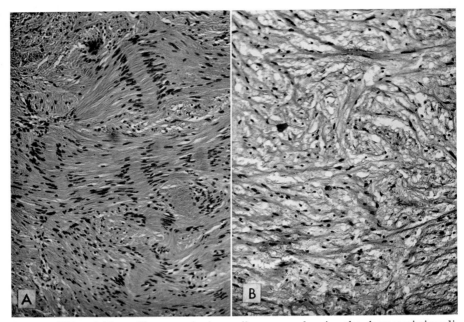

FIG. 107.   *A*, Neurofibromatosis. A neurilemmoma showing the characteristic pali-sading of cells to form Verocay bodies. This is the Antoni type A. (× 180.) *B*, A neurilemmoma illustrating the myxomatous character of the Antoni type B lesion. (× 180.)

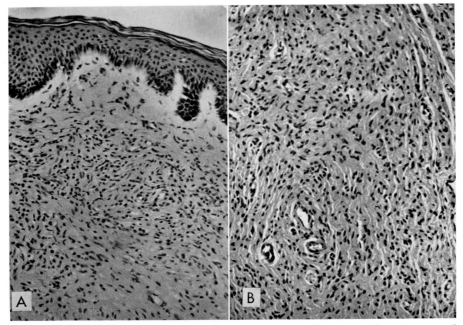

FIG. 108.   *A*, Neurofibromatosis. Section through a fibroma molluscum covered with epiderm. (× 130.) *B*, Section from a lesion in bone. The same collagenoblastic proliferation is seen here as that found in the soft tissue lesions. (× 130.)

benign and malignant, have been described in the central nervous system.

The fibroma molluscum (Fig. 108 A) in the skin consists of masses of spindled cells which might be either Schwannian or fibrous in origin. They are smaller and more firmly woven than the components of the usual skin fibroma.

PROGNOSIS

Neurofibromatosis (von Recklinghausen) may be of any degree of severity. There may be only a few neurofibromas or café-au-lait spots or the process may involve almost every system with hideous skeletal deformity, fantastic skin lesions and death with a glial tumor of the brain. There is a tendency for the progress of the disease to slow and sometimes stop at about the time of cessation of normal growth. The condition may then remain latent for the remainder of a normal life span or it may be reactivated at any time and go on to death. Perhaps 10 per cent of the neurofibromas undergo a change to frankly malignant neoplasms. The rate of growth increases, they become more invasive and metastasize by way of the blood stream. It has been suggested that repeated biopsying of these lesions in the various clinics that these patients eventually enter, seeking help, predisposes to malignant change. Since biopsy is not usually necessary for diagnosis, and assists in no way in therapy, it should not be done for teaching purposes or to satisfy the curiosity of the clinician.

PSEUDARTHROSIS

Pseudarthrosis is a pathologic entity characterized by deossification of a weight-bearing long bone, bending, pathologic fracture and inability to form normal callus in healing. Approximately half the cases reveal at least some evidence of an accompanying neurofibromatosis of which café-au-lait spots are the most common. The condition is hereditary, congential and familial.

Ducroquet[15] reported 11 cases of pseudarthrosis in 1937. Of these, nine had accompanying café-au-lait spots including one with neurofibromas. There was evidence of neurofibromatosis in one of the parents of four of this series. Barber[16] was the first to report the condition in the American literature. He emphasized the association with von Recklinghausen's disease. Until the paper of Holt and Wright[17] in 1948, it was generally believed that the pathologic fracture was the result of weakening of the bone due to the presence of a neurilemmoma. This belief was supported by the finding of nerve fibers within

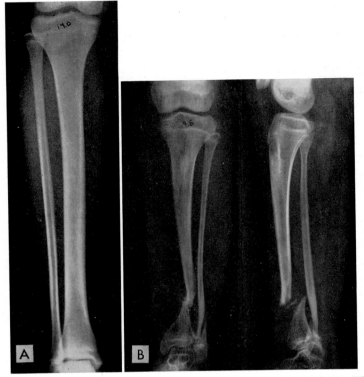

FIG. 109.   Pseudarthrosis. The left tibia and fibula are involved (B). There is a discontinuity of these bones which too are shorter than the right tibia and fibula (A). The bone at the site of the abnormality is tapered and delicate. The cortices are thin and a radiolucent area representing fibrous tissue separates the bones at the site of the pseudarthrosis. Deformity is apparent.

cortical bone. Aegerter[18] pointed out that if the clinical aspects of the disease are considered from the beginning it will be noted that the fracture site is only a part of a much wider area of diffuse deossification and that the fibro-osseous tissue interposed between the bone ends is the result and not the cause of the fracture.

The early stages of pseudarthrosis, or even fracture, have been noted at birth. More attenuated cases develop during childhood or occasionally in adolescence. Pathologic fracture is the event which usually calls attention to the condition, though roentgenographic studies will frequently reveal a more diffuse process than is represented by the fracture site. The tibia in its lower two thirds is the most commonly affected bone, though the fibula is frequently involved and other long bones are not excepted. The softening of the cortices appears to be a gradual lysis, probably physiologic, with an inability to replace the bone that is lost. Instead, there is a fibrous proliferation which does not accept the calcium salts and, therefore, remains pliable. There is an attempt at callus formation with indifferent success. Usually the bone ends are welded together but the failure to form rigid bone leaves the region flexible. Sometimes there is sufficient fibro-osseous metaplasia to simulate normal repair but when weight-bearing is resumed, the bone that has been formed melts away and "refracture" occurs. This sequence may be repeated indefinitely until the limb becomes distorted beyond functional practicability. The formation of a "false joint" has given rise to the name "pseudarthrosis."

MICROSCOPY

If tissue is removed from between the bone ends and sectioned, a monotonous pattern of purposeless fibrocytes is seen (Fig. 110). The spindled cells are rather small and there is little evidence of organization into a pattern of trabeculation. Collagen formation is usually ample but there is no more than a half-hearted attempt to form osteoid. There seems to be no deficiency in mineralization, once the organic matrix is produced. Cartilage formation is entirely lacking or very scant. There is often an extension of the fibroblastic proliferation out around the external cortical surfaces of the area.

It has been suggested that the members of the primitive cell mass are incapable of differentiation into normal osteoblasts. This inability is apparently a part of a more generalized mesenchymal derivative

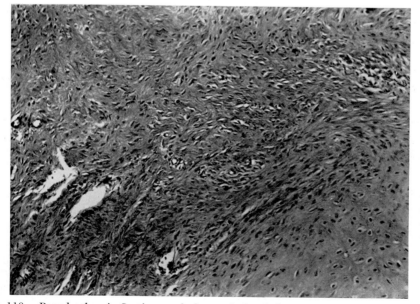

FIG. 110.   Pseudarthrosis. Section made from a lesion in bone. In the lower right-hand corner there is evidence of fibro-osseous metaplasia. ($\times$ 130.)

defect and when the manifestation is more florid the other aspects of neurofibromatosis become apparent.

PROGNOSIS

The inability to heal a fracture sustained in childhood may persist throughout life if orthopedic attention is inadequate or unsuccessful. The patient usually has periods of limited function interspersed with longer episodes of complete disability of the part. There is a tendency for the condition to improve upon skeletal maturation but by this time deformity may be so extensive that complete function is never regained.

REFERENCES

ENCHONDROMATOSIS

1. Mahorner, H. P.: J. Pediat., *10*:1; 1937.
2. Ollier, M.: Bull. Soc. de Chir. de Lyon., *3*:22; 1899.

HEREDITARY MULTIPLE EXOSTOSES

3. Jaffe, H.: Arch. Path., *36*:335; 1943.
4. Jansen, M.: Dissociation of Bone Growth, Rob't Jones Birthday Volume. Oxford University Press, London, 1928.

FIBROUS DYSPLASIA

5. Schlumberger, H. G.: Military Surgeon, *99*:504; 1946.
6. Freund, E., and Moffert, C. B.: Surg., Gynec. & Obst., *62*:541; 1936.
7. McCune, D. J., and Bruch, H.: Am. J. Dis. Child., *54*:807; 1937.
8. Albright, F., Butler, A., Hampton, A., and Smith, P.: New England J. Med., *216*: 729; 1937.
9. Lichtenstein, L.: Am. J. Surg., *36*:874; 1938.
10. Lichtenstein, L., and Jaffe, H. L.: Arch. Path., *33*:777; 1942.
11. Thannhauser, S. J., Medicine, *23*:105; 1944.
12. Stauffer, H. M., Arbuckle, R. K., and Aegerter, E.: J. Bone & Joint Surg., *23*:323; 1941.

NEUROFIBROMATOSIS

13. Aegerter, E., and Smith, L. W.: Am. J. Cancer, *31*:212; 1937.
14. Holt, J. F., and Wright, E. M.: Radiology, *51*:657; 1948.

PSEUDARTHROSIS

15. Ducroquet, R.: Mém. Acad. de Chir., *63*:863; 1937.
16. Barber, C. G.: Surg., Gynec. & Obst., *69*:618; 1939.
17. Holt, J. F., and Wright, E. M.: Radiology, *51*:647; 1948.
18. Aegerter, E.: J. Bone & Joint Surg., *32A*:618; 1950.

9

Functional Disturbances

of the

Reticuloendothelial

System

HAND-SCHÜLLER-CHRISTIAN DISEASE

Hand-Schüller-Christian disease, sometimes called lipoid granuloma-
tosis, cholesterol reticuloendotheliosis or histiocytosis, is a condition
in which multiple, microscopically characteristic, non-bacterial, focal
granulomas develop first in relation to bones, in more severe cases
extending to the extraosseous reticulum deposits and skin and in some
invading the viscera. The cause is unknown but a highly characteristic
and peculiar part of the mechanism is the deposition of a variety of
lipids, preponderantly cholesterol and its esters, within macrophages.

Hand,[1] in 1893, was the first to report descriptions of the lesions
as an entity. The etiology was presumed to be tuberculous though at
the time he expressed doubt as to the correctness of this presumption.
He later recognized it as a non-tuberculous entity and published his
opinion as such.[2] In 1915, Schüller reported three cases of the disease,
and in 1919 Christian made his report[3] in which appeared the first
description of the triad of exopthalmos, diabetes insipidus and multiple focal areas of deossification. Rowland[4] in 1928 recognized the condition as a disturbance in lipid metabolism with phagocytosis of

excessive macromolecules of lipid by the reticuloendothelial system. It had previously been thought, because of the hypophyseal involvement in the reported cases, that the lesions were an expression of pituitary dysfunction. Rowland's report shifted opinion to a systemic disturbance of lipid metabolism and related the condition to Gaucher's disease and Niemann-Pick disease.

With the concept that the reticuloendothelial system played a secondary role in merely accumulating the lipids at fault the disease was classified with the xanthomatoses. When Farber, in 1941,[5] directed attention to the similarity of the lesions of Hand-Schüller-Christian disease and those of eosinophilic granuloma, a condition which was presumed to be caused by an unknown infectious agent, opinion swung back again to approximately where it had started.

Today, most will admit that the cause of Hand-Schüller-Christian disease is unknown. It appears to result from the inability on the part of the reticuloendothelial components of certain regions to process several of the complex lipids, principally cholesterol. This inability may arise from a congenital enzymatic lack or from an alteration of metabolic capacity of the cells whose function it is to handle these lipids. Or it might be caused by an outside agent, perhaps infectious in nature, such as a virus, though none has been isolated even though sought for.

The former association with the hypercholesterolemic and hyperlipemic xanthomatoses seems to have dissolved with a better understanding of the physiology of these processes. The relationship to the other lipid reticuloendothelioses is uncertain since they often show hereditary features which are lacking in Hand-Schüller-Christian disease. It may be that an enzymatic deficiency is the basic difficulty in all these conditions, but the cause of this deficiency and the cells involved may be variable.

Hand-Schüller-Christian disease usually begins in infancy or early childhood. Less often it appears in adolescence and rarely it is first diagnosed during adult life. The earlier the onset, the more grave the prognosis is apt to be. Before x-ray therapy was generally used for this disease, cases beginning in childhood or earlier usually terminated fatally in from two to four years. With the benefit of proper roentgen therapy most patients now survive well into adult life. In some series there has been a preponderance of males, in other series this sex predilection has been lacking.

The commonest site of origin is the intraosseous reticulum and its derivatives. When manifestations are minimal, the skeleton is apt to be the only structure involved. In somewhat more florid cases the spleen, liver and lymph nodes may be the sites of granulomatous lesions and the skin is often affected. In the cases that begin early in life and run a malignant course most of the tissues of the body are involved, including the lungs, brain, heart, kidneys, mucous membranes, tendon sheaths, fascia and serous surfaces. Rarely the disease may remain latent as a solitary lesion for a long period and then progress into typical multicentric Hand-Schüller-Christian disease. A few cases are reported to run a fairly classic course for several months and then develop into a fulminant terminal phase which is identical with that of Letterer-Siwe disease.

The fundamental lesion of Hand-Schüller-Christian disease is a focal granuloma which grows peripherally to agglomerate with other granulomas until a large irregular mass is formed. The blood supply to the normal tissue of the site is obstructed, normal structures degenerate and the granulomas replace them. Thus, the lesion compresses, pushes aside or destroys the normal tissue where it develops.

Actively hematopoietic marrow is most commonly involved and so flat bones are the most frequently affected. Long bones are not spared, however. The affected areas may give rise to pain. In cylindrical bones, unlike most of the bone tumors, the lesion of Hand-Schüller-Christian disease may begin in any region. The metaphysis is no more frequently involved than the mid-diaphysis. Bone-supportive fibrous tissue is also frequently involved so that the lesions may begin in the periosteum or, when in the head, beneath the dura or the scalp tissues. They begin as miliary lesions which enlarge and coalesce. Cancellous and cortical bone in their path melts away leaving sharply delineated areas of deossification. This tissue is moderately firm, has a yellow or yellowish gray color and may show inconspicuous areas of hemorrhage or cystic degeneration in its active phase.

The bones of the head are most frequently involved (Fig. 111). The calvarium may become riddled with circular holes which may be palpated through the scalp. Involvement of the base and the sella causes pituitary dysfunction in about one third of the cases. If the posterior pituitary lobe is affected there may be polydypsia and polyuria—diabetes insipidus. If the anterior lobe is involved there may be delayed somatic and sexual growth with infantilism, dwarfism, adiposogenital syndrome or Simmonds' disease. Compression on the base of the brain may result in hydrocephalus with symptoms of headache and vomiting. The jaw is frequently involved causing swelling of the gums and loosening of the teeth.

The spleen, liver and lymph nodes are not affected in the very mild cases and are never greatly involved. The reticulum of the marrow is frequently sufficiently invaded to cause an anemia.

The skin is involved in less than one third of the cases. The

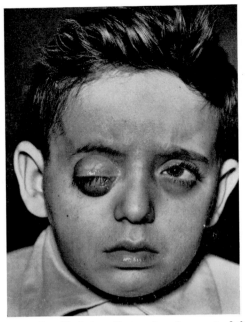

FIG. 111.   Hand-Schüller-Christian disease. Involvement of the bones of the orbit cause proptosis. This, plus pituitary dysfunction due to involvement of the sella, and x-ray rarefaction of other skull bones constitutes a common and classic triad of the disease.

typical lesions are yellow nodules and plaques in the corium covered with a thin layer of epiderm. At times the latter ulcerates and chronic, ragged craters persist complicated by an indolent infection.

Hypercholesterolemia and hyperlipemia have been frequently reported, particularly in the earlier papers, but most authors now agree that alterations in the serum lipids are unusual and are probably not characteristic. Eosinophilia has been reported in a few cases, particularly since an association with eosinophilic granuloma has been stressed. The eosinophilic leukocyte count has never been high and is probably of no significance. A mild fever and leukocytosis have been mentioned in a few instances.

For Roentgenographic Manifestations see page 177.

MICROSCOPY

The diagnosis of Hand-Schüller-Christian disease can be made with finality only by examination of involved tissue under the microscope. Even with this evidence it is frequently necessary to supplement the microscopic picture with clinical and roentgenographic evidence since the microscopy varies and in some stages is entirely non-specific.

The typical lesion of Hand-Schüller-Christian disease suggests that the reticulum and its derivatives of a more or less circumscribed area have become unable to process certain lipid substances with which they have come in contact. It is a popular concept that these lipids are normally processed by these cells but that owing to a fault in their metabolic activities the cells can now only absorb them into their cytoplasmic substance where, instead of being processed and passed on, the lipids accumulate and eventually cause cell death and rupture with a spilling of the lipids into the supportive tissues of the area. The hypothesis that the disease is a systemic fault in lipid metabolism resulting in the circulation of an excessive amount of this material, which is eventually picked up by the phagocytic reticulum elements, lacks support in that if this were the case and the reticulum were healthy one might expect all units of the normal reticulum to be affected equally. Universal involvement is seen in only the most florid cases of lipid reticuloendotheliosis.

For a proper concept of the microscopic features of the lesion of Hand-Schüller-Christian disease one must realize that the cells specifically involved are those of the reticulum and its derivatives, particularly the motile, phagocytic cells, and that the elements of this system have the capacity of morphologic and apparent functional interchange. Thus the lesion seems to undergo a series of changes throughout its life cycle and the terminal phase is quite different in appearance from the early stage. It should be kept in mind also that cells other than the specifically affected reticulum elements are usually involved, so that the character of the lesion may vary depending upon the tissue site. Thus it is small wonder that the pathologist frequently misses the diagnosis unless he maintains a high level of suspicion for this rather rare disease or unless he has the benefit of the roentgenologic and clinical data when he examines his sections.

The exact sequence of events in the early stages of the lesions of Hand-Schüller-Christian disease is probably not known with certainty, though in all instances there appears to be a migration or proliferation of large macrophages, monocytes or histiocytes in the affected area. Before the other events of the cycle take place, large fields of these cells may closely simulate neoplasm and one must guard against the temptation to diagnose the lesion as Ewing's tumor (Fig. 112). At some time during the early stages of the cycle there is an influx of eosinophilic leukocytes, lymphocytes, plasma cells and neutrophils, their numerical incidence being approximately in the order named. At times the inflammatory reaction is more apparent than the histiocytic nature and a diagnosis of non-specific osteomyelitis may be made. In at least some lesions the eosinophilic leukocytes may completely dominate

FIG. 112.   FIG. 113.

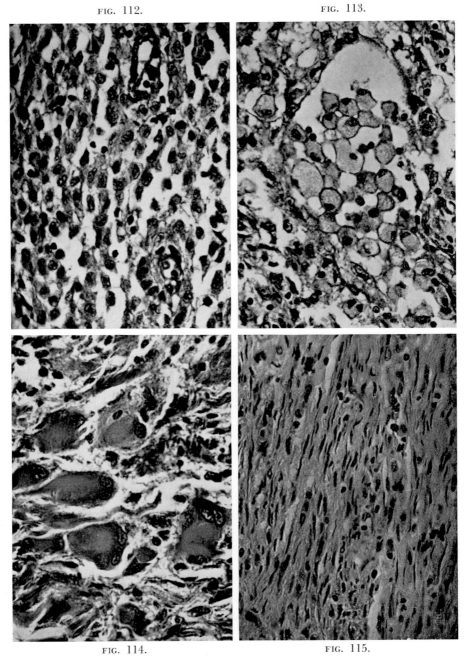

FIG. 114.   FIG. 115.

FIGS. 112–115.   Hand-Schüller-Christian disease.

FIG. 112.   The early lesion may consist largely of macrophages (histiocytes or epithelioid cells). The nuclei are large, pale and often have irregular or reniform outlines. Abnormal amounts of fat may be hard to demonstrate at this stage. The uniformity of the cells may suggest neoplasm. This type of lesion cannot be differentiated from eosinophilic granuloma. (× 450.)

FIG. 113.   At some time (usually early) the macrophages begin to fill with lipid.

the picture and unless the lesions are known to be multiple a diagnosis of eosinophilic granuloma is quite understandable. At some time in the course of the cycle, collections of lipids are noted within the cytoplasm of the histiocytes. At first the cytoplasm is granular, then vacuolated and finally swollen and foamy. Many of the nuclei appear to shrink and become more pyknotic (Fig. 113). Tissue necrosis occurs and there is an admixture of detritus among the cell components. Eventually some of the histiocytes rupture and the lipid material collects in the intercellular spaces. In hematoxylin-eosin stained preparations one finds sharply pointed clefts in the tissue, the sites of crystals of cholesterol before they were dissolved in the processing fluids. A foreign body reaction is engendered by the presence of the lipids and multinucleated giant cells make their appearance. This is the cytologic picture that one usually thinks of as characteristic of Hand-Schüller-Christian disease (Fig. 114). The background is composed of histiocytes, many of them lipid-bearing, exudative inflammatory cells, particularly eosinophilic leukocytes, necrosis, intercellular cholesterol crystals and giant cells. Soon the inflammatory reaction becomes less apparent and the exudative cells may disappear entirely. Fibroblasts appear and gradually dominate the picture, probably as a transition of the histiocytes which were not too damaged by their lipid content. Eventually the lesion may be converted to a collagenizing fibrous scar showing crystals of cholesterol and perhaps some foreign body reaction (Fig. 115).

The differentiation of Hand-Schüller-Christian disease and eosinophilic granuloma cannot be made on a cytologic basis alone. The great majority of solitary lesions occurring after the age of ten years will turn out to be the latter though occasionally even one of these cases may run a course with the development of multiple lesions that is much more like a mild Hand-Schüller-Christian disease. The lesions of Letterer-Siwe disease are usually quite unlike those described above. The histiocytic aggregates are present and often an exudative inflammatory reaction, but the lipid element is usually considerably less evident and sometimes cannot be found at all, leading to the term "non-lipid histiocytosis." The foreign body reaction usually does not appear.

There is usually very little attempt at regeneration of the destroyed bone in Hand-Schüller-Christian disease. This may possibly

---

The cytoplasm becomes swollen with pale granules or vacuoles. The nucleus shrinks and becomes pyknotic. (× 450.)

FIG. 114.   Giant cells soon form and these with the other elements plus lymphocytes and eosinophilic cells constitute the characteristic picture of the disease. (× 450.)

FIG. 115.   Following degeneration, the lesion is converted to collagenizing fibrous tissue which remains as the scar of the active lesion.

be accounted for on the basis of an interruption of the blood supply. If fracture occurs, there is apt to be callus formation with spicules of new bone and islands of cartilage. Then the picture may be exceedingly difficult to interpret.

Much of the lipid material which appears in the lesions of this disease can be stained with Sudan III or Scharlach R. It is doubly refractile with polarized light and analysis has shown it to consist largely of cholesterol and cholesterol esters. However, it is almost certain that the lipids involved constitute a group in which, though cholesterol is most abundant, there are traces of a variety of other complex lipoid substances. This is another reason to suggest that the fault lies not in the systemic metabolism of a specific lipid but rather in a cellular defect involving a group of related chemical substances.

PROGNOSIS

Approximately one half of the cases of Hand-Schüller-Christian disease have terminated fatally though with proper roentgen therapy many patients have survived over a period of years and as yet no one knows what the eventual prognosis will be. In the florid cases, beginning early in life, the outcome is dubious no matter what the therapy, though since a few cases of Letterer-Siwe disease have responded to antibiotic and other agents it is probable that this field has not been fully exploited as yet. Visceral involvement is a bad prognostic omen and if the infiltration is extensive, death is apt to occur within two years.

EOSINOPHILIC GRANULOMA

Eosinophilic granuloma of bone is a disease entity in which one or more focal areas of bone are destroyed by a granulomatous process of unknown etiology. The striking similarity of the microscopy of these lesions to those of Hand-Schüller-Christian disease has led most observers to consider the two conditions variants of the same process.

On January 13, 1940, Otani and Ehrlich[6] submitted for publication a paper entitled "Solitary Granuloma of Bone" and on January 19 of the same year Lichtenstein and Jaffe[7] submitted a paper entitled "Eosinophilic Granuloma of Bone" to the same journal. The first was published in July and the second in September of that year. These were the first papers to report this common condition as a pathologic entity though both papers credit the Italian and German literature with earlier descriptions of the disease. In April, 1941, Farber, Green and McDermott read a paper[8] before the American Association of Pathologists and Bacteriologists in which they stated that they believed that eosinophilic granuloma (using the name suggested by Lichtenstein and Jaffe), Hand-Schüller-Christian disease and Letterer-Siwe disease were all variants of the same process and in 1942 they published a series of ten cases[9] in support of this hypothesis. Today, most observers subscribe to this opinion since enough data have been accumulated, both clinical and pathologic, to corroborate the original observations.

Most cases of eosinophilic granuloma are seen in childhood, adolescence or early adult life and there is a considerable male predominance, when the reported cases are pooled. In almost half the cases there are two or more lesions. The most common site is in one or both frontal bones though lesions have been described in almost every bone of the skeleton. They rarely, if ever, occur in the small bones of the hands and feet. When they involve the vertebrae they may cause vertebra plana.[10]

Extraosseous, soft tissue eosinophilic granulomas have been reported but when unassociated with bone lesions they constitute a vague group, the identity and significance of which is difficult to evaluate. Recently, multiple nodules within the lungs have been found[11] accompanying typical bone lesions. The author has had the opportunity of examining material from one such case.

Eosinophilic granuloma usually causes some pain though as a rule this is not severe. When it occurs in the vicinity of a joint the symptoms may suggest the diagnosis of arthritis. Sometimes the onset is relatively sudden which is hard to explain in terms of the underlying tissue alterations.

Unlike most of the true neoplasms of bone, eosinophilic granuloma has no predilection for any particular area within the bone, appearing within the diaphysis of long bones as often as the metaphysis. Since it is an osteolytic process it does not cause cortical expansion nor is there apt to be overlying subperiosteal osteophytic bone production. The contiguous cortex melts away and the granuloma frequently extends out into the soft tissue. The surgeon may be surprised, having curetted an eosinophilic granuloma of one of the skull bones, to find that he has exposed the dura or even the brain. The lesion is usually small when discovered, often not more than a few millimeters in diameter, but they may enlarge up to 2 or even 3 centimeters. The curetted tissue is soft, nondescript red or mottled gray and rarely contains bone fragments. The area of bone destruction is usually found to be sharply limited. Its vascularity is not remarkable. Cultures of the tissue are sterile.

FIG. 116.

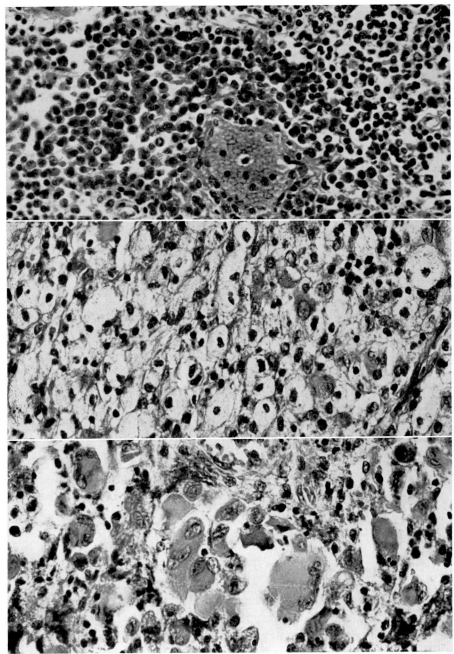

FIG. 118.

FIGS. 116, 117 and 118.   Eosinophilic granuloma.

FIG. 116.   Illustration of a mass of eosinophilic leukocytes. In the section this nodule of cells stands out in vivid contrast to the surrounding tissue but in the photograph it appears only as a rounded aggregate of cells the cytoplasm of which is darker. Some plasmacytes and neutrophils are intermixed with the eosinophils. ($\times$ 450.)

A few cases have manifested a moderately elevated eosinophilic leukocyte count in the peripheral blood but this finding is so inconstant that it is of little diagnostic value.

For Roentgenographic Manifestations see page 177.

MICROSCOPY

The term "eosinophilic granuloma" is an admirably descriptive one for the majority of these lesions when examined through the microscope. The matrix usually consists of a reticulated mass of histiocytes infiltrated with eosinophilic leukocytes. The latter may be so numerous that they form solid masses occupying a good portion of the low power field, staining the area a deep brick red. The eosinophilic cells may be filamented forms but usually they are younger and often are eosinophilic myelocytes. When these cells are present in considerable numbers the diagnosis can hardly be missed (Fig. 116). At times, however, the eosinophilic cells may be scant or lacking. There may be a prevalence of lymphocytes, of plasma cells or even neutrophilic granulocytes, all types may be represented, or there may be no leukocytes at all. Occasionally the lesion may consist entirely of masses of rather immature histiocytes (Fig. 117). Such lesions have led to the histologic diagnosis of myeloma in the past.

As the process matures, lipid material can be demonstrated within the cytoplasm of the phagocytic histiocytes (Fig. 117). Eventually this substance may become quite obvious even with routine hematoxylin-eosin stains though in the very early lesions it may be entirely lacking. Necrosis soon takes place and the histiocytes pick up nuclear fragments and debris. Apparently the lipid content of the macrophages becomes so great that they die and contribute this material to the detritus. Giant cells are formed (Fig. 118), probably by the agglomeration of histiocytes, and these too act as phagocytizing agents. The lipid accumulates in crystals to form slit-like, pointed clefts. Gradually the exudative inflammatory reaction subsides and fibroblasts begin to dominate the section. We assume that the lesion eventually becomes completely fibrosed. Much of the lipid material can be stained with Scharlach R and it will be seen to be doubly refractile when examined with polarized light. It has been identified as cholesterol and cholesterol esters.

FIG. 117 (*Center*). Macrophages have picked up large amounts of pale-staining lipid which swells the cytoplasm and causes the nuclei to become pyknotic. Some of the cells show evidence of bursting with escape of the lipid contents. ($\times$ 450.)

FIG. 118. Eventually giant cells characterize the lesion. They probably arise as a result of the lipids which are spilled into the tissue. Exudative inflammatory cells are the result of degenerative changes. ($\times$ 450.)

When one examines a series of sections of eosinophilic granuloma of varying stages and compares the microscopy with that of Hand-Schüller-Christian disease, one is impressed with the similarity, within the broad range of the varying pictures of the two conditions. It is probable that the former is a focal and often solitary manifestation of the latter. The clinical findings in a number of cases support this thesis.

PROGNOSIS

Eosinophilic granuloma is usually considered an innocuous condition, completely cured by curettage or x-ray therapy. In a few cases, however, the condition has progressed to a state which cannot be differentiated from Hand-Schüller-Christian disease. If the lesions are multiple, begin in early childhood and especially if there is accompanying visceral involvement, the prognosis should be guarded.

LETTERER-SIWE DISEASE

Letterer-Siwe disease, which has been called non-lipid reticulo-endotheliosis, is a fulminant, usually fatal disturbance of the total body reticulum apparatus with manifestations referable to the principal reticulum stations, the bone marrow, spleen, lymph nodes and liver and often the skin. It will be described only briefly here since it can be construed as orthopedic pathology only by virtue of its relation to Hand-Schüller-Christian disease and eosinophilic granuloma.

This condition as originally described by Letterer[12] and later Siwe[13] is a disease of infants. The onset is usually quite sudden, often with symptoms of an acute infection. In the course of a blood analysis it is usually found that there is an anemia, a thrombocytopenia and often a leukopenia. It becomes obvious that there is a disturbance in marrow function. The patient develops pallor and bleeding phenomena with petechial hemorrhages in the skin (Fig. 119) which become macular and finally confluent. Resistance to infection is lost. The spleen and liver become greatly enlarged and lymphadenopathy of peripheral and deep nodes usually becomes prominent. Until relatively recently all cases terminated fatally, usually within one to three months. In 1940, Glanzman[14] suggested that Letterer-Siwe disease is a fulminant variety of Hand-Schüller-Christian disease, and in 1941 Farber[15] expressed his belief that these two conditions and eosinophilic granuloma are all different manifestations of the same disease process. Since the last named is a granuloma and was thought at that time to

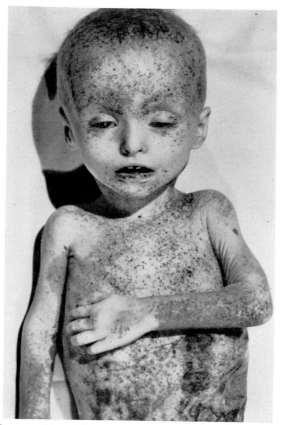

FIG. 119.   Letterer-Siwe disease. Replacement of bone marrow induces a mye-lophthisic anemia and bleeding phenomena. Petechial and macular hemorrhages are highly characteristic findings.

be of probable infectious origin, massive doses of antibiotics were given in a few cases diagnosed as Letterer-Siwe disease with survival.

Today, the etiology of Letterer-Siwe disease remains unknown and the question of correct diagnosis must of necessity arise in any cases which survive. Most observers believe that the disturbance represents an incapacity of the reticulum apparatus to process certain lipids, of which cholesterol and its esters appear to predominate.

ROENTGENOGRAPHIC MANIFESTATIONS

The radiographic manifestations of Hand-Schüller-Christian disease, eosinophilic granuloma and Letterer-Siwe disease will be considered together. The osseous lesions of all are secondary to granulomatous proliferation of the intraosseous reticulum and its derivatives, and radiographically have similar patterns. Radiographs

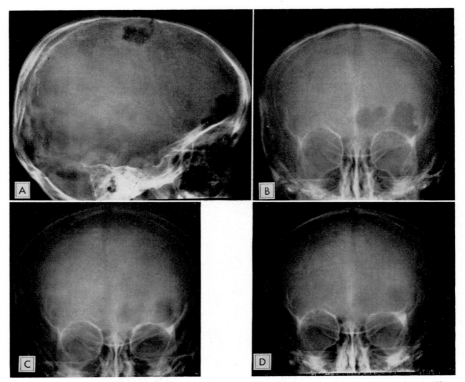

FIG. 120.   Multiple lesions of the cranial bones secondary to Hand-Schüller-Christian disease in a 5-year-old white male. Exophthalmos on the left was the presenting complaint. *A* and *B* represent the initial radiographs; *C*, a radiograph six months later and *D*, a radiograph exposed twelve months after the original examination. The initial lesions have sharply defined, although irregular, margins. Three large defects are evident, probably the result of confluence of multiple smaller ones. Healing, as shown in *C*, is manifest by an indistinctness of the borders of the lesions and a diminution in their size. In *D*, healing has progressed even further and the medial of the two defects is barely visible.

may reveal hepatosplenomegaly and pulmonary infiltrates which are the result of systemic reticulum involvement.

A sharply defined radiolucent defect is the characteristic bony lesion. It is round or oval with no surrounding sclerosis and may be described as "punched out." The defect represents a granuloma which has destroyed bone and is of the density of soft tissue. There is no bony reaction to the destructive process. Flat bones are more frequently involved than cylindrical bones.

Cranial bones are probably the most commonly affected and often small lesions will enlarge and coalesce to form a large irregular defect. Periosteal new bone is not a feature of the cranial lesions, and both inner and outer tables may be destroyed.

The area of destruction in a cylindrical bone initially involves

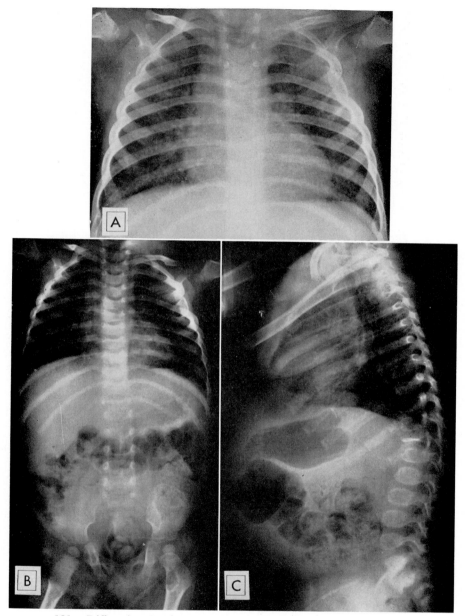

FIG. 121.   Diffuse involvement of the reticuloendothelial system in a white male, aged fifteen months. The skin was involved as were numerous lymph nodes, the liver and spleen. The disease was fatal. The histologic findings were compatible with Letterer-Siwe disease, as were the clinical and radiographic manifestations. *A* illustrates miliary-like involvement of the lungs which may simulate tuberculosis. Such involvement may also be seen in Hand-Schüller-Christian disease and eosinophilic granuloma. *B* and *C* show deformity of the twelfth dorsal vertebra as well as lesions of the proximal left femur, the right pubic bone and the fourth left rib. The peculiar vertebral deformity may be seen as an isolated lesion and may be the result of an eosinophilic granuloma. Note the preservation of the intervertebral disc spaces, above and below the involved vertebral body.

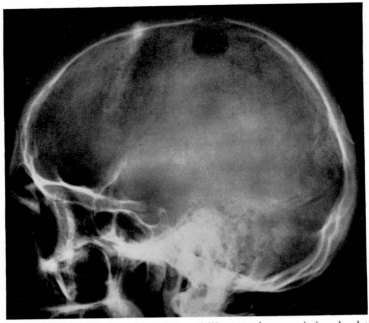

FIG. 122.   The solitary lesion of eosinophilic granuloma as it involved the skull of a 22-year-old white male. A soft tissue mass was present over the defect in the parietal bone. The lesion is punched out but does present a sequestrum in its center. This latter is an unusual finding, but has been documented in the literature. There is no sclerosis about the round radiolucent defect.

the medullary canal in most instances. As it enlarges, the inner aspect of the cortex may be eroded and periosteal new bone may result if the erosion progresses. Periosteal new bone is evident if fracture occurs through a lesion.

When a vertebral body is affected, it loses stature. It may present as a thin dense plate. The intervertebral disc spaces above and below maintain their normal width. Such an affected vertebra, when seen as an isolated lesion, should be considered as being due to eosinophilic granuloma until proven otherwise.

Healing of the osseous lesions starts at the periphery of the defect and proceeds centrally. The margins become indistinct and somewhat dense, and gradually the lesion fills in with new bone. There are no residual manifestations in the majority of instances.

It must be recognized that the osseous defect is not an empty space but is occupied by a soft tissue mass. This mass of tissue causes secondary effect such as exophthalmos when bones of the orbit are involved. Mandibular involvement may destroy tooth sockets and be responsible for the extrusion of teeth. Mastoiditis may be suspected when the temporal bone is involved. In few diseases is the correlation of all data so important for the establishment of a diagnosis.

MICROSCOPY

Knowledge of the cytologic aspects of this disease has come from needle aspiration biopsies of the bone marrow and spleen and from several thorough necropsy studies.[16]

The bone marrow (Fig. 123) is almost completely replaced by a proliferation of the reticulum and its derivatives. This proliferation so packs the medullary regions that it may cause a diffuse demineralization and thinning of the cortex. At the ends of cylindrical bones where hematopoietic tissue predominates the deossification may be so accentuated as to resemble tumor. The sections are composed largely of young histiocytes. In some cases lipid material was searched for and not found and this led to the term "non-lipid histiocytosis." In most instances, however, the lipid, though not as obvious as in Hand-Schüller-Christian disease, is quite apparent and its presence can be surmised even with hematoxylin-eosin technique.

The same type of cell dominates the sections of spleen, lymph nodes and liver (Figs. 124 and 125). In the first, large areas of necrosis and hemorrhage are apt to occur because of interference with the blood supply. There may be myeloid metaplasia and occasional megakaryocytes occur. Unless the pathologist maintains a high index

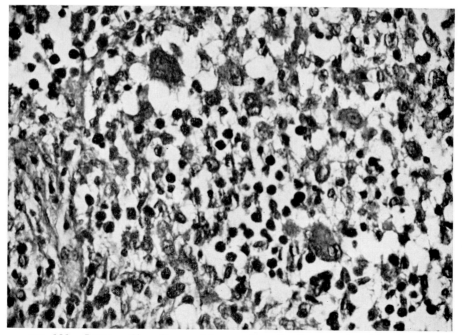

FIG. 123.   Letterer-Siwe disease. Marrow tissue has been replaced by a proliferation of reticulum. Note the large cells, some of them with multiple nuclei, and the lymphocytes which infiltrate the lesion. (× 450.)

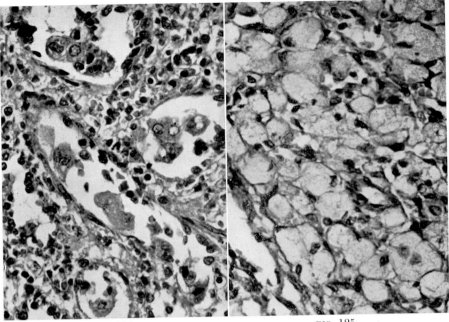

FIG. 124.   FIG. 125.

FIGS. 124 and 125.   Letterer-Siwe Disease.

FIG. 124.   A section from the spleen reveals numerous lipid-filled macrophages within the sinusoids. ($\times$ 450.)

FIG. 125.   Section taken from a lymph node. The fibrous trabeculae are infiltrated with lipid-filled macrophages. ($\times$ 450.)

of suspicion for the lipid reticuloendothelioses the sections may be misinterpreted as atypical leukemia. If the clinical aspects of the case are known the diagnosis should be apparent.

PROGNOSIS

Typical Letterer-Siwe disease always occurs in infants, usually under one year of age. The originally reported cases all terminated fatally within a period of a few weeks or months. More recently some cases, treated with massive doses of antibiotics or cancerocidal chemotherapy or both, have survived. A few have developed a clinical picture not unlike that of Hand-Schüller-Christian disease. It is still unproven that either of the above agents has been curative since the doubt must always arise in the unautopsied case as to whether it was true Letterer-Siwe disease. If it can be shown that the antibiotics will cure a reasonable proportion of the cases, this would be strong evidence for an infectious agent as the cause of the three related cholesterol reticuloendothelioses. On the other hand, if nitrogen mustard or another of the cancer chemotherapeutic agents can be shown to benefit Letterer-Siwe disease it would suggest that this is the malignant neoplastic form of a granulomatous process, something akin to the sarcomatous and granulomatous forms of Hodgkin's disease.

GAUCHER'S DISEASE

Cerebroside reticulocytosis, usually called "Gaucher's disease," is a disturbance in which there is an excessive production of histiocytes, most of which become filled with a complex lipid, a cerebroside known as kerasin. Aggregates of these cells accumulate in the spleen, liver, bone marrow and skin. Symptoms are referable to enlargement of the spleen and liver, interference with marrow function and destruction of bone.

The disease was described in the French literature by Gaucher in 1882. Since then the condition has been extensively discussed by Pick[17] and others. It is stated that there are two forms, an infantile variety which runs a fulminant course and is fatal within eighteen months and a more chronic form, the initial symptoms of which may appear at any period of life though usually before the age of forty. Clinically, the two types are completely different since in the infantile variety the brain is prominently involved and, therefore, the course is much like that of Niemann-Pick disease. Indeed, it is usually impossible, apparently, to distinguish the two except by chemical analysis of the involved tissues. Since in the fulminant, infantile types of lipid reticuloendothelioses a variety of complex lipids are usually involved one might question whether, on the basis of the few analyses which have been done in these rare cases, a separate entity—acute, infantile Gaucher's disease—actually exists.

The usual form of the disease begins insidiously. The older literature states that Gaucher's disease usually begins during the first decade but more recent reports[18] describe the onset of symptoms occurring quite equally scattered along the first half of the life span. This discrepancy may arise from the possibility that incipient cases are frequently discovered today in the older age group by more efficient diagnostic tools such as x-ray and liver and spleen puncture.

A familial and hereditary incidence is found in approximately one third of the cases. There appears to be a somewhat higher incidence in the Jewish race though about half are found among the Caucasian groups in the United States. The most common site of involvement causing symptoms is the spleen, though if the bone marrow is carefully searched the characteristic tissue changes will be found in possibly every case.

The spleen may reveal a very moderate enlargement for many years. In most cases it eventually becomes huge and may fill practically the entire abdominal cavity. The small spleens are symptomless but, as they enlarge, they give rise to pain and a sense of dragging discomfort. These symptoms in themselves may necessitate splenectomy.

Enlargement of the liver in Gaucher's disease does not usually give rise to symptoms though in a few cases mildly altered liver function tests have been recorded.

Changes in the skin and conjunctivae will be noted in a high percentage of the cases if they are looked for. Irregular, poorly delineated, light tan areas appear in the skin of the exposed parts. It is uncertain what causes this pigmentation though it is assumed that the color is due to excessive lipochrome pigment within the reticulum elements of the corium. Brownish tan pingueculae may appear in the sclerae. These lesions have led some authors to classify Gaucher's disease with the idiopathic xanthomatoses, unjustifiably since the offending lipid of the xanthoma is cholesterol.

Symptoms of bone marrow involvement are usual though they may not appear until the disease is well advanced. These findings arise from a marrow depression due to replacement of hematopoietic tissue. All three elements are involved. The anemia is of the hypochromic type and is usually not more than moderately severe. The fall in erythrocyte count is usually accompanied by a leukopenia. A thrombocytopenia may be suspected in a high percentage of patients who complain of ecchymoses on mild trauma. The blood picture is apt to return toward normal, at least for a considerable period, following splenectomy. The lymph nodes are usually not prominently involved until the late stages of the disease and then often only the deep nodes become enlarged.

The changes in the skeleton are usually found by a roentgenographic skeletal survey, done only after the diagnosis is suspected because of an enlarged spleen or a depressed marrow function. Since it is the marrow reticulum which is involved any bone bearing hematopoietic tissue may be affected; thus, depending upon the age, any or all bones may show the lesions. A particularly high incidence has been reported in the femurs, the vertebrae, ribs, sternum and flat bones of the pelvis. It is said that the cylindrical bones of the lower extremity are involved more often than those of the arms. Masses of lipid-bearing macrophages may pack the intramedullary spaces causing erosion of the cortices from the inside. Since the process is very slow, appositional bone is laid down on the outer cortical surfaces of the involved areas and thus an "expansile" lesion is produced at the ends of long, cylindrical bones, particularly at the lower ends of the femurs. The process does not involve cartilage so that the epiphyses are spared except by extension from nearby centers of hematopoiesis. When this occurs there may be collapse of the head not unlike that of epiphyseal osteochondritis. This may lead to symptoms of arthritis and severe disability. The cortices may be so extensively eroded and weakened that pathologic fractures result. Compression fractures of the vertebrae are relatively common in the advanced stage of the disease. Fractures of the ribs and long bones of the extremities are also reported.

The focal lesions develop so slowly that, like enchondromas, they usually do not cause bone pain. Occasionally pain is the presenting symptom but it is probable that in these cases there has been infraction or the joint is affected.

The blood chemistry reveals no alterations of diagnostic significance.

Several analyses have been done of the lipid material which appears to be the offending agent in Gaucher's disease. All are in accord that the lipid in greatest abundance is a cerebroside, i.e., a lipid linked carbohydrate with nitrogen. Here agreement ends. The carbohydrate of normal kerasin is galactose. Some chemists have isolated galactose, others glucose, and still others a combination of both. Phospholipids and cholesterol in smaller amounts have also been found. It has been suggested that there may be two types of Gaucher's disease, one with a cerebroside containing galactose and the other with glucose. Since, as yet, there is no evidence that the clinical course is influenced by the chemistry of the lipid at fault, it is probably wiser to accept the concept that Gaucher's disease is a disturbance resulting in the inability of the reticulum and its motile derivatives to process certain carbohydrate-linked lipids. Because a variety of cerebrosides are found, along with other lipids, in an acute process of infancy, a disease which is quite different clinically from Gaucher's disease, this does not necessarily make it belong to this group.

GROSS PATHOLOGY

The spleen may enlarge to a huge mass weighing as much as 5000 grams. The consistency usually remains about normal or somewhat softened. The capsular surface of the large spleens usually shows areas of necrosis or hyalinized scars of healed necrotic portions. Throughout the parenchyma one usually finds mottled areas of pale yellow or gray, often intermixed with areas of necrosis and hemorrhage. The latter resemble irregular infarcts.

The enlarged liver may or may not reveal the aggregates of lipid material to the naked eye. Small pale areas against a red background may be identified in the bone marrow. These may coalesce to form large patches and streaks of obviously abnormal tissue.

ROENTGENOGRAPHIC MANIFESTATIONS

When abnormal reticulum cells accumulate in marrow the osseous lesions of bone destruction may become evident radiographically. The proliferation of Gaucher cells may involve the marrow cavity of one or more bones either in a diffuse or localized manner. In either instance the lesions are predominantly radiolucent, although some observers feel that sclerosis about the lesions is common, the result of the formation of new bone. Any bone may be affected, but involvement of cranial bones and those of the hands and feet is rare.

Diffuse involvement of the marrow cavity results in a wide medullary canal, a thin cortex and sparse trabeculae. Femoral involvement is usually of this type and expansion of the distal diaphysis is common (Erlenmeyer flask deformity). Localized radiolucent defects may occur in any portion of a bone and pathologic fracture of weight-bearing

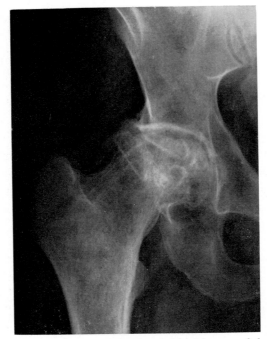

FIG. 126.   Gaucher's disease involving bone. Involvement of the femoral head has resulted in destruction with deformity that may be confused with osteoarthritis. In the child, involvement of the femoral capital epiphysis will mimic aseptic necrosis. Note the radiolucent areas with irregular sclerosis about them.

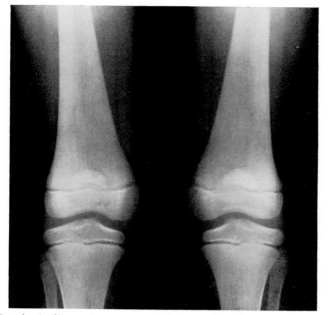

FIG. 127.   Gaucher's disease in a young girl as manifest by wide distal femora, thin trabeculae and narrow cortices.

bones so involved, particularly the femurs, and vertebrae is not uncommon. Epiphyseal destruction will cause growth disturbance.

The radiographic manifestations of Gaucher's disease may, therefore, present great variability, depending on the extent of osseous involvement, the speed with which the process progresses and the effects of bone destruction. Pulmonary infiltrates have been reported and splenomegaly may be recognized.

MICROSCOPY

The diagnosis of Gaucher's disease may be made by aspiration biopsy of the bone marrow, the spleen or the liver. A careful search of the smears from the marrow may be necessary but usually the pathognomonic cells will be found.

These cells are motile reticulum derivatives. They are often huge, measuring up to 50 to 75 microns. The substance of the cytoplasm is pale with the hematoxylin-eosin technique. It may have a crackle-glaze or crushed tissue paper appearance. These have been called "foam cells." The appearance is due to the presence of the kerasin which has accumulated within the cytoplasm. The nucleus is somewhat smaller and more heavily stained than that of the normal macrophage or histiocyte. This pyknosis is probably due to the altered intracellular metabolism. The nuclei may be multiple.

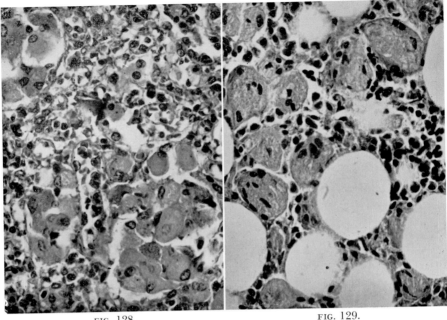

FIG. 128.   FIG. 129.

FIGS. 128 and 129.   Gaucher's disease

FIG. 128.   In the spleen one may find the sinusoids filled with lipid-containing macrophages (Gaucher's cells). It is this accumulation which causes splenomegaly. (× 450.)

FIG. 129.   Large lipid-filled macrophages can be identified between the normal fat cells (the circular clear spaces) in the bone marrow. (× 450.)

The foam cells may occur singly though they are usually found in aggregates which may coalesce into huge sheets. In this event their appearance is monotonously similar. In the spleen (Fig. 128) they are found in the spongiosa between and often compressing the follicles. In the liver they infiltrate the portal areas and in the intramedullary regions they replace the marrow (Fig. 129).

PROGNOSIS

The prognosis of the chronic form of Gaucher's disease is less grave than any of the other types of idiopathic lipid reticuloendotheliosis with the exception of eosinophilic granuloma or some cases of xanthomatosis. The earlier the symptoms appear the more extensive the disease is apt to be, and the patient may succumb after a period of years because of the interference with marrow function. Splenectomy should alleviate these symptoms. It has been said that splenectomy increases the rate of bone involvement. When the reports

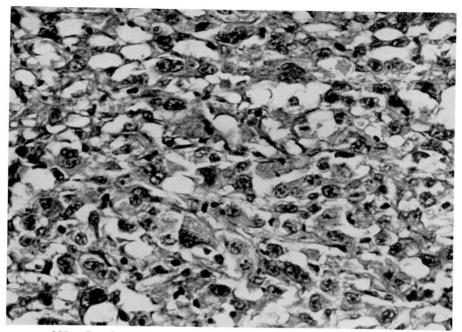

FIG. 130.   Gaucher's disease. In this unusual case the terminal phase of the disease behaved as a reticulum cell sarcoma. The section is composed of tumor reticulum cells. ($\times$ 450.)

of large numbers of cases are reviewed this does not appear to be true. Most patients, properly treated, lead a comfortable and uncurtailed life.

The author has seen one patient in whom, after a number of years of Gaucher's disease, a sarcoma apparently of reticulum cell origin (Fig. 130) arose in the involved areas and rapidly metastasized, killing the patient. This event must be exceedingly rare since no account of a similar behavior can be found in the published reports.

NIEMANN-PICK DISEASE

Niemann-Pick disease is a disturbance in which abnormal quantities of the phospholipids and cholesterol are deposited in most of the mesenchymally derived tissues of the body and some of epithelial derivation. A brief account is given here only because the marrow is involved and because of the relation of this disease to the other lipoid reticuloendothelioses.

The condition is rare. Members of the Jewish race are affected in about half the cases. Parental consanguinity has been noted in several of the cases in Gentiles. The disease practically always occurs in infants of less than eighteen months of age though three cases of a very similar nature have been reported in adults. The disease is probably always fatal, usually within a year of onset.

The reticulum of the spleen, liver and lymph nodes is most dramatically involved though deposits of lipid-bearing macrophages have been found in most other tissues. The cause of the disease is unknown though there is a strong familial incidence. Several siblings may be affected and in some series the adult blood relatives have shown non-symptomatic enlargement of the spleen and liver.

Both fixed and motile phagocytic cells become engorged with a variety of lipids of which sphingomyelin predominates. These deposits of phosphosphingosides cause the remarkable enlargement of all the normal reticulum stations and typical cells have been found in the circulating blood. Marrow involvement eventually causes a hypochromic anemia. The serum neutral fat, cholesterol and phospholipid may be elevated.

Niemann-Pick disease is frequently associated with amaurotic familial idiocy (Tay-Sachs disease). It was originally thought that the cerebral involvement was merely an extension of the generalized process but analysis of the brains of some cases has shown a predominance of lecithin rather than sphingomyelin in the nerve tissue. When the brain is involved the cherry-red macula and mental deterioration are to be expected. It is probable that the difference in the predominating phospholipid in the systemic tissues and the brain is due to native metabolic variation in the cells involved, since it seems highly unlikely that two such rare entities would occur in the same patient if their mechanisms were distinctly different.

Abnormal pigmentation has been noted at the normal sites of lipochrome pigment and a brownish discoloration has been described in the skin of the extensor surfaces of the joints.

The cells which store the involved lipid become swollen to many times their normal size, ranging from 20 to 60 microns. The material is seen within the cytoplasm with the Lorrain Smith and Weigert techniques and by routine methods the cells have a foamy appearance. The striations which characterize the "foam cells" of Gaucher's cells are not seen and the Niemann-Pick cells are more finely vacuolated.

The reticulum of the bone marrow is probably always involved and the diagnosis may be corroborated by marrow aspiration. Since the disease is of relatively short duration, the bone itself may not be affected. In some cases a diffuse halisteresis has been noted and in at least one reported case there was said to be delay in the development of the ossification centers.

LIPOCHONDRODYSTROPHY

Lipochondrodystrophy (Hurler's disease, gargoylism) was recognized at least as early as 1916, but was not fully described until Hurler's report[19] in 1919. She recognized it as a hereditary disease and supposed it to be a primary skeletal growth disturbance.

Classically, the disease begins in early childhood causing skeletal deformity, failure of mental development, blindness and enlargement of the liver and spleen.

The disease is rare, there being less than one hundred cases reported. The first symptoms may be noted soon after birth and it is entirely probable that in most instances the disease begins in utero. The condition is probably hereditary of the recessive type and if all cases in the literature are true lipochondrodystrophy it may be familial. In one family apparently only males were involved, suggesting dependence upon a sex-linked recessive gene.

Ellis, Sheldon and Capon[20] coined the term "gargoylism" because of the strikingly repulsive appearance and the fancied resemblance to the well known architectural device. The condition progresses through early childhood but, since it is not incompatible with life, the patient may live to middle age.

The peculiar facies may be noted soon after birth. The head may be large, the forehead low and covered with fine hair, the nasal bridge sunken, the nostrils flared. The interocular distance is increased, the ears set low and far back on the head. The distance between the posterior margins of the mandibles may be increased to cause a widening of the lower portion of the face. The tongue is large and thick. Frequently the metopic suture line between the frontal bones is prominently ridged. The teeth are widely separated and poorly formed. The neck is short. The belly is protuberant because of an enlarged liver and spleen and the intra-abdominal pressure may result in umbilical and inguinal hernias (Fig. 131). Peripheral lymph nodes may be enlarged. A dorsolumbar kyphosis usually appears early. The hands show a trident deformity.

Retardation of sitting, standing, talking and walking is noted in time and some time within the first to third year the cornea begins to show clouding. At first there may be no impairment of vision but as the clouding increases there is progressive loss of sight.

Mental retardation should be noted early if looked for, and usually development progresses no further than the stage of idiocy.

After six months the disturbances in skeletal growth become more and more apparent. There is failure to attain normal stature with resultant dwarfism. The poorly formed, narrow vertebral bodies and

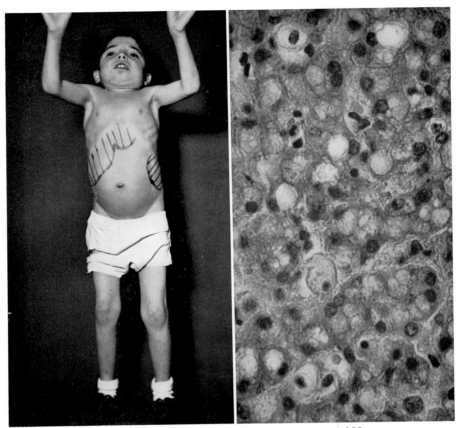

FIG. 131.   FIG. 132.

FIGS. 131 and 132.   Lipochondrodystrophy

FIG. 131.   The liver and spleen margins have been outlined on the skin. There are an umbilical hernia and an enlargement of cervical lymph nodes.

FIG. 132.   The offending material, whatever its chemical nature, accumulates in both mesenchymal and epithelial tissue. In the liver it replaces the cytoplasm of the hepatic cells. ($\times$ 450.)

kyphosis cause collapse of the trunk. Flaccidness of joints has been reported but usually there is extension disability. The arms may not be lifted above shoulder level nor the forearm completely extended. There is often a flexion deformity at the hips and knees.

ROENTGENOGRAPHIC MANIFESTATIONS

The skeletal changes in lipochondrodystrophy (gargoylism) vary from those of a mild degree to marked severity; they may develop slowly, requiring a considerable period of time. In the typical case, generalized skeletal changes are evident early in life and are of diagnostic significance. Lesions other than osseous ones are sometimes evident radiographically, such as hepatosplenomegaly and umbilical hernia.

The cranial vault is characteristically enlarged in its anterior-posterior dimension and the bones are often thick and dense. In many instances, the sella is shallow and elongated anteriorly beneath the anterior clinoids. The nasopharynx tends to be small and obstructed by lymphoid tissue.

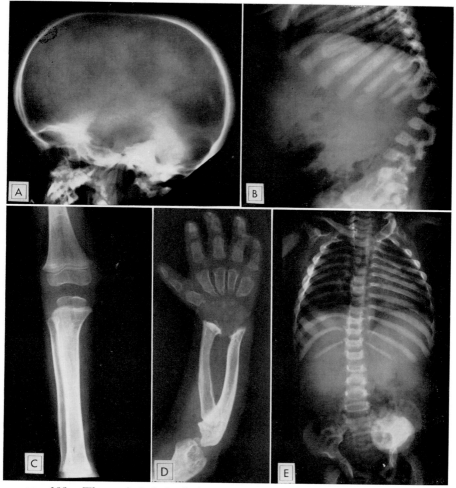

FIG. 133. The typical skeletal changes in gargoylism. The lateral projection of the skull (*A*) shows the increase in the anteroposterior diameter, the thickness of the cranial bones and the elongation of the sella turcica. The small size of the nasopharynx may be appreciated. A gibbus with vertebral deformity is evident in *B*. Proximal pointing of the metacarpals and the angulation and deformity of the distal radius and ulna are evident in *D*. Contrast the relative lack of abnormality of the bones of the lower extremity (*C*) with the deformed, short and thick bones of the forearm (*D*). The pelvis, proximal femora, ribs and clavicles are to be noted in *E*. The round, somewhat dense shadow overlying the left ilium represents a large umbilical hernia.

The broad ribs narrow at their vertebral ends and are blunt anteriorly. The clavicles are short and thick. There is a characteristic gibbus at the low dorsal or high lumbar region occasioned by deformity of one or more vertebras. The affected vertebral bodies are hypoplastic, have an anterior inferior beak and are displaced posteriorly. The intervertebral disc spaces are maintained.

The bones of the upper extremity are more abnormal than those of the lower extremity. The medullary canals are widened and the epiphyseal centers are flat and often irregular. The humerus is short and thick, bulges in its mid-portion and may taper toward its distal end. The radius and ulna too are short and thick and taper distally where the articular surfaces face one another. The metacarpals tend to be narrow proximally and the phalanges are short and broad. The bones of the feet show changes similar to those of the hand. The bones of the lower extremity are not affected as to length but valgus deformity of the femurs is common. The acetabula are shallow, the ilia flared and the ischia thick.

Gross irregularity of the growing ends of the long bones is not as marked as in achondroplasia and other osteochondrodystrophies. The radiographic manifestations of typical gargoylism are of importance in establishing the diagnosis but become meaningful when correlated with clinical and pathological data.

MICROSCOPY

Lipochondrodystrophy appears to be a storage disease. Very little tissue has been available for examination but in the past two decades all investigators have agreed that deposits of some alien substance are found in both parenchymal and mesenchymal tissues. The senior author had the rare opportunity of autopsying and studying one case,[21] an eight and one-half year old male. The heart was large, pale and firm and the mitral, aortic and tricuspid valves were sites of heavy, yellow-orange deposits with calcification. There was evidence of generalized cardiac insufficiency. The liver was immensely enlarged and greasy. There were splenomegaly and an enlarged brain. The cells of the anterior pituitary, the brain, the liver and the adrenal medulla contained globules of some unstained substance as did practically all the derivatives of mesenchyme including the cells of the peripheral blood (Fig. 132).

Dawson,[22] in a later report, expresses the belief that the substance found in the cerebral neurons is a combination of a mucopolysaccharide with a phosphatide and cerebroside which is insoluble in the usual fixatives. He believes the other cells contain a soluble muco-polysaccharide.

Zellweger[23] and co-workers have found coarse, deeply staining, violet granules in the neutrophils, lymphocytes and eosinophilic leuko-cytes of the peripheral blood stream with Wright's stain. They believe that this finding may be present in patients without clinical manifesta-tions of the disease and perhaps those who will later develop the disease in an abortive form.

Several authors have examined sections of epiphyseal tissue in cases of lipochondrodystrophy. Apparently some cases (as the author's) fail to show significant alterations in morphology, others reveal a lack of chondroblastic activity and presumably stasis of enchondral bone growth, and a third group has shown irregularity and distortion in the maturation zone and a transverse plate of bone across the metaphysis.

From the material presently at hand it may be that lipochondro-dystrophy is not a primary disturbance in enchondral bone growth. Rather, the skeletal distortion is probably the result of interference in normal function of mesenchymal derivatives secondary to an in-ability to metabolize certain substances, perhaps a mucopolysaccharide. Another possibility which comes readily to mind is that the infiltra-tion of endocrine glands, particularly the anterior lobe of the pituitary, so perverts their function that necessary hormones are unavailable for normal bone formation. A superficial resemblance to cretinism supports this hypothesis.

Because of the very close similarity, both clinically and radio-logically, of lipochondrodystrophy to Morquio's disease, the two condi-tions have been confused in some reports. Abnormal storage substance has not been reported in bona fide cases of the latter and if the former is a storage disease, as it now appears to be, this confusion should be eliminated in the future.

PROGNOSIS

The victims of Hurler's disease may die in childhood or they may live well into adult life, but the appalling skeletal deformity, the mental deficiency and blindness make them helpless and hopeless members of society.

REFERENCES

HAND-SCHÜLLER-CHRISTIAN DISEASE

1. Hand, A.: Transactions of the Philadelphia Pathological Society, *16*:1891–1893.
2. Hand, A.: Pennsylvania M. J., *9*:520; 1905–1906.
3. Christian, H. A.: Contributions to Medical and Biological Research. Paul B Hoeber, vol. 1:390; 1919.

4. Rowland, R. S.: Arch. Int. Med., *42:*611; 1928.
5. Farber, S.: Am. J. Path., *17:*625; 1941.

EOSINOPHILIC GRANULOMA

6. Otani, S., and Ehrlich, J. C.: Am. J. Path., *16:*479; 1940.
7. Lichtenstein, L., and Jaffe, H. L.: Am. J. Path., *16:*595; 1940.
8. Farber, S., Green, W., and McDermott, L. J.: Am. J. Path., *17:*625; 1941.
9. Green, W., Farber, S., and McDermott, L. J.: J. Bone & Joint Surg., *24:*499; 1942.
10. Compere, E., Johnson, W., and Coventry, B.: J. Bone & Joint Surg., *36A:*969; 1954.
11. Childers, J., Middleton, J. W., and Schneider, M.: Ann. Int. Med., *42:*1287; 1955.
11a. Wilson, R. G., Minteer, D. M., and Hayes, J. D.: Am. J. Roentgenol., *69:*936; 1953.
11b. Avery, M. E., McAfee, J. G., and Guild, H.: Am. J. Med. *22:*636; 1957.

LETTERER-SIWE DISEASE

12. Letterer, E.: Frankfurt. Ztschr. f. Path., *30:*377; 1924.
13. Siwe, S.: Ztschr. f. Kinderh., *55:*212; 1933.
14. Glanzman, E.: Ann. Paediat., *155:*1; 1940.
15. Farber, S., Green, W., and McDermott, L. J.: Am. J. Path., *17:*625; 1941.
16. Levinsky, W.: Arch. Path., *48:*462; 1949.

GAUCHER'S DISEASE

17. Pick, L.: Med. Klin., *18:*1408; 1922.
18. Medford, A. S., and Bayrd, E. D.: Ann. Int. Med., *40:*481; 1954.

LIPOCHONDRODYSTROPHY

19. Hurler, G.: Ztschr. f. Kinderh., *24:*220; 1919.
20. Ellis, R. W. B., Sheldon, W., and Capon, N. B.: Quart. J. Med., *29:*119; 1936.
21. Kressler, R. J., and Aegerter, E. E.: J. Pediat., *12:*579; 1938.
22. Dawson, I. M.: J. Path. & Bact., *67:*587; 1954.
23. Zellweger, H., Giaciai, L., and Fuzli, S.: Am. J. Dis. Child., *84:*421; 1952.

10

Disturbances in Vitamin Metabolism

RICKETS

Rickets is a disturbance in the formation of bone in the growing skeleton caused by a failure of deposition of bone salts within the organic matrix of cartilage and bone. This failure is the consequence of an inadequate supply of calcium or phosphorus ions or both in the fluid which perfuses the matrix tissue. The inadequacy is due to a deficiency in the dietary intake or to a failure of adequate absorption through the gut wall. In an attempt to maintain a normal serum calcium level, salts may be withdrawn from the portions of bone which were mineralized before the onset of the disease with resultant softening of the previously normal skeleton. The ability to produce hyalin and osteoid organic matrix is retained. The effects of the disturbance are manifested in the growing skeleton and so do not pertain to bones after their secondary ossification centers have closed, though the distortions resulting from defective enchondral bone mineralization and secondary bone softening may persist for the life of the parts involved.

The earliest reports of a condition which can be indubitably identified as rickets come from England in the seventeenth century. It is almost certain that rickets must have existed among the ancients, but it may not have been common or severe enough to arouse general concern. Since most rickets results from insufficient vitamin D to maintain normal calcium absorption and since vitamin D is synthesized in vivo by the action of sunlight on the cholesterol supplies of the skin, it may be presumed that the geography of civilization played an important role in the incidence of the disease. The regions around the

Mediterranean owe a considerable part of their enviable climatic reputation to the quantity and quality of their sunshine. England and especially Scotland are not so fortunate in this respect. There, where fog and industrial smoke filter out most of the sunlight, and where cold and the niceties of civilization necessitate a covering of the body surfaces, there is too little naturally synthesized vitamin D to prevent the condition.

Since the work of Mellanby[1] and Park[2] the civilized world has learned that it is possible to prevent rickets even among its poorer populations. In lieu of sunshine, fish liver oils and the more accurately controlled synthetic preparations supply the necessary vitamin D. Both calcium and phosphorus are fairly ubiquitous minerals in most populations because of their high content in milk and dairy products. Consequently, the incidence of symptomatic rickets has diminished in most areas until now it is difficult to obtain adequate material for teaching purposes. Only in unenlightened areas, starvation populations and races and cults with dietary eccentricities does the fully advanced disease occur in numbers.

Most rickets today is caused by an inadequate intake of vitamin D in infancy and early childhood. Dietary calcium, normal in amount, is excreted in the feces because of failure of absorption. It is quite unusual for the infant diet to be deficient in either calcium or phosphorus. Rarely severe fibrocystic disease of the pancreas and more often idiopathic steatorrhea (celiac disease), because of the disturbance in fat metabolism at the intestinal level, may interfere with calcium absorption. This result is probably largely due to incomplete vitamin D utilization since it is a fat-soluble vitamin. The presence of excessive fatty acids which may combine with calcium to form non-absorbable soaps and the resultant diarrhea which does not allow sufficient time for mineral absorption may play some part in the diminished absorption of calcium. It is probable that all three mechanisms combine in this type of rickets.

Since active rickets is manifested only in the growing skeleton, its most obvious expression is seen in the period of most active growth, between six months and three years, though its effect may be encountered earlier and the less florid late rickets may manifest itself in the prepubertal years.

In infancy, the brain is the most rapidly growing organ of the body and the bones which surround it must keep pace. The enlargement of the cerebral cavity is accomplished by the intramembranous apposition of osteoid along the flat-bone edges within the fibrous sutures. The molding is the result of osteolysis of the inner table in areas which result in a flattening of the curve and apposition on the outer table to maintain thickness. Since in rickets osteoid production is not impaired and osteolysis continues until the bone surface is covered with a more resistant but unmineralized and, therefore, soft osteoid, the calvarium enlarges, but it is thin and more pliable, the outer contours expressing more intimately the shape of the brain. When to this conformation there is added the external osteoid apposition in areas of normal bone growth together with the lag in antero-posterior growth at the base, the frontal areas become prominent and box-like. This frontal bossing and thinning are called craniotabes.

The softening of the normally mineralized vertebral bodies allows the intervertebral discs to expand and the stress of weight-bearing results in further compression so that the spine becomes twisted and bent. The lumbar spine and sacrum telescope into the softened pelvis which must bear the weight of the trunk, head and upper extremities. The acetabular roofs are pushed upward and inward to further narrow the pelvic outlet. The resultant pelvic distortion, making parturition impossible, is one of the most serious consequences of the disease. The loss of rigidity of the weight-bearing long bones of the lower extremities leads to a characteristic bowing. If the progress of the disease is arrested before skeletal deformity due to softening is too far advanced, remodeling in the normal stress lines during uncomplicated skeletal growth will erase much of the distortion. But, if the effects of rickets are severe and if the disease is active even though slowed through childhood and adolescence, the abnormalities harden into permanent deformities.

In the areas of enchondral bone growth the inadequate mineral supply interferes with bone formation and conformation. Length growth is inhibited so that the bones fail to achieve normal stature. If there is an inadequate supply of mineral salts the band of provisional calcification in the epiphyseal plate cannot form. This interferes with cartilage cell maturation and utilization. The bars which make up the mineralized lattice of the metaphysis are not produced. Consequently, there is no scaffolding for the deposition of osteoid. Moreover, the tufts of metaphyseal granulation are not properly guided in their invasion of cartilage. The result is that their course is erratic and masses of cartilage cells which should have been used in the process of provisional calcification are isolated and overtaken by the advancing frontier of bone formation until they eventually come to lie deep within the metaphysis. The osteoblasts provoke osteoid formation as they are intended, but there is no preformed pattern to guide this process. Since the unmineralized osteoid remains flaccid, there can be no modeling due to normal stress stimuli. The useless osteoid

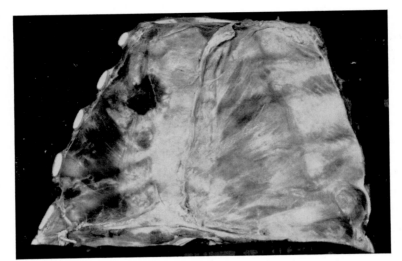

FIG. 134.   Rickets in a child. Plastron removed at autopsy. Internal surface. Along the right-hand side of the specimen one notes the prominent nodules at the costochondral junctions. This is the cause of the "rachitic rosary" which is often seen on the external surface.

piles up about islands of still viable cartilage cells and eventually fills the entire metaphyseal region.

It appears that mineralization of the layer of hyalin matrix which supports the columns of mature osteocytes, the line of provisional calcification, plays an important curbing function in cartilage cell proliferation. In rickets the formation of a provisional line of calcification cannot occur and the columnated cartilage cells behave as though a restraining influence had been removed. They proliferate and persist until large, irregular masses of cartilage widen the epiphyseal line and extend into the metaphysis, there to mingle with the patches of osteoid in an irregular, patternless aggregate.

The normal flaring of the diaphyseal ends cannot be reduced by the modeling process, perhaps because of a lack of rigidity or because of the abnormal deposits of cartilage and osteoid. Consequently, the ends of long bones reveal the graduated widening which has been so aptly called "trumpeting." This metaphyseal widening produces the enlarged joints which are so characteristically seen at the wrists, knees and ankles. It also produces a bulbous enlargement of the costochondral junctions and when marked this results in the "rachitic rosary." Sometimes this row of subcutaneous bumps will fail to appear on the external thoracic surface, but will be quite apparent on the pleural side of the plastron (Fig. 134). The negative intrathoracic pressure which sucks the sternum inward while the ribs are being raised in inhalation expansion may produce a deep, midline furrow down the anterior chest. The pull of the diaphragm along its line of attachment creates a second, coronal furrow with flaring of the lower thoracic margins called "Harrison's groove." These various deformities of the chest may persist throughout adult life and stamp the owner as a victim of rickets in his early childhood.

One would expect the serum calcium level to be below normal in the actively rachitic patient, since the disturbance here is in the dietary supply or more often the failure of absorption. As long as the parathyroid function remains intact, the inadequate extrinsic supply of calcium is compensated by the stored calcium in the skeleton. Thus the serum level is usually on the low side of normal even though the bones must be demineralized to maintain it. Examination of the parathyroid glands usually reveals a moderate secondary hyperplasia. The low calcium levels apparently stimulate the parathyroid glands to excessive secretion and their hormone affects the distal convoluted tubules of the kidney to inhibit reabsorption of the phosphorus which has passed the glomerular filters. Consequently, the serum phosphorus level is usually low. The sacrifice of the normally mineralized bone to this end causes excessive activity of the osteoblasts in an attempt to keep abreast of the eroding skeleton and so the alkaline phosphatase in the serum is apt to rise.

ROENTGENOGRAPHIC MANIFESTATIONS

Rickets, or osteomalacia, involving growing bone is manifest radiographically by alterations secondary to a deficiency of mineral salts associated with alterations in the maturation and proliferation of cartilage. The relationship of the radiographic changes to the altered physiology is best illustrated in the long bones. Although generalized osseous alterations occur, these are first and are most apparent at those sites where the growth of bone is most rapid, e.g., the wrists, knees and costochondral junctions.

The earliest radiographic sign is haziness of the zone of provisional calcification, which is soon followed by disappearance of this zone. This reflects the failure of deposition of mineral salts within the organic matrix of the degenerated cartilage cells. Failure of degeneration of the cells of the epiphyseal cartilage results in irregularities in the metaphysis and in the epiphyseal center; the changes in the latter site are less apparent, however, since the growth of bone is very slow in the epiphyseal center as compared with the metaphyseal zone. Failure of degeneration of cartilage cells results in an actual increase in the width of radiolucent cartilaginous matrix interposed between the epiphyseal center and the metaphysis, and on radiographs this zone is

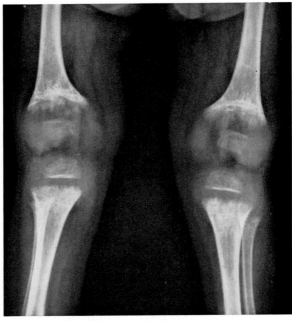

FIG. 135.   Rickets. The alterations are marked. The coarses trabeculae are evident and the zone of provisional calcification is absent. There is irregularity of the metaphyses, widening of these areas and an apparent increase in the distance between the epiphyseal centers and the metaphysis. Radiolucent streaks are visible in the cortices.

further increased in width as a result of failure of calcification of cartilaginous matrix as well as of osteoid tissue. Since the failure of degeneration is not complete along the line of ossification, but occurs in a patchy, irregular manner, any osteoid which is deposited is laid down along this irregular line of ossification in the metaphyseal zone. Attempts at ossification of the irregularly deposited osteoid enhance the irregularity of the metaphyseal region, which results in a radiographic appearance which has been compared to the bristles of a paint brush. Cupping of the ends of the bones probably results from mechanical effects acting upon the soft, non-mineralized osteoid tissue at the metaphysis which in addition resists modeling.

In the shaft, resorption of bone continues, possibly at a faster rate than is normal as a consequence of increased parathyroid activity. The smaller trabeculae may be completely devoid of mineral salts and blend with the soft tissue of the marrow cavity. The larger trabeculae appear prominent and are often arranged longitudinally. The cortex is deceptively thick. It is made up of poorly ossified osteoid and radiolucent streaks may be seen within it. This undermineralization of the cortex contributes to the ease with which the larger trabeculae

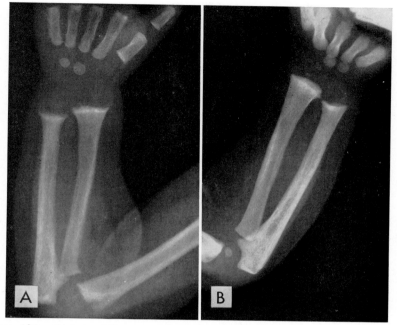

FIG. 136.   Rickets. *A* illustrates the early changes of rickets at the wrists. The zone of provisional calcification is hazy and irregular. Mild widening of the ends of the bones is evident. The cortex is not well defined and the trabecular pattern is coarse. After two months of therapy (*B*), the cortex is more dense as are the zones of provisional calcification. The epiphyseal center for the distal radius has appeared.

are seen radiographically and hence to the coarse trabecular pattern.

Greenstick fractures are common and the soft osteoid predisposes to bowing. Sharply defined, focal areas of decreased density may be seen traversing the shaft of the long bones. The origin of these "umbauzonen" has never been completely understood but their radiolucency is related to the fibrous tissue and osteoid present at these sites.

When healing of the rachitic process begins, the zone of provisional calcification appears at the site it would normally occupy if there had been no interference with mineralization. Later, the radiolucent metaphysis fills in with new bone. At this time, concavity of the ends of the bones may be most marked.

MICROSCOPY

The most characteristic microscopic picture is obtained by making a longitudinal section through the epiphyseal and metaphyseal areas of a long bone in the rachitic infant. The cartilage cells and their hyalin matrix deeply situated in the epiphyseal chondral plate are

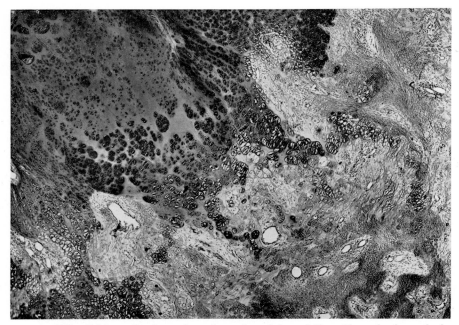

FIG. 137. Rickets. Section taken through epiphyseal line. Note the irregularity because of a lack of rigidity due to a failure of deposition of calcium salts. Stress probably causes the deformity. (× 28.)

normal in morphology and pattern. Maturation begins on schedule, but the cells, having obtained their normal component of glycogen and enzymatic potentialities, are not used so they persist while new cells are added at the top of the column. Depending upon the degree of calcium and phosphorus paucity, there is usually some attempt at mineralization of the hyalin in contact with the mature cells, but a continuous line of provisional calcification is not formed (Fig. 137). The persistence of unused chondrocytes which are pushed farther and farther into the metaphysis creates the impression that the fingers of vascularized granulation invade farther than normal into the chondral plate. The failure of the appearance of the calcified hyalin bars allows this granulation to progress along unguided routes so that the normal vertical pattern is destroyed and islands of cartilage cells drift into the metaphysis. The islands as well as fragments of imperfectly mineralized, primitive bone serve as foundations for the apposition of newly formed osteoid (Fig. 138). The latter also remains uncalcified so that there can be no alignment of lamellae and therefore no haversian system formation. In its full-blown state, there is no condition which exactly duplicates this picture. Several of the congenital disturbances of enchondral growth result in poor columnation, scaffolding formation and spicule production, but there is never an

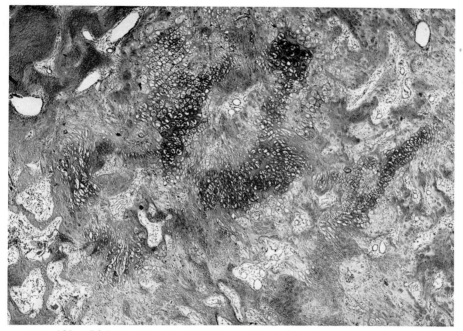

FIG. 138. Rickets. Islands of hyalin and cartilage cells are pushed into the metaphysis where they serve as nuclei for the deposition of osteoid. The latter remains unossified because of a lack of mineral salts. ($\times$ 30.)

excessive cartilage cell persistence plus abnormal amounts of osteoid without mineral deposition.

PROGNOSIS

The addition of an adequate amount of vitamin D to the diet is usually all that is required to halt the progress of the disease. In the rare instances in which this is not effective, the diet should be critically examined and the bowel habits and stools analyzed. In the case which obstinately persists, the fault will almost surely be found to be in the function of the kidney. These cases have been called refractory rickets.

VITAMIN D REFRACTORY RICKETS

In their monograph on the parathyroid glands and metabolic disease,[3] Albright and Reifenstein mention and give a follow-up on their originally published case (1937) of rickets which was resistant to ordinary doses of vitamin D but which responded to massive therapy. Since that time, numerous reports have appeared describing cases of severe rickets which can be controlled only by giving enormous doses of vitamin D. Since the symptoms, signs and bone changes are the same as those of ordinary rickets, it was almost inevitable that this condition should receive the name of vitamin D refractory rickets. It was assumed that the tissue threshold for vitamin D effect was higher in these patients than in the normal and indeed, since the several facets of vitamin D activity have not yet been certainly delineated, this cannot be denied. There is ample evidence to show that the main activity of this vitamin in physiologic amounts is the mediation of the absorption of calcium through the gut wall. Massive doses over a long period result in a generalized deossification of the skeleton and it has been assumed that its action is directly upon the bone, very similar to that of the parathyroid hormone. For some time it has been suspected that massive amounts of vitamin D also have a controlling action upon the kidney tubules. This suspicion has been strengthened by several recent reports[4] and though definitive evidence is still wanting, the available facts best fit this hypothesis.

In 1946 Albright and co-workers[5] published a paper concerning several cases of Milkman's syndrome and the mechanism by which this type of osteomalacia was produced. They believed that a decreased ability of the kidney tubules to form ammonia and excrete an acid urine created an expenditure of serum base calcium and produced a hypocalcemia. They noted the low serum phosphorus level and the abnormal amounts of phosphates in the urine and believed this to be due to a stimulation of the parathyroids by the low serum calcium level and a resultant phosphorus diuresis due to inhibition effect of excess parathormone upon phosphate reabsorption by the tubules.

Fanconi had already reported a condition in which abnormal quantities of numerous amino acids occur in the urine with normal or slightly elevated blood levels. These patients frequently have systemic acidosis. Albright proposed the same mechanism of serum base calcium expenditure in these cases.

Dent[6] in reviewing this work states that the kidney tubules may be incapable of reabsorbing a large number of substances from the glomerular filtrate, including phosphates, glucose, amino acids, water and potassium, singly or in combination. He groups six of these types, all of which show an abnormal reabsorption of phosphates, into three categories. In one group, there is defective phosphate and potassium reabsorption and, in addition, an inability to excrete acid urine and, in some, decreased ammonia formation. This is the group that Albright called "tubular insufficiency without glomerular insufficiency." It has since been known as the Albright-Butler syndrome. In another group there is defective phosphate, glucose and amino acid reabsorption. These types are known as the Fanconi syndrome or Debre-de Toni-

Fanconi syndrome. In the third group there is primarily an inability to reabsorb phosphates with abnormal phosphorus excretion. These cases fall in the classification which has been known as refractory rickets in children and Milkman's syndrome in adults.

In all groups, Dent believes it is essentially the phosphate loss by failure of tubule reabsorption which depletes the serum phosphorus, thus making unavailable a sufficient amount of phosphorus for mineralization of osteoid. The result in relation to the skeleton is the same as that in vitamin D deficient rickets.

In addition, he further states that massive doses of vitamin D cause phosphate retention, probably through stimulation of tubule reabsorption, and thereby alleviate the rickets. He emphasizes that this type of rickets is identical with vitamin D deficient rickets, but somewhat different from the rickets found in longstanding cases of nephritis, renal rickets. He would call the latter glomerular renal rickets and the other tubular renal rickets.

In rickets due to renal tubule disease, manifestations of the rachitic state appear early and the patient is apt to suffer from the disease for the remainder of his life, though progress appears to decrease after closure of the epiphyseal growth centers. Because of the long duration of the disease, the skeletal deformity is apt to be more severe than that found in ordinary rickets. The serum chemistry is characteristic of that of rickets, i.e., a low serum phosphorus, low normal serum calcium and an elevated serum alkaline phosphatase. Because the disease is present throughout the growth period, dwarfism is the usual result. This is most notable in the failure of length growth of the lower extremities. All the other deformities which characterize rickets are also seen.

Pedersen and McCarrol[7] reported 25 such cases and found involvement in 10 parents. They concluded that there is a strong hereditary and familial incidence. Since dwarfism is the outstanding feature of the disease and since these patients do not respond to average doses of vitamin D, it is possible, as they suggest, that numerous cases of refractory rickets are masked at present as congenital chondrodystrophic dwarfism. These cases may be diagnosed, when suspected, by blood chemical analysis and therapeutic trial. Doses of as high as one million units of vitamin D daily have been used though considerably smaller doses are usually effective.

ROENTGENOGRAPHIC MANIFESTATIONS

The radiographic manifestations of vitamin D refractory rickets are those of osteomalacia in a growing bone. The zone of provisional

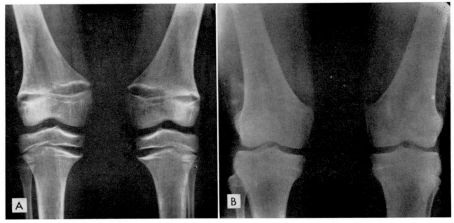

FIG. 139.   Vitamin D refractory rickets. The wide metaphyseal zones and coarse trabecular pattern are evident in *A* (age 10 years). At age 14 years (*B*), the epiphyses are seen to be uniting but the coarse trabeculae are apparent as well as the over-all radiolucency of the bony structures. This patient received large doses of vitamin D for many years.

calcification is indistinct and hazy and the metaphysis is widened. There is a coarse trabecular pattern and cortices that appear normal in thickness but within which radiolucent streaks may be seen. The alterations are most marked where bone growth is most rapid. Deformities of the long bones may be marked, particularly bowing.

MICROSCOPY

Sections through the metaphyseal areas of bones in refractory rickets are quite like those in vitamin D deficient rickets except that all the abnormal features are apt to be exaggerated. There is a failure of formation of the line of provisional calcification and a persistence of the unused mature cartilage cells. The latter form irregular masses deep in the metaphysis. Without hyalin mineralization there can be no normal lattice formation so that osteoid is laid down around anything in the metaphysis which will serve as a scaffolding. Irregular fields of unmineralized osteoid in patternless masses are the result. The lack of rigidity results in distortion of the epiphyseal line and the metaphyseal cortices. This is most notable in the areas of greatest stress, namely in the lower extremities.

PROGNOSIS

If cases of refractory rickets are properly treated, the deformities may be arrested. The minimum dosage of vitamin D to cause phosphate retention and roentgenographic healing must be calculated.

Toxicity may be avoided by carefully watching the serum calcium level and decreasing dosage when it rises above 11.5 mg. per 100 ml. Maintenance requires periodic blood chemical analysis. It is thought that the "refractory rickets–Milkman's syndrome" and the "Fanconi syndrome" groups are due to a genetic fault and tend to improve or recover early in adult life. The "Albright-Butler syndrome" groups are apparently caused by postnatal renal damage. The progress may be arrested by substituting a base ion such as sodium citrate for those in the blood, especially calcium, which are being dissipated. So treated, the basic defect remains but may be controlled in a state of health throughout life.

HYPERVITAMINOSIS D

Hypervitaminosis D is a clinical entity caused by an excessive intake of vitamin D, usually D_2, resulting in a high serum calcium level and eventual deossification of the skeleton. The latter occurs usually without symptoms, but the prolonged high serum calcium level produces (1) symptoms referable to its effect on peripheral nerves, muscles, both skeletal and visceral, and probably the brain, and (2) metastatic calcification of numerous tissues, particularly the kidneys.

The term "hypervitaminosis D" is probably inexact since almost all cases reported have been due to an excess intake of vitamin D_2, though vitamin D_3 has caused the condition in infants.[8]

The disease is rarely encountered now because of the general awareness that vitamin D is a toxic agent in massive doses and because more effective therapy has been found for the conditions in which it was used. A decade ago, vitamin D in daily doses of 50,000 I.U. and up was commonly used in the treatment of rheumatoid arthritis, tuberculosis, Boeck's sarcoid and certain allergic conditions. With the discovery that irradiation and electrical activation of such substances as ergosterol produced therapeutic agents of great potency, it became possible to prescribe massive doses of vitamin D at relatively small expense and inconvenience to the patient.

The variation in dosage and in the time required to produce the disease are considerable, ranging from 50,000 to one million I.U. daily and from a few days to six years.[9] Since in very few of the reports is the specific type of the offending preparation noted, it is impossible to be sure whether these variations are due to the chemical constituents of the agent or the resistance of the patient. There is some evidence to show that if a high calcium diet accompanies the excessive vitamin D dosage, the disease is brought on more rapidly. It might be presumed that if the diet contains large amounts of a chelating agent such as the phytates found in the roughage cereals, the opposite might be true.

A knowledge of this disease helps to understand the mechanisms of the action of vitamin D. The enhancement of the absorption of calcium through the gut wall is indicated and is accepted now almost universally. The action of vitamin D upon the renal tubules is still debated. The evidence garnered from study of cases of vitamin D toxicity suggests that this agent, in large doses at least, increases reabsorption of phosphates from the glomerular filtrate. It does not negate the possibility that smaller doses may inhibit phosphate re-absorption.

The possibility that vitamin D has a parathormone-like action directly upon the bone, causing deossification, has long been suspected. Massive doses of vitamin D in the human cause a sustained, high serum calcium level even with a low calcium intake. This seems to verify the above suspicion, particularly since the source of the calcium is apparently the skeleton which synchronously undergoes demineralization.

The symptoms of an abnormally high serum calcium content are much the same as those in hyperparathyroidism and the latter condition is the most difficult to differentiate. The sense of profound fatigue and weakness is often the first to manifest itself and probably reflects the action of calcium ions upon the peripheral nerves and myoneural junctions. The diarrhea, abdominal pain, anorexia, nausea, vomiting and eventual weight loss are doubtless due to comparable effects on the smooth muscle of the gastrointestinal tract. Paresthesias are sometimes encountered. The mental depression, psychoses, headache and vertigo may be the direct effects of the excessive calcium in the fluid which perfuses the nerve cells of the central nervous system, or they may be caused by the cerebral edema which has been reported in hypercalcemia. The altered electrocardiograph, with a shortened QT interval, also may be a neuromuscular phenomenon.

Metastatic deposits of calcium salts within collagen are particularly common in hypervitaminosis D. This incidence is presumably the consequence of the combined high levels of both calcium and phosphorus. It is found in hyperparathyroidism also but less constantly, perhaps because here there is a parathormone action upon the renal tubules which causes a phosphorus diuresis, thus maintaining a normal or low serum phosphorus content. In vitamin D poisoning, calcium deposits have been reported in almost every conceivable area[10] including the corneas, the meninges, the skin, the capsules of joints and bursae, tendon sheaths, blood vessels, gastric mucosa, heart, lungs, thyroid, pancreas and kidneys. Deposits in the skin may give rise to pruritus, in the cornea to a "band keratitis."

Nephrocalcinosis is the most important sequel of the disease since it may lead to permanent kidney damage, uremia and eventual death. The evidences of kidney insufficiency are found in a rising non-protein nitrogen and albumin, casts and red cells in the urine. The specific gravity remains low. Polydypsia and polyuria have been severe enough to arouse the suspicion of diabetes insipidus. Eventually, there is a normocytic, normochromic anemia.

The calcific deposits in the periarticular tissues are considered characteristic though they have also been reported in the various types of hyperparathyroidism. The joint capsules, tendon sheaths and bursae are particularly prone to calcification. Because most cases of vitamin D toxicity have occurred in treatment of rheumatoid arthritis, the question is pertinent whether the regional selectivity involving the joints may be due to the changes in the collagen incident to the disease being treated. These masses of calcium may be very large, measuring up to 10 cm. in diameter. When opened, they are found to contain a pale grumous material not unlike that found in gout, or they may be cystic and contain a fluid which closely resembles milk. The calcium salt deposits have been of particular interest to the roentgenologists.

The skeletal demineralization which occurs is generalized, resembling that of osteoporosis. In early or mild cases this change may not appear. In some instances focal areas of bone destruction have occurred, but it is likely that this finding was the result of the disease that was being treated and not of the action of vitamin D. The occurrence of deossification strongly suggests a direct action of vitamin D upon the bone, since the parathyroid glands are not involved and the high serum calcium level forestalls any need for withdrawal of the calcium stores.

Chemical evaluation of the serum is most helpful in hypervitaminosis D. The calcium content should be above 12 mg. per 100 ml. and has been reported as high as 16. The phosphorus is often normal but is more apt to be slightly elevated. The serum alkaline phosphatase is usually high normal or slightly raised, depending upon the stage of activity and degree of severity of the disease. The phosphorus level may be particularly helpful since usually the most difficult differential problem is hyperparathyroidism, which should produce a low normal or subnormal level.

Other differential possibilities are nephritis, diffuse bone tumor (myeloma) or neoplastic bone metastasis, myelogenous leukemia and certain cases of osteopetrosis. All of these with the exception of nephritis should have accompanying signs and symptoms which are foreign to vitamin D toxicity. An accurate history with specific questioning concerning the taking of vitamin D is, of course, of the greatest help. It is not enough to know that the patient is not taking vitamin D at the moment. Cases have been reported in which termination of therapy had occurred as long as two months before the patient presented himself for diagnosis.

ROENTGENOGRAPHIC MANIFESTATIONS

The radiographic manifestations of hypervitaminosis D in the adult are those of demineralization of skeletal structures, focal or diffuse, and soft tissue calcification. Since the demineralization produces the picture of osteoporosis and osteoporosis of disuse may result from the disease for which vitamin D was administered, this manifestation may be difficult to appreciate except when focal. The soft tissue calcification may present as periarticular, irregular masses of opaque material. Joint capsules or vessels may be visible by virtue of calcification. Renal calcification is often evident.

In contrast with the above, the radiographic manifestations of excessive vitamin D intake in an infant consist of an increase in the opacity of skeletal structures. The ends of long bones show alternating transverse bands of radiolucency and opacity, the epiphyseal centers

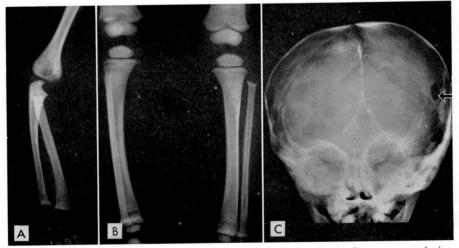

FIG. 140.   Hypervitaminosis D. This child received an excessive amount of vitamin D over many months. The bones at the base of the skull are dense and thick and there is calcification of the falx and tentorium (C). A surgical defect is present in the left parietal region (arrow). Alternating bands of opacity and radiolucency are evident at the ends of the long bones (A and B). The patient ultimately developed the osseous lesions of rickets as a result of renal failure. (Courtesy of John W. Hope, M.D., The Children's Hospital of Philadelphia, Philadelphia, Pa.)

may be ringed by a dense opaque band and the bones at the base of the skull may be more opaque than the normal. Calcification of soft tissues, such as the kidneys, falx cerebri and tentorium, may be seen. When renal damage occurs, rickets may complicate the total picture.

MICROSCOPY

Nothing is known of the microscopic appearance of the bone in hypervitaminosis D. The so-called "calcium cysts" have been removed surgically and examined. The masses of calcium salts apparently cause tissue necrosis. The area may break down and liquefy, producing a milk-like fluid, or it may remain as an inspissated, chalky mass which is positive with the calcium stain. There is a stimulation of a fibrous reaction around the calcium deposits to form a heavy, collagenous capsule. There is usually a giant cell foreign body reaction in this capsule and in contiguous tissues.

PROGNOSIS

The condition is treated by withdrawal of vitamin D and placing the patient on a low calcium, high fluid diet. There is a gradual but progressive dissolution of the calcified areas, though if they are massive they may not completely disappear. Cases of well defined kidney insufficiency have been reported to recover normal function over a period of months on this regimen.

SCURVY

Scurvy is the result of (1) an inability on the part of the finer ramifications of the vascular tree to hold blood and (2) an inability to manufacture adequate normal intercellular collagen and organic bone matrix. One is strongly tempted to link the two inabilities as a part of the same mechanism, and it has been hypothesized that the capillary extravasations are due to a failure in the production of a normal cement substance, supposedly of the same chemical order as collagen and osteoid, which binds the vascular lining endothelial cells and makes the vessel walls impervious. Factual proof of such cement substance and its lack in scurvy is still undemonstrated, though all recent studies do show a lack of osteoblastic activity with failure of osteoid production and there are some data which suggest a similar inactivity of fibroblasts in stimulating collagen production.

The disease is caused by a deficiency in vitamin C. This substance was isolated by Szent-Györgyi in 1928 and is known to be levo-hexuronic acid, now known as ascorbic acid.

The history of scurvy is a long and romantic one since in the past it was a disease of peoples who because of distant travel or siege were forced to accommodate their dietary intake to stored supplies. Since adequate quantities of ascorbic acid are found only in fresh dairy products, fruit and vegetables and since in its raw state the vitamin cannot be adequately stored, adult scurvy played an important role in the history of exploration, war and frontier life. Accounts of the condition which is now recognizable as scurvy were recorded during the thirteenth century crusades by de Joinville and later by others, until Lind proved in his unique experiments on twelve sailors that the disease was caused by a deficiency of a factor which resided in citrus fruits, and so reported in 1753 in his "Treatise of the Scurvy."

Until the latter nineteenth century, though adult scurvy was adequately diagnosed and treated, the incidence and importance of infantile scurvy was unappreciated largely because it is symptomatically different (the disturbances in bone growth obviously can be manifested only in younger patients) and because of the prevalence and similarity of rickets, with which it was confused, in the same age group. In 1883 Sir Thomas Barlow[11] separated infantile scurvy from rickets and since that time the condition frequently has been called "Barlow's disease." Other important contributions were made by Hess,[12] who in 1917 called attention to and stressed the importance of latent infantile scurvy, and by Szent-Györgyi who isolated ascorbic acid in 1928.

In the world of today, there is practically no incidence of full-blown adult scurvy except in those who are accidentally deprived of fresh food and medical supplies. Recently, however, there have been reports[13] of latent adult scurvy brought on by a too casual consideration of dietary requirements in a harassed business population. The symptoms of fully developed scurvy in the adult are due largely to hemorrhages in soft tissue and to a lesser extent in bone and subperiosteal tissues. The gums are especially involved. They become greatly enlarged, soft, spongy, edematous and discolored. They bleed upon pressure. Macular hemorrhages appear in the various mucous membranes and eventually in the skin. Hemorrhages into the joint spaces cause arthralgia and those in the muscles and beneath the periosteum make movement painful and eventually impossible. An anemia develops and eventually there may be frank hemorrhage from the mucosa of the gastrointestinal tract and even the conjunctivae. If ascorbic acid is not soon introduced into the diet, death may result from a variety of infections which the body is unable to resist.

Latent scurvy may be suspected in adults who complain of weakness, weight loss, poor appetite, diarrhea, bleeding from the gums, hypermenorrhea and a hemorrhagic perifollicular skin rash. An anemia which is resistant to therapy with iron, vitamin B_{12} and folic acid yields to ascorbic acid. This is a nutritional type of anemia which may be due to the limitation of conversion of pteroylglutamic acid to the citrovorum factor.[15] The diagnosis is made by finding a positive tourniquet test and a blood ascorbic acid level of less than 0.8 mg. per 100 ml.

In modern medical practice the term scurvy usually refers to infantile scurvy unless otherwise designated. The condition almost always develops between the sixth and eighteenth months. It is rarely seen after the second year. The onset is insidious with a loss of appetite, listlessness and a failure of normal weight gain. The gums become swollen and ecchymotic, hemorrhages appear in the oral mucous membranes and the skin. Bone pain becomes manifest when the child is lifted. A laxness of the muscle tone may be noted. A swelling of the ends of the long bones occurs and the costochondral junctions become prominent. If the condition is allowed to continue there is a retardation of growth. Hematuria may occur and the capillary resistance test will be found to be positive. Laboratory examination will reveal subnormal levels of serum alkaline phosphatase and ascorbic acid.

ROENTGENOGRAPHIC MANIFESTATIONS

The radiographic manifestations of infantile scurvy are a reflection of osteoporosis and hemorrhagic phenomena. Alterations are first apparent and are most marked where the growth of bone is most rapid, e.g., the wrists, knees and costochondral junctions. Because there is a disassociation of chondroblastic and osteoblastic activity, the changes are first manifest at the growing ends of the bones. The zone of provisional calcification is normally formed. An increase in the opacity and the width of the zone of provisional calcification occurs as a result of failure of resorption of the calcified cartilaginous matrix. Lack of osteoid production results in a deficiency of new trabeculae of bone in the metaphysis, and hence a radiolucent band is found adjacent to the zone of provisional calcification, the so-called scorbutic zone.

Epiphyseal centers are altered in the same way as is the metaphysis. The zone of provisional calcification around the centers becomes thicker than normal and, combined with the thin, sparse trabeculae of the center, results in a radiographic appearance described as "ringing of the epiphyses."

The trabeculae of bone become small as a result of continued resorption of bone combined with defective formation of new bone. Many of the finer trabeculae disappear altogether. Thus the bone of

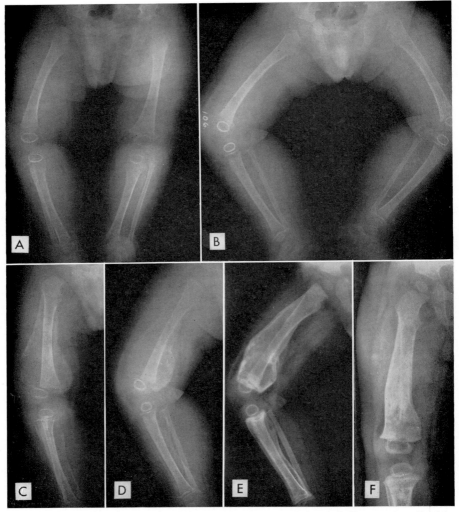

FIG. 141.   Infantile scurvy. The uniform opacity of the medullary cavity, the thin cortices, the metaphyseal rarefaction and the opacity of the zone of provisional calcification around the epiphyseal centers and at the ends of the shafts are illustrated in *A* and *B*. A vague soft tissue shadow is evident around the distal diaphysis of the right femur. Anterior-posterior (*C*) and lateral (*D*) projections of the right femur made ten days later and after the initiation of therapy demonstrate anterolateral displacement of the distal femoral epiphyseal center and zone of provisional calcification and calcification in subperiosteal hematoma. Such calcification is also evident about the right tibia. *E* and *F* are radiographs of the same area seven weeks and six months later. These demonstrate progressive calcification of the subperiosteal hematoma and remodeling of the femur.

the spongiosa offers little contrast to the soft tissues of the marrow cavity and the medullary cavity therefore appears almost uniformly opacified, the so-called "ground glass" appearance. The cortex becomes thin as a consequence of bone resorption and deficient periosteal new bone production.

The opacity of the zones of provisional calcification does not connote strength, but rather these areas are brittle and multiple impaction fractures occur within these zones. These are evident radiographically as irregularity of the zone of provisional calcification. The metaphyseal area, weakened as a consequence of hemorrhage into the area, deficient production of osteoid (trabeculae) and persistence of unutilized calcified cartilaginous matrix and cells, is readily separated from the adjoining diaphysis. Such fractures through this zone superficially suggest epiphyseal separations, but are really subepiphyseal. They are responsible for lateral spurring at the end of the shaft.

Subperiosteal hemorrhage may be recognized at times only as a vague, irregular shadow of the density of soft tissue adjacent to the shaft. When healing begins, calcification in the subperiosteal hematomas is seen and is probably one of the earlier signs of healing.

That the osteoporosis associated with scurvy may in part be the result of disuse is probable. In any event, the radiographic alterations in infantile scurvy can be correlated with the histopathology, and when this is done the alterations become meaningful.

MICROSCOPY

Scurvy is essentially a matter of blood extravasation from the capillaries and a failure of osteoid and collagen production. Examination of the vasculature of scorbutic tissues fails to reveal the cause of the multiple hemorrhages which occur, especially into the mesenchymal tissues. Since an intercellular cement substance between the endothelial lining cells is difficult to demonstrate, the explanation involving its deficiency must be regarded as hypothetical. Adequate studies of the endothelial cells themselves and of the subendothelial wall have not been done. It is still quite possible that a failure in the maintenance of the vascular collagen supportive substance may be at fault for this aspect of the disease.

In respect to the skeletal system, the hemorrhages occur in the metaphyses, in the central portions of the epiphyses and beneath the periosteum, particularly at the ends of the cylindrical bones. In the metaphysis the extravasations interfere with normal bone growth and hematopoiesis. About the vessels in the center of the epiphysis they delay the appearance of the osseous nucleus. In the juxtacortical region they lift the periosteum in a collar about the metaphysis, and gradually dissect it toward the mid-shaft until the periosteum may become virtually detached from the diaphysis, except at the point where it merges with the perichondrium. The latter is never raised from the cartilaginous epiphysis.

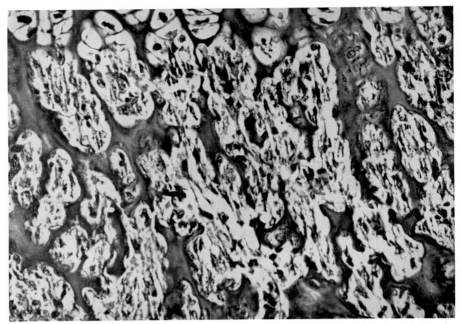

FIG. 142.   Scurvy. The epiphyseal line is seen along the upper border of the picture. The scaffolding of hyalin has been laid down in good order and is now mineralized. No osteoid seams appear around the hyalin bars because there is an inability to produce osteoid. ($\times$ 396.)

Ascorbic acid is apparently not required for the normal growth and maturation of chondroblasts and the formation of hyalin. But it is necessary for the production of osteoid. Thus, in scurvy there is the rare disassociation of chondroblastic and osteoblastic activity. This same disassociation is seen in osteogenesis imperfecta. Combined with the failure of osteoid production, there is a deficient growth in the metaphyseal granulation. These two factors appear to cause most of the disturbance in the regions of enchondral bone formation.

The chondroblasts of the epiphyseal plate reproduce normally and align themselves in columns. Intercolumnar hyalin bars are formed and a line of provisional calcification appears since there is no disturbance in mineral supply or deposition. At this point the normal process is interrupted. There is inadequate penetration of the bases of the cartilage cell columns by the fingers of granulation (Fig. 142) and thus, as in rickets, the mature cartilage cells are not utilized and so persist and are pushed downward into the metaphysis. This creates a widened zone of hyalin which mineralizes and causes the white line of Fraenkel seen on the roentgenograms.

In the complete scorbutic state osteoblasts do not emerge from the multipotent cell mass. Follis has noted that osteoblasts which can be identified lose the basophilic quality of their cytoplasm. By special staining methods he concludes that this is due to a loss of ribose nucleic acid. There is also a disappearance of intracytoplasmic phosphatase and cytochrome oxidase activity. It is quite possible that cells so disabled are incapable of maturing as osteoblasts and of producing organic bone matrix. If osteoblasts actually contribute a cell-synthesized substance to osteoid, this would seem to be a tenable hypothesis. It is noteworthy that electron microscopic studies of scorbutic osteoid show an alteration in the number and quality of the collagen fibers. Since these fibers in both osteoid and fibrous collagen have been shown to consist largely of protein, this fault may be linked to the altered enzymatic activity of the cells concerned. It remains to be shown that ascorbic acid is an essential building block for this particular metabolic activity.

The persistence of unutilized cartilage cells, the lack of osteoid production and the hemorrhage into the metaphysis all contribute to a weakening of or, rather, a failure of development of a strong, stress-bearing metaphyseal area. Infractions occur in the regional cortices and it is quite usual to find fractures through the entire region with displacement of the epiphysis and its epiphyseal line. It is notable, however, that with realignment and proper antiscorbutic therapy, enchondral bone formation may proceed without permanent scarring.

The failure in production of organic matrix precludes the deposition of mineral salts in this region. This accounts for the zone of subnormal x-ray density which lies shaftward from the widened line of provisional calcification. The central area of the bony epiphyseal nucleus is translucent and its periphery, the widened zone of provisional calcification, is denser than normal. This presents the roentgenographic picture which has been called "ringed epiphysis."

Extravasations of blood within tissues normally induce fibrosis. In scurvy there is an inability to produce normally collagenized fibrous tissue. The hematopoietic marrow of the metaphyseal area is replaced by a primitive type of connective tissue, sometimes called areolar connective tissue, with very little or no intercellular collagen. The extent of this marrow replacement is probably not sufficient to cause the anemia which is seen in scurvy. This appears to be a nutritional type which results from a metabolic defect similar to that which causes an inability to form normal osteoid and collagen. The collagen-forming defect likewise may be reflected in the diminished tensile strength of tendons and fascia which is reported.

Roentgenologists long ago emphasized the curious diffuse loss of density which occurs throughout the skeleton. It is difficult to explain this phenomenon without involving the principle of disuse atrophy. It is quite true that pain greatly limits activity, and pediatricians frequently mention listlessness and refusal to move the extremities as early signs of the disease. It is quite probable that this is at least an important factor in the etiology of this finding.

PROGNOSIS

Scurvy is a preventable disease and one which is readily amenable to dietary adjustment. Moreover, massive dosage with vitamin C does not produce toxicity. Unless the fully developed ascorbic state has persisted for a very long time all the signs of its presence will be erased by adequate therapy. Even the evidence of retarded growth may eventually disappear.

HYPERVITAMINOSIS A

Hypervitaminosis A, almost always caused by the taking of excessive amounts of certain proprietary agents, is manifested by changes in the skin and mucous membranes, the skeleton and the central nervous system. Acute and chronic forms have been reported in both children and adults. Since the bone changes are similar to those of infantile cortical hyperostosis (Caffey included two cases of hypervitaminosis A in his early series of cortical hyperostosis), a discussion of the subject is germane to the consideration of orthopedic pathology.

We are indebted to the studies of Wolbach[16] for our knowledge of the action and mechanisms of vitamin A in the growth of bone in the experimental animal. He showed that this substance is necessary for the normal reproduction, growth and maturation of the epiphyseal chondroblasts and, therefore, plays an important role in enchondral bone growth. He believed that vitamin A is also a factor in the modeling of bone, stimulating osteoclastic activity in areas where changes in conformation of bone mass is taking place. We have almost no data regarding a deficiency state and bone formation in the human and it is unknown whether such deficiency affects the growth of bone. It is apparent, however, that an excess of vitamin A causes an abnormal subperiosteal bone proliferation, one of the principal findings in vitamin A toxicity.

Arctic explorers have known for nearly a century that the liver of the polar bear contains a toxic substance which, when eaten, induces an acute episode of headache, nausea, vomiting, dizziness and drowsiness. In 1943, it was shown[17] that the substance in the liver responsible for these symptoms is vitamin A, concentrated to the extent of 18,000 U. per gram. In 1944, Josephs[18] reported a case of hypervitaminosis A in a child. Following this, numerous cases in children have been reported, including a series of five by Caffey[19] and an extraordinary case in an adult[20] reported in 1954.

Chronic hypervitaminosis A has been reported most commonly in children between the ages of one and three years, a period when they are dosed with vitamins and when less attention is paid to the exact measurement. It has not been reported in infants under one year, probably because the infant does not absorb the oily medium as efficiently and because some time must elapse to establish high storage levels and development of the symptoms. Acute hypervitaminosis A may occur at any age from the ingestion of a million or more units. Frontal headaches, bulging fontanels in infants and drowsiness indicate the sudden increase in intracranial pressure. Desquamation may begin within thirty-six hours and become severe. There are no changes in the bones.

Chronic hypervitaminosis A begins with anorexia, weight loss and finally causes nausea and vomiting. There are numerous signs and symptoms referable to the nervous system, most of which can be accounted for on the basis of an elevated intracranial pressure due to an increase in the amount of cerebrospinal fluid. It is not known whether this increase is due to an excessive formation or a decreased absorption. Headache appears early and is severe. Irritability, dizziness, fatigue and insomnia have been reported. Signs referable to the eyes are exophthalmos, strabismus, nystagmus and papilledema.

The skin becomes dry and there is a furfuraceous desquamation. Eventually the palms may become thickened, cracked and scaly. Pruritus may be a troublesome feature. The mucous membranes are dry and fissures appear in the lips. The hair becomes dry and coarse and there is epilation of both scalp and body areas including the eyebrows and the lanugo hair.

Bone pain is a constant finding in chronic hypervitaminosis A. This has been severe enough to cause complete invalidism. Firm tumefactions may be noted over the mid-shaft regions of the long bones and ribs. Almost any bone may be affected though there are no reports of involvement of the mandible. Roentgenograms reveal a subperiosteal proliferation of bone which is thickest in the center of the diaphysis and fades off toward the epiphysis, giving the shaft a fusiform shape. The metatarsals and the ulna are the bones most commonly reported affected.

The serum calcium and phosphorus levels are normal. The serum alkaline phosphatase may be moderately elevated. The serum vitamin A and carotene levels must be high to confirm the diagnosis.

Because of the roentgenograms these cases are frequently misdiagnosed as cortical hyperostosis. Caffey[19] notes the following distinguishing features. In cortical hyperostosis the onset is within the first six months of life, there is accompanying fever, the x-ray outline of the lesion is more irregular, lesions of the jaw are usual and in the metatarsals rare, there are no accompanying signs of skin and central nervous system involvement.

The most helpful finding is, of course, a history of excessive vitamin A ingestion. It is usually taken in the form of one of the proprietary agents such as oleum percomorphum. Because the concentrations are high, large doses may be taken in a relatively small amount of medium. These accidents usually occur because the patient or his parents have not been instructed that overdosage with vitamin A can result in a state of toxicity.

MICROSCOPY

Very little is known of the tissue changes which are produced by hypervitaminosis A. Biopsies of the skin and bone were made in the adult case reported by Gerber, Raab and Sobel.[20] The skin showed hyperkeratosis and parakeratosis. There was appositional new bone formation by the periosteum.

PROGNOSIS

The treatment for hypervitaminosis A is withdrawal of the causative agent. When this is done, the bone pain is relieved within a week and the patient becomes asymptomatic in about a month. The roentgenographic changes fade more slowly but in children the skeleton resumes a normal appearance within a year.

REFERENCES

RICKETS
1. Mellanby, E.: J. Physiol., 52:11, 1918.
2. Park, E. A.: Physiol. Rev., 3:106, 1923.

VITAMIN D REFRACTORY RICKETS
3. Albright, F., and Reifenstein, E. C.: Parathyroid Glands and Metabolic Disease. Williams and Wilkins Co., Baltimore, 1948.
4. Harrison, H. E., and Harrison, H. C.: J. Clin. Invest., 20:47, 1941.
5. Albright, F., Burnett, C. H., Parson, W., Reifenstein, E. C., and Roos, A.: Medicine, 25:399, 1946.
6. Dent, C. E.: J. Bone & Joint Surg., 34B:266, 1952.
7. Pedersen, H. E., and McCarrol, H. R.: J. Bone & Joint Surg., 33A:203, 1951.

HYPERVITAMINOSIS D
8. Christensen, W. R., Liebman, C., and Sosman, M. C.: Am. J. Roentgenol., 65:27, 1951.

9. Chaplin, H., Clark, L. D., and Ropes, M. W.: Am. J. M. Sc., *221*:369, 1951.
10. Adams, F. D.: New England J. Med., *244*:590, 1951.

Scurvy

11. Barlow, T.: Med. Chir. Trans., *66*:159, 1883.
12. Hess, A. F.: J.A.M.A., *68*:235, 1917.
13. Morris, G. E.: Am. Practitioner & Digest of Treatment, *5*:658, 1954.
14. Jandl, J. H., and Gabuzda, G. J.: Proc. Soc. Exper. Biol. & Med., *84*:452, 1953.
15. Follis, R. H.: Bull. Johns Hopkins Hosp., *89*:9, 1951.

Hypervitaminosis A

16. Wolbach, S. B.: J. Bone & Joint Surg., *29*:171, 1947.
17. Rodahl, K., and Moore, T.: Biochem. J., *37*:166, 1943.
18. Josephs, H. W.: Am. J. Dis. Child., *67*:33, 1944.
19. Caffey, J.: Am. J. Roentgenol., *65*:12, 1951.
20. Gerber, A., Raab, A. P., and Sobel, A. E.: Am. J. Med., *16*:729, 1954.

Disturbances in the Normally Formed Skeleton

11

The Repair of Fractures

An understanding of fracture healing is a prerequisite of successful fracture treatment. It is regrettable that the physiology of the commonest of bone ailments cannot yet be completely described. We know a good deal about the formation of new bone and somewhat less about the lysis of dead bone, but the accounts of the chronologic order of the several stages in bone healing and the stimuli which direct their order find little agreement among authors who have written on the subject. The detailed examination of the entire pathologic structure at multiple intervals over the healing course in the experimental animal demands techniques which are unavailable to most. Such studies in man are obviously impossible and so much of our knowledge consists of fragments derived from animal experimentation pieced together with what fortuitous biopsies of human bone the surgeon has produced. The danger of application of findings observed in the experimental animal to human physiology need not be emphasized here, but it is hardly out of place to remark that the processes of bone healing in the cat and in the dog are little more alike than their temperaments and are probably quite as different from the process as it occurs in the human.

Several modern writers[1] regard the hematoma consequent to fracture as an inactive by-product of no importance, an incidental occurrence which affects callus formation neither positively nor negatively. This opinion is apparently derived by observation of fracture healing in the animal. One should not contradict such opinions without carrying out the same experiments, but the experienced pathologist finds it hard to believe that the hematoma of fracture can be so innocently innocuous when elsewhere in the body hematoma plays a very important role in the response to trauma. Moreover, the meager bits of

227

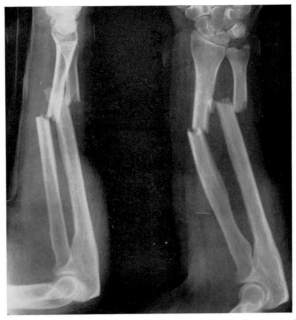

FIG. 143.   Transverse fracture of both bones of the forearm. A fracture line is radiolucent by virtue of discontinuity in the bone. Deformity is best described as the distal fragment relates to the proximal fragment.

tissue which we have been able to retrieve from human fractures of various ages strongly suggests that the hematoma does organize and that from the collagenous tissue which is thus provoked comes certain important elements which eventually constitute the callus.

Some writers[2] state that all or most of the bone tissue of callus is produced by the osteoblasts of the viable cambium and the endosteal lining cells. Thus the callus is said to develop by the formation of two collars, one about the end of each fragment, which grow toward each other and eventually unite to form a bridge over the hiatus produced by the fracture. Examination of sections of fracture material leaves little doubt that these cells do produce bone and perhaps the preponderant part of the callus, but the ability of collagenoblasts to change into osteoblasts and chondroblasts in the callus medium is equally striking, and the bone and cartilage therefrom appear to be very important components of the healing process. Since healthy osteoid is mineralized and therefore becomes opaque to x-rays within a matter of hours to days after formation, if the collar or bridge hypothesis were correct one should be able to follow the progress of the advancing margins as these collars approach each other by a series of correctly timed roentgenograms. But such roentgenograms do not support this theory. Instead one perceives the full-blown callus as

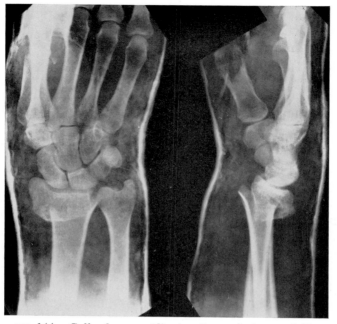

FIG. 144.   Colles fracture (distal radius and ulnar styloid).

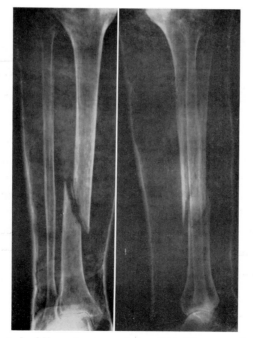

FIG. 145.   Comminuted, oblique fracture of the tibia. The comminuted fragment lies
adjacent to the medial aspect of the end of the proximal fragment.

soon as its opacity is greater than the surrounding soft tissue, and though it increases in x-ray density as it collects osteoid and mineral, this density is diffuse rather than polar concentrations which eventually merge.

There has been a tendency recently to minimize the proclivity of collagenoblasts to form bone and cartilage by metaplasia. The experienced general pathologist who examines tissues from all parts of the body is not surprised to find this phenomenon in the most unexpected places. More often than not, fragments of newly formed bone are found in the vicinity of abnormal calcium deposits in mesenchymal tissues. It is as though the presence of calcium salts induces a change in collagen so that it now accepts mineral just as does osteoid. Whether the influence is upon the collagenoblasts or on their intercellular product is not known, or indeed, whether the mineral is the initiating agent or merely a by-product of some unknown force which induces both metaplasia and calcification. The entire subject of cell induction[3] is fascinating but it seems unnecessary to imagine some mysterious agent passed from one cell to another to comprehend fibro-osseous metaplasia. The collagen of connective tissue, the hyalin of cartilage and the osteoid of bone are all remarkably similar substances despite the obvious differences in their physical properties. They are elaborated in the presence of three types of cells, the collagenoblast, the chondroblast and the osteoblast, all of which arise from a common stem cell, the fibroblast. The factors which induce the fibroblast to differentiate into one of these three types are unknown but they are related to environmental circumstance and probably have to do with pH, the amount of blood supply, motion, the presence of mineral salts, stress and perhaps other factors as yet unsuggested. A specific humoral substance may be the dominant agent but as yet none has been isolated, and explanations based on its presence sometimes sound like the older theories based on the Galenic humors.

The repair of fractures is like the reparative processes elsewhere in mesenchymal tissue except that the end product is bone rather than collagenous scar. The differences between osteoid and collagen are largely chemical and can probably be accounted for on the basis of environmental factors. It is the author's contention that the osteoblast forms osteoid because of its metabolic resources. If we knew more about its metabolic habits we would probably find that it can produce hyalin or collagen with equal facility.

Bone fracture heals by the production of a callus. This callus tends to immobilize the bone fragments. When immobilization is once achieved, stress trajectories are established and further bone production is directed by the principle of the attainment of the greatest strength with the least mass. Bone production takes time. The greater the amount of callus necessary to reestablish continuity of the fragments, the longer will be the healing time. Thus the principles of fracture treatment are obvious. Reduction should bring the ends as close together as possible in the nearest approximation of normal alignment in order that the smallest possible callus may suffice. Immobilization should be designed to control motion to a degree that will prevent any disturbance in the rigid callus structure. In most instances immobilization should be as complete as possible. Muscle tension and movement of the part as a whole should provide sufficient stress to stimulate osteoblastic action. Finally, the multiple factors in callus and normal bone production should be kept constantly in mind with every effort to provide these factors when they are deficient. Splints, casts, plates, pins and nails as well as traction appliances should be used where necessary with the least interference to blood supply. Adequate caloric intake with sufficient ascorbic acid and vitamin D should be maintained. If endocrine deficiencies are apparent, especially estrogen, they should be corrected. Under optimum conditions from 1 to 3 cm. of large cylindrical bone tissue should be formed within a year.

If bone production is deficient and the healing process delayed substantially beyond a year, especially in those areas where there is repeated motion, a pseudarthrosis is likely to be formed. The organism is slow in bridging with rigid bone an area where motion is constant. Instead the callus remains fibrous and pliable. Eventually a bursa-like sac develops in the region and its walls may undergo cartilaginous metaplasia. This is a marvelous imitation of a joint with articular plates covering the bone ends, an illustration of the adaptability of tissues to new environmental conditions.

The factors which cause non-union and delayed union may be exceedingly complex and difficult to determine. A discussion of these factors and of the mechanics of fracture treatment is not pertinent to the subject matter of this text. These subjects belong to the experienced orthopedist and none other should try to explain them.

When fracture of a bone occurs, the soft tissues on either side of it are lacerated. The periosteum is usually torn and the vascular channels of the parosteal and endosteal soft tissues are opened. Arterial blood flows out into the tissues to produce a hematoma. The continuity of the small channels within bone that carry nutrient material to the lacunar osteocytes is interrupted and these cells die. Thus the edges of the fragments, back as far as the junction of collateral channels, consist of dead bone. The hematoma forms within and outside the cortical walls. Within a matter of hours a network of fibrin is

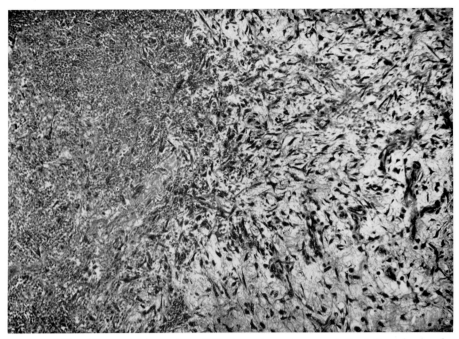

FIG. 146.   The central portion of the hematoma is seen at the left and granulation at the right. At the junction of the two zones fibroblasts and capillary buds are entering the former, thus converting it to the latter. (× 180.)

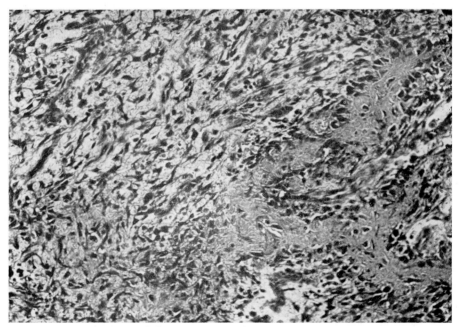

FIG. 147.   A spicule of recently formed fiberbone (on the right) ensheathed with osteoblasts is found in a mass of granulation which was probably formed from hematoma. Thus the hematoma enters indirectly into the formation of bone. (× 180.)

precipitated, first at the edges and then into the center of the clot. Soon collagenoblasts penetrate the hematoma from the labile mesenchymal tissues surrounding the injured area. As these climb through the network of fibrin strands the torn capillaries send endothelial buds after them, and soon the hematoma is organized (Fig. 146) and gradually becomes converted to a mass of granulation. The hyperemia thus induced probably plays a role in the lysis of the ragged fragments of dead bone which constitute the fracture edges, surcharging the intercellular fluids with mineral salts. As the inflammatory reaction subsides the pH probably is altered.[4] During this time the viable osteoblasts begin to produce osteoid and new fibroblasts within and without the cortex mature into osteoblasts (Fig. 147) and chondroblasts (Fig. 148). As the collagenoblasts lay down collagen the recently formed vascular channels are squeezed out of existence and the blood supply is consequently diminished. Osteoid is laid down wherever a nidus of solid tissue will serve as a base: on fragments of old bone (Fig. 149) and on islands of newly formed cartilage (Fig. 150). Mineralization follows close on the heels of osteoid production. Throughout the area one can find small masses of cartilage surrounded by

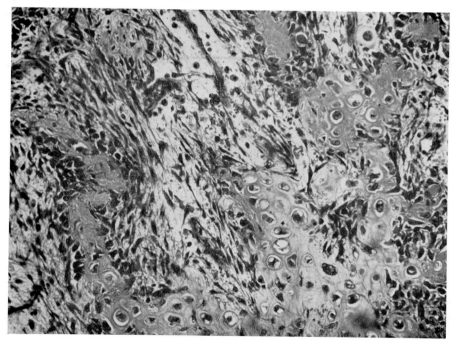

FIG. 148.   An island of young cartilage cells is surrounded by granulation. These cells appear to have been derived from the fibroblasts of granulation about the periphery of the cartilaginous island. Osteoblasts are laying down fiberbone. This combination of central cartilage and peripheral bone in a field of granulation is seen wherever callus is formed. The material has been called osteochondroid. ($\times$ 180.)

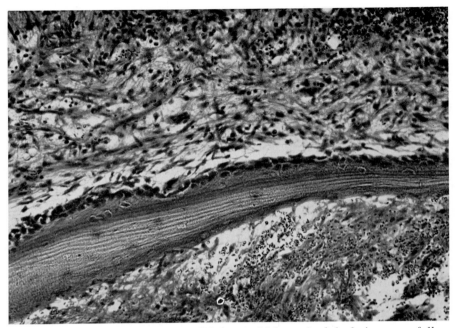

FIG. 149.   A spicule of normal adult bone which survived the lytic process following fracture. It acts as a nidus for the apposition of new bone. Along its upper surface
a layer of osteoblasts can be seen laying down a seam of new osteoid. (× 180.)

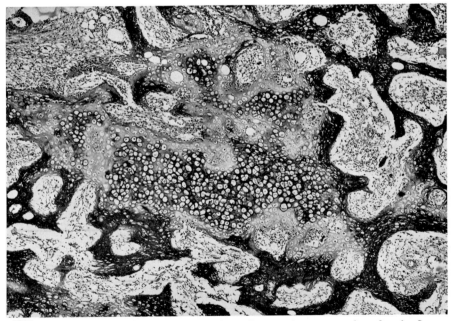

FIG. 150.   An island of newly formed cartilage acting as a nucleus for the formation of bone at its periphery. There is apparently a normal progression; hematoma to
granulation to fibroblasts to cartilage to bone. (× 40.)

fiberbone, osteochondroid (Fig. 151). The osteoid at the periphery appears to merge into the cartilaginous centers and some observers have interpreted this as the direct transition of cartilage into bone. A more plausible explanation to the writer is that fibroblasts first mature into chondroblasts and produce hyalin. As the lesion ages, fibroblasts become osteoblasts which continue the laying down of intercellular substance which eventually becomes recognizable as osteoid. Where a large cartilage island persists, usually at the periphery of the lesion, the chondroblasts mature and columnate just as in the enchondral plate and a line of provisional calcification is laid down. At this point the irregular cartilage edge takes on the appearance of an epiphyseal line, producing a scaffolding of mineralized hyalin for the deposition of osteoid. This manner of enchondral bone formation is apparently neither necessary nor exceedingly common, judging from the number of times it turns up in sections made of callus tissue.

Why cartilage is produced in some areas and bone in others remains a mystery to the writer. Some authors have proposed the theory that cartilage thrives in ischemic areas that are too barren for osteoid to survive. If variation in oxygen tension is the reason, then the theory is hard to support on morphologic grounds since these areas are scrambled in a patternless array.

The metaplasia of fibroblasts into bone and cartilage-forming

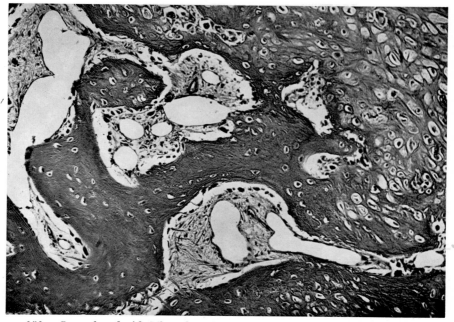

FIG. 151.   Osteochondroid. The edge of a cartilaginous nucleus is seen in the right upper corner. About it new bone is being formed. ($\times$ 180.)

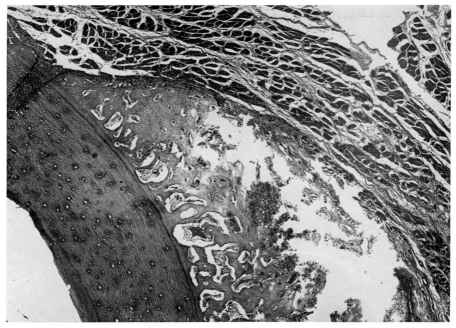

FIG. 152.   A segment of the cortex of a cylindrical bone is shown in the left lower portion. The muscle and periosteum in the right upper half of the picture have been detached by the fracture. The cambium has laid down a thick layer of new bone between the periosteum and the external cortical surface. (× 28.)

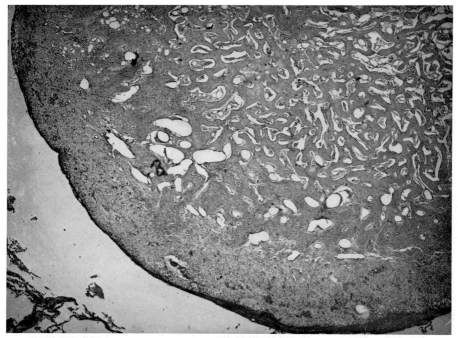

FIG. 153.   A segment of the cortex of a fractured bone. The medullary tissues have been replaced by a solid core or plug of callus which is annealed to the inner cortical surface. (× 16.)

elements is by no means the whole explanation for callus formation. Where the cambium is torn from the compacta one can see the diligent production of new bone between the periosteum and old cortex (Fig. 152). A solid mass of bone also replaces the marrow tissue, forming a plug or core which merges through the cortical hiatus with the outside callus (Fig. 153). Thus the shaft of a cylindrical bone is braced both within and without. All of this cellular activity constitutes a composite, the callus. This again is an illustration of the ability of the organism to adapt itself by cellular activity and metaplasia to the circumstances of a new environment.

The bone of the callus consists largely of fiberbone which must be replaced with adult bone if it is to withstand the stress of normal function. Trajectories of stress determine the shifting of bone without diminishing mass and thereby strength. New adult bone is laid down on one side of a piece of fiberbone while the other side is undergoing lysis (Fig. 43, Chap. 5). Thus, strong, adult bone moves into the areas where strength is needed and the weaker fiberbone melts away. The organism is able to straighten the angulations of malposition even though side-to-side rather than end-to-end approximation resulted from poor reduction (Fig. 154). As adult bone is exchanged for fiberbone the need for bulk is diminished and so the callus is

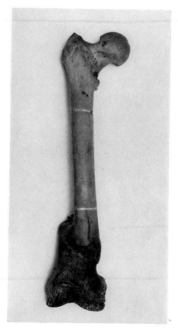

FIG. 154.   A femur with old fracture through the lower third and side-to-side approximation. Callus annealed the two fragments allowing full weight-bearing although with considerable shortening.

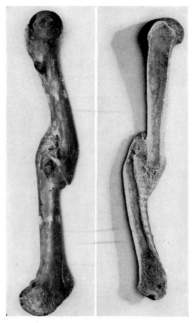

FIG. 155.   Picture of the outer surface and the cut surface of a femur with old fracture and healing. Note how the callus persists along the trajectory lines but has disappeared within the medullary areas of the two fractures. Because there was side-to-side rather than end-to-end apposition the continuity of the medullary spaces of the two fragments was never reestablished.

reduced in size. If the fragments are perfectly aligned, the need for extracortical callus disappears and it melts away leaving a perfectly smooth cortex. Since stress is borne through the cylindrical cortex, the medullary core of callus is no longer needed and it undergoes lysis, allowing a reestablishment of communication between the medullary cavities of the two fragments (Fig. 155). Should infection complicate an open fracture the normal sequence of healing events is disturbed, as one might expect it would be. The callus is prevented from performing its normal function and an imperfect result is inevitable (Fig. 156).

Organized tissues, like organized societies, respond in an astonishing fashion to emergencies. Callus may form in response to a fracture in a bone which was poorly constructed in the beginning—osteogenesis imperfecta—or normally constructed but unable to maintain itself—fibrous dysplasia and pseudarthrosis. One might reason that the newly formed bone in these instances is the product of the osteoblasts which are recently formed from the emergency fibroblasts. It is said that muscle cells will undergo atrophy to supply to the emergency tissues the building blocks with which to construct callus. It is of interest that the bone formed under such circumstances is not durable. Once

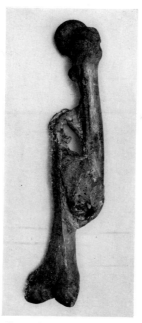

FIG. 156.   Osteomyelitis complicated this fracture so that repair was inhibited and the callus developed numerous sinuses.

the emergency is past, this bone responds in the same manner as the original bone of the fragments.

REFERENCES

1. Ham, A. W., and Harris, W. R.: In Bourne, G. H.: Biochemistry and Physiology of Bone. Academic Press, Inc., New York, 1956, p. 475.
2. McLean, F. C., and Urist, M. R.: Bone. University of Chicago Press, 1955, p. 139.
3. Spemann, H.: Embryonic Development and Induction. Yale University Press, New Haven, 1938.
4. Schram, W. R., and Fosdick, L. S.: J. Oral Surg., *1*:191, 1943

12

Circulatory Disturbances

BONE INFARCT

Sudden and complete obstruction of the arterial blood supply to bone results in death of the tissue supplied—an infarct—in much the same manner that infarction occurs in such soft tissues as the heart, spleen and kidney. In the diaphysis, cancellous tissue is involved and the overlying cortex spared so that there is no change in the external aspect of the bone. Since the periosteum is not involved, the infarct is without symptoms. When the infarction involves the epiphysis, the support for the articular cartilage may be destroyed and then the condition poses as osteoarthritis or rarely as epiphyseal ischemic necrosis (epiphyseal osteochondritis). For these reasons, bone infarct was quite neglected until Kahlstrom, Phemister and Burton[1] published their paper in 1939. The condition had been recognized in 1878 when Bert described the lesion in patients who had worked in a high atmospheric pressure. A few subsequent reports appeared emphasizing the arthritic aspect and describing roentgenographic features.

Because all of the early reported cases were associated with increased atmospheric environments, the condition has long been known as caisson disease. Kahlstrom and Phemister[2] reported the disease in a patient in 1946 who denied ever doing caisson work and numerous other cases are now known. They contend that bone infarct occurs as often in non-caisson workers as in those who are exposed to high pressure. They state that if a high index of suspicion is maintained the diagnosis will be made much more frequently. Such has not been the experience of some, who though on the alert for the condition have been able to make the diagnosis only in rare instances.

The history of caisson disease should cause one to explore the possibility of bone infarct as a part of the complex of multiple infarction of soft tissues. The caisson worker is exposed to atmospheric pressures of from 25 to 50 pounds. As the worker is compressed, gas is absorbed by the blood. Fat has a greater affinity for nitrogen than does the blood, estimated at about five-fold. Tissues composed largely of lipids, the omentum and mesentery, the subcutaneous tissue and the marrow of long bones, absorb large quantities of nitrogen under conditions of compression. As the worker is decompressed, this nitrogen is released into the blood but the lungs are unable to clear the latter as fast as it is released so that it accumulates in minute bubbles which may coalesce to form pockets of intravascular nitrogen. This unabsorbed nitrogen causes gas embolism in the vicinity where the gas is released.

In the skin and subcutaneous tissue there are usually flushing, areas of lividity and pruritus. Bleeding occurs from the mucosa of the gastrointestinal, respiratory and urinary tracts. Cramp-like pains may occur in the abdomen due to multiple small infarcts of the viscera. If enough small bubbles are delivered to the lungs there may be dyspnea. Infarcts occurring in the spinal cord and brain may cause a variety of signs including visual disturbance, tinnitus, hypesthesias, motor paralysis and even collapse and death. Most of the symptoms occur while decompression is being accomplished or within three hours but in a few cases they have appeared as late as twenty-three hours after.[3]

It is probable that bone infarcts occur in the majority of these cases, but because there are no immediate symptoms they are missed. The long bones are involved almost exclusively, the upper end of the femur most commonly and then the lower femur, upper tibia and upper humerus. These areas are doubtless most vulnerable because of their proximity to fat stores and because they are supplied by long arteries with few collaterals. Spongy tissue is involved while the overlying cortex escapes. The infarct may occur at any point in the bone, but the incidence is highest at the bone ends. The lesion varies in size from a few millimeters in diameter to involvement of the entire half of the shaft. If the infarct is restricted to the diaphysis, symptoms may never develop and the area is noted only when roentgenograms are made for other reasons. When the epiphysis is involved, the supportive columns of the articular plate eventually give way resulting in unevenness or actual collapse of the latter. Symptoms of arthritis usually develop within six months to a year.

When an area of bone tissue is deprived of its arterial blood supply it dies. The soft, fatty marrow undergoes coagulation and liquefaction necrosis. In the bone spicules the osteocytes die and leave

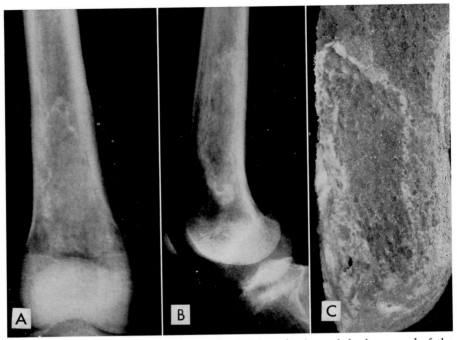

FIG. 157.   *A*, Anteroposterior and *B*, lateral projections of the lower end of the femur; *C*, a sagittal section through the bone. This area is the site of a large infarct which in *C* is outlined by a sclerotic margin of hard, white, mineralized collagen.

their lacunae empty. As long as there is no circulation through the area, it must remain, more or less intact, as dead tissue. But at the margins of the infarct, where it adjoins healthy tissue, there is circulation and here phagocytes enter to clean up the debris and dead bone can be absorbed. Vessels sprouting from the healthy area surround the infarct with a capsule of granulation tissue. Fingers of the latter insert themselves as far into the dead tissue as its vasculature will support it. It is probable that small infarcts are completely absorbed and replaced by new and healthy cancellous tissue. In larger lesions, the aging granulation collagenizes before it completes its task and soon the vessels are choked off by shrinking scar tissue. The fibrous capsule calcifies, perhaps because of the abundance of calcium salts in the area or possibly because of its chemical make-up. The calcified collagen frequently goes on to ossification. Thus, the area of dead bone and marrow is surrounded and isolated by a layer of dense fibrous scar (Fig. 157), of calcified collagen, of new bone or, as in most cases, of a combination of these tissues. The encapsulated infarct may be suspended in cancellous tissue or it may abut against the cortical wall. Here it remains indefinitely, usually unsuspected unless some unrelated event leads to roentgenographic or surgical investigation. When these areas turn up on a roentgenogram, they introduce a serious diagnostic problem. Though the radiologist may surmise their true nature, if there is no history of caisson exposure the diagnosis can be confirmed only by biopsy.

Infarcts in the epiphysis usually run an entirely different course. Here, failure of the support of the articular plate leads to impairment of the weight-bearing surface and joint disease of a type similar to osteoarthritis sets in. Pain, deformity, disability and even ankylosis may occur. The gross appearance of the infarct is altered by the motion and pressure of usage and eventually even large amounts of dead tissue may be converted to granulation and then to new bone. But by this time the normal anatomy is so distorted that function may be impossible without surgical repair.

It is certain that the nutrient vessels of bone uncommonly are closed by agents other than the nitrogen emboli of caisson disease. There appears to be no reason why thrombosis and thrombus embolism cannot occur in the vessels of bone just as they occur in those of soft tissue. Yet, unless diaphyseal infarction is missed because there is no history of caisson disease or unless these events play an etiologic role in epiphyeal osteochondritis and osteochondritis dissecans, there appears to be little clinical evidence of these vascular accidents. If thrombosis or embolism is an important cause of the aseptic necrosis of epiphyseal osteochondritis, it has never been sat-

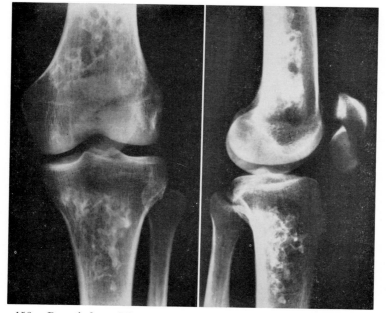

FIG. 158.   Bone infarct. The spongiosa of the distal femur and the proximal tibia is involved. The cortex is spared. The irregular opacities within the marrow cavity are evident, a reflection of calcified or ossified collagen about and within the infarcted areas. The radiolucent areas are the residual of areas of necrosis.

isfactorily explained why this lesion occurs with such constancy in its particular age range.

MICROSCOPY

Sections taken from the center of a well established bone infarct show spicules of dead bone with empty lacunae (Fig. 159). The intervening marrow has been converted to an amorphous mass of tissue debris. There are areas of liquefaction necrosis surrounded by irregular patches of fibrous collagen in which may be embedded crystals of cholesterol. With the routine hematoxylin and eosin technique these appear as fusiform clefts with sharply pointed ends. Coarse granules of deep blue calcium salts are scattered about and there is usually evidence of old hemorrhage with finer hemosiderin particles. In some areas there is coagulation necrosis and a retaining of the architecture of masses of fat cells. Elsewhere, the sections take a washed-out bluish stain indicating the partial splitting of neutral fats.

About the periphery of this region one should find fields of mature fibrous tissue (Fig. 160), and often this will be so densely infiltrated with mineral that it may require decalcification for sectioning (Fig. 161). There is usually some bone formation about the periphery where circulation has been reestablished.

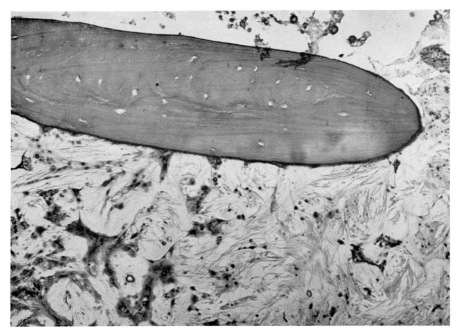

FIG. 159.   A spicule of dead bone lying in a mass of necrotic medullary soft tissue. The osteocytes have disappeared from the lacunae. Surrounding the bone is an oily mass of necrotic tissue containing only a few fibroblasts. ($\times$ 180.)

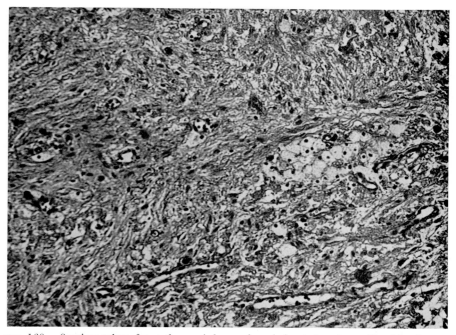

FIG. 160. Section taken from the periphery of an infarct showing a fibroblastic proliferation. (× 180.)

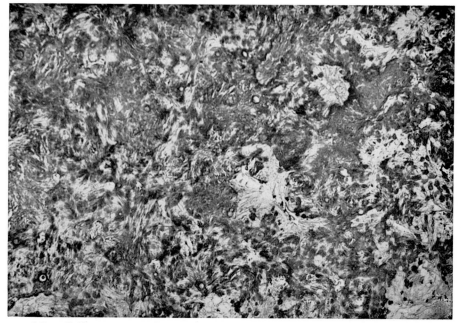

FIG. 161. Collagenous margin of an infarct with massive deposition of mineral salts. (× 180.)

PROGNOSIS

Bone infarcts in the diaphysis have been known to exist for years without giving any symptoms. Their chief importance is the diagnostic problem they introduce when turned up as an incidental finding. Infarcts in the epiphysis cause severe arthritis and crippling. It may be necessary to reconstruct an articular surface and its support to reestablish function.

EPIPHYSEAL ISCHEMIC NECROSIS

By this term we refer to the condition which is variously called osteochondritis deformans juvenilis, the osteochondroses, epiphyseal osteochondritis or epiphyseal aseptic necrosis. When the process involves the capital epiphysis of the femur it is usually called Perthes' disease or Legg-Calvé-Perthes disease or simply coxa plana. When it involves the secondary or less frequently the primary epiphyses of other bones, it is often designated by an eponym such as Osgood-Schlatter disease (tibial tubercle), Köhler's disease (tarsal navicular and sometimes the patella), Freiberg's disease (second metatarsal head), Scheuermann's disease (vertebral bodies), Panner's disease (capitellum of the humerus) and others, depending upon the site. Today most orthopedists agree that the pathogenesis of these lesions is the same and that the benumbing array of eponyms should be discarded in the name of clarity and common sense.

The process is essentially a degeneration and eventual replacement of the osseous nucleus of an epiphysis, almost certainly the result of an interference with its blood supply. In a sense, it is an infarct of the bony epiphysis which then collapses under pressure and causes distortion of the surrounding healthy tissues which it is supposed to support. To use the term "osteochondritis" is to imply that inflammation is an important factor, which in most cases it certainly is not. While there is a very convincing array of data to support the ischemia hypothesis, the offending vessels have not yet been conclusively demonstrated in all cases. In addition, since a few cases have yielded positive bacterial culture, the name "aseptic necrosis" is untenable.

Most types of the disease occur more commonly in males, coxa plana in a ratio of about four to one. Since the more important types occur in the unclosed epiphysis of a growing bone it is usually seen in the younger age groups, most often children, with some of the less common types appearing in adolescents and adults. The primary epiphyses are apt to be involved at an earlier age than the secondary. Thus, the primary epiphysis of the tarsal navicular is usually affected between the ages of four and six years, whereas the secondary epiphyses of the vertebral bodies show involvement during adolescence. In certain types in which the vessel damage is probably caused by repeated trauma, the head of the second metatarsal and the carpal lunate reveal the characteristic changes, as a rule, in adult life. Two of the most important types of epiphyseal aseptic necrosis occur in the superior epiphysis of the femur in children between three and twelve years old and in the tibial tubercle during adolescence. Other less common types include osteochondrosis deformans tibia or tibia vara, which too may be due to an ischemic necrosis of the medial proximal epiphysis of the tibia, resulting in an idiopathic type of lateral bowing of the tibia. The same process in the epiphyses of the proximal phalanges has been called Thiemann's disease.

The cause of epiphyseal ischemic necrosis has been the subject of polemic debate since Osgood and Schlatter each wrote their separate papers on the condition in 1903. It would be entertaining to review the various theories, their authors and the authors' supportive arguments, but such a review would probably do little to enhance one's understanding of the disease. It will suffice to list the more popular theories such as embolism, acute and chronic repeated trauma, congenital and hereditary factors, infection and endocrine disturbances. It is probable that most of these causes have played a role in the vasculature and blood supply of the affected epiphyses in the past, but it is the resultant ischemia that is the common denominator of all the lesions. All the acceptable, well documented facts support this hypothesis. In brief, the vessels may rarely be closed by emboli (supported by cases in which embolism occurs in other soft tissue vessels), the vessels may be torn or thrombosed by trauma (aseptic necrosis has occurred in those cases of trauma in which all vessels were involved), and the lesion has yielded indubitably positive cultures in a very few cases. A dysgenesis of the superior femoral epiphysis which has much the same appearance as epiphyseal ischemic necrosis occurs in cretinism. The failure of true coxa plana to occur after puberty is probably due to the change in vasculature which is incident to epiphyseal ossification. The excessive incidence of this lesion in boys conceivably may be due to their propensity for traumatizing activity. Though papers[4] still appear, associating epiphyseal ischemic necrosis with hypothyroidism, there is little beyond the slender substance of which they are composed to convince one. The congenital and hereditary hypotheses probably stem from the similarities of lesions in such conditions as Morquio's and Hurler's disease which have been mistaken for epiphyseal ischemic necrosis.

The most important member of the epiphyseal ischemic necrosis group from the standpoint of both incidence and morbidity is the process in the capital epiphysis of the femur, commonly called coxa plana or Perthes' disease. Since the morbid physiology of the various members of the group is the same, only the clinical and radiologic aspects differing with the various sites, a detailed discussion of coxa plana will serve to illustrate the process in general.

Before discussing ischemic necrosis of the superior femoral epiphysis, an understanding of the vasculature of the head and neck of the femur is essential.[5] The epiphysis is almost completely supplied by two arteries: the lateral epiphyseal artery arises from the medial femoral circumflex and is the dominant source of blood for the epiphysis; the medial epiphyseal artery is a continuation of the artery which courses through the ligamentum teres which in turn rises from the acetabular branch of the obturator. These vessels anastomose with each other and send branches toward the articular cartilage. These branches form single large capillaries which occupy the zone immediately beneath the articular plate. To date no vascular channels have been demonstrated within the substance of the articular cartilage. The metaphysis of the femoral neck is supplied by two groups of vessels. The inferior metaphyseal arteries supply the greater portion of fresh blood and the superior metaphyseal arteries, from two to five in number, supply the lesser portion.

Until ossification of the enchondral plate, there is little communication between these two sets of vessels. Following closure of the epiphyseal line, anastomosing branches between the epiphyseal and metaphyseal groups have been demonstrated. Neither group is intimately associated with the main nutrient artery of the femoral shaft.

Until 1910, ischemic necrosis of the superior femoral epiphysis was confused with other diseases of the hip joint, principally tuberculosis. In that year, there appeared three separately authored papers in the American,[6] French,[7] and German[8] literature distinguishing the condition as an entity. Though Perthes originally suggested the ischemic nature of the condition, the realization that it is an example of a process which may affect any epiphysis was not general until many years later.

Coxa plana is a relatively common orthopedic disease. It affects males more often than females in a proportion of about four to one. The peak age incidence is about six years though it may occur between the ages of three and twelve. It probably never starts, at least in its typical form, after twelve years though the regenerative stage may progress well into adolescence. It is bilateral in perhaps 10 per cent of cases.

The symptoms may be insidious in onset or sudden, the latter frequently associated with trauma. Pain of varying degrees of severity, limp and limitation of motion are usually the presenting complaints. The pain frequently starts in the knee region and may persist here for weeks or even months, obscuring the actual source. The pain may be referred to the inner thigh or the groin following the distribution of the obturator nerve. It is usually worse on activity and relieved by rest. Motion is often limited, particularly on internal rotation and in flexion and abduction. There may be anterior and posterior tenderness. Eventually the pain disappears spontaneously and motion is restored. If a limp persists it is due to mechanical factors rather than pain. At this time one may note minimal atrophy of the thigh muscles and eventually slight shortening (growth failure) of the involved extremity. Having run its course, the disease may leave a crippled hip, the patient adjusting his activity to the amount and type of joint impairment. In later adult life, an osteoarthritis often sets in because of the altered stress trajectories and weight-bearing surfaces.

Ischemic necrosis of the capital femoral epiphysis runs its morbid course in from two to six years. The earlier the onset the more severe the course and the greater the residuum are apt to be. It is usually divided into three active phases and a fourth or healed period of static altered joint and bone structure.

The first stage lasts from two weeks to two months. Because weeks or even months elapse before the changes in bone consequent to deprivation of its blood supply occur, the changes of the first period are those which appear in the soft tissue. There is swelling and a low-grade inflammatory reaction in the joint synovia and capsule. Eventually fibrosis with thickening intervenes.

During the second phase the predominant feature is a necrotizing process within the osseous nucleus and underlying chondral plate. The articular plate derives almost all of its nourishment from the joint fluid, and though there is edema and congestion of the soft tissues of the joint incident to the epiphyseal ischemia, the articular cartilage usually survives intact until its osseous support collapses. Then surface irregularities, flattening and spreading occur. The osseous nucleus dies in toto or in part. Since the enchondral plate derives its blood supply from the same vessels, it too usually softens. Enchondral growth is inhibited or stops completely. The second phase, that of necrosis, persists for from six to eighteen months or somewhat longer. Since the osseous nucleus is small and is supplied by more than one vessel, it is rare that the entire epiphyseal blood supply is lost. Thus, though the bone and contiguous cartilage die, granulation can still generate from the persisting mesenchymal cells. Deltas of new arterioles and capillaries bring in sufficient blood to partially demineralize the bone and weaken its supportive strength. It collapses and becomes condensed owing to stress pressures. It may fragment or give the appearance of fragmentation because of the inroads of granulation.

In the third phase the predominant feature is the replacement of dead tissue by new bone and cartilage. Its duration varies from a year to several years depending upon the size of the area affected, the availability of a new supply of vessels and the extent of the distortion which occurs in the second phase. If the original epiphyseal vessels are completely lost, the area must await granulation to penetrate from the metaphysis and during this period the lesion appears to be static. Eventually the debris of the dead bone, cartilage and marrow is removed and replaced by new bone, or by densely collagenized fibrous tissue. The flattened head, the shortened and thickened neck and the corresponding modeling changes which occur in the acetabulum remain as the residuum, sometimes referred to as the fourth phase.

ROENTGENOGRAPHIC MANIFESTATIONS

The radiographic manifestations of epiphyseal ischemic necrosis parallel the alterations in anatomy and physiology. These are the same no matter which epiphyseal center is involved, so that a discussion of the process as it involves the femoral capital epiphysis will apply to other epiphyses. The radiographic recognition of this process as it involves the hip is important because of the desirability of early treatment.

During the first stage of the disease there may be only meager radiographic changes, consisting of a bulging of the joint capsule, as a result of synovial thickening and fluid within the joint. The capsule

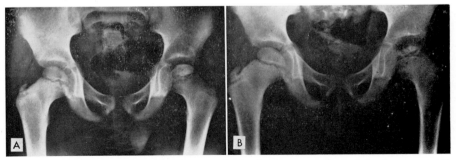

FIG. 162.   Epiphyseal ischemic necrosis. In the latter portion of the first stage (*A*) the opacity of the left femoral capital epiphysis is evident. The surrounding bony structures are demineralized which accentuates this opacity. The joint space is widened, the metaphysis is broad and more radiolucent than is normal and the femoral neck is deformed. One year later (*B*) fragmentation is evident and dead bone (opaque) may be seen. The joint space is wide. This radiograph represents the second stage of the process.

may be visualized by virtue of more radiolucent fat contiguous to it. At this time, minimal lateral displacement of the proximal femur in relation to the acetabulum may be appreciated. Later the femoral capital epiphyseal center appears more opaque than is normal. This does not represent a real increase in mineral content. Instead, it is caused by demineralization of the surrounding bony structures as a result of disuse secondary to pain or immobilization or hyperemia coupled with persistent mineralization of the epiphyseal center. This cannot demineralize because its blood supply is lost. The radiolucent epiphyseal line widens and becomes irregular, often showing frank cystic changes. The epiphyseal line undergoes such alteration because its blood supply is absent; it is supplied by the same vessels that nourish the epiphysis.

The second stage is characterized by opacity, fragmentation and flattening of the epiphyseal center. These changes reflect the invasion of the necrotic epiphyseal center by granulation tissue and the effects of stress on this weakened structure. The increase in opacity of the epiphyseal center now is probably real and reflects the collapse of the center and apposition of its fragments.

In the third stage or healing stage, new bone is formed and the outline of the epiphyseal center again becomes regular and intact. Often the process will appear to be completely healed on radiographs made in the anterior-posterior projection, but when the hip is examined in the lateral projection radiolucent areas may be evident.

In addition to the changes in the epiphyseal center itself, alterations occur in the metaphysis as a result of which the femoral neck becomes broad and short. The acetabulum must adapt itself to the flat, broad femoral head. Thus, the fourth stage is represented by a short, broad femoral neck which is often angled anteriorly more than is normal; a flat, broad head; and an enlarged acetabulum that cor-

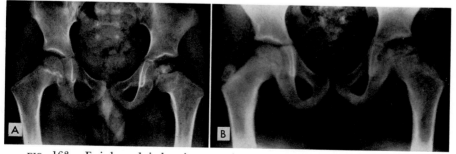

FIG. 163.   Epiphyseal ischemic necrosis. *A* illustrates the second stage of the process. In *B,* 28 months later, the femoral capital epiphyseal center is nearly reconstituted. It is flat and adaptive changes in the acetabulum and deformity of the femoral neck are apparent. This represents the third stage of the disease process.

responds roughly in shape to the femoral head. The fourth stage is represented by the final deformity of the hip joint.

PATHOLOGIC MORPHOLOGY

Pathologists have had little opportunity of studying the lesion as a whole since the disease is not fatal and rarely has the orthopedist resorted to resection of the entire head and neck as a means of therapy. Since modern treatment with reasonably early diagnosis is entirely conservative and without surgery, adequate material, even fragments, has rarely been available for conclusive studies. Our information has been picked bit by bit from a number of sources. When this is fitted together and correlated with the clinical and roentgenographic details, the lesion emerges as an area of bone and cartilage which has been deprived of a blood supply adequate for continued life and health.

Gall and Bennett[9] had the opportunity of doing an autopsy study on a patient with coxa plana who died of secondary parathyroid hyperplasia and kidney failure. The head of the femur was flattened and though the articular surface was widened and irregular it was still intact. The osseous nucleus was necrotic, compressed and fragmented. There was evidence of old hemorrhage, cystic degeneration and replacement fibrosis. The enchondral plate was softened and distorted, the epiphyseal line irregular and, in the central portion, completely replaced by fibrous granulation growing in from the metaphysis.

The paper of Zemansky[10] gives one of the most complete descriptions of the microscopy. The cytologic findings depend upon the phase in which the lesion is sectioned. In the first phase, the bone and cartilage are intact though one may note changes in or death of the osteocytes. The vessels are dilated and filled with static blood. Degenerative changes soon become apparent in the marrow. The contiguous soft tissues reflect the altered physiology of the vascular accident. The synovial membranes and capsule are thickened by congestion and edema (Fig. 164). The dilated vessels may be circled by small aggregates of lymphocytes. If the stasis persists long enough, a fibroblastic action eventually takes place. In the second phase one finds irregular fragments of well preserved dead bone interspersed with areas of necrotic bone which is undergoing lysis. Between and around the fragments there is granulation. The cartilage of the enchondral plate may show enlargement of its lacunae and distortion of the cellular pattern. The soft interspicular tissue is converted to an amorphous mass (Fig. 165) of extravasated red cells, degenerating fat and marrow cell debris. Shadow cells may be discernible such as those that appear

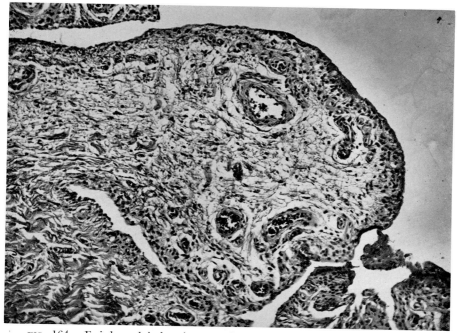

FIG. 164.   Epiphyseal ischemic necrosis (Perthes' disease). Section through the synovial lining of the joint. A villous process is pictured. It is thickened by edema and a mild inflammatory process. (× 180.)

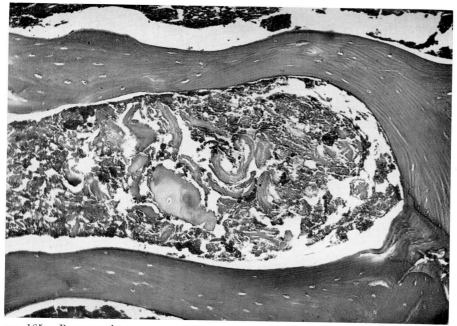

FIG. 165.   Between the two arms of this bone spicule there is a mass of necrotic debris with flakes of bone and soft tissue intermixed. (× 180.)

in soft tissue infarcts. Osteoclasts are in evidence and there may be occasional giant cells. Masses of tissue with a microscopic resemblance to giant cell tumor have been described. Such an extravagant giant cell reaction has never occurred in our material and it is rarely noted in the literature.

During the third phase there is a gradual lysis of dead bone and cartilage by newly formed granulation. The rate of granulation formation is dependent upon the extent to which a healthy vascular bed has been retained around the necrotic nucleus. If all the blood supply to the epiphysis has been obliterated, the necrotic center may have to wait until granulation grows up from the metaphysis before a sufficient blood and macrophage supply can accomplish lysis. Irregular masses of cartilage and bone may be found. It is difficult to be certain whether these are newly formed as a part of the repair process or the residuum of areas whose blood supply was less severely jeopardized than the necrotic fragments. In some cases the destroyed area is eventually replaced by a densely collagenized mass which extends from the under surface of the remaining articular cartilage to, and to merge with, the fibrous tissue of the metaphyseal medullary area. In some cases this area is converted to bone and then resembles a closed, albeit deformed, epiphysis.

PROGNOSIS

The course and ultimate deformity of coxa plana depend upon the age of onset, the number of vessels occluded and, thereby, the size of the epiphyseal infarct and finally the amount of usage to which the injured member is put. In general, the damage is apt to be greater in the younger age group, from three to six years. Most orthopedists agree that some motion in the healing stage acts as a stimulus to new bone growth. The stress must be so calculated that it will encourage and not distort the newly formed epiphyseal structures. Sometimes surgery is necessary to remove large areas of dead tissue which might never resolve or to reshape a deformed articular plate or femoral neck which would handicap normal motion when healing is at last achieved.

OSTEOCHONDRITIS DISSECANS

Osteochondritis dissecans is essentially a type of epiphyseal ischemic necrosis in which only a peripheral segment of the bony epiphysis is involved. Since in the unclosed epiphysis of childhood its blood supply and that of the metaphysis is almost entirely separate, usually the entire bony nucleus or a considerable portion is involved when the epiphyseal vessels are affected because there is insufficient collateral circulation from the metaphysis. This results in epiphyseal ischemic necrosis. Consequently, though osteochondritis dissecans can occur at any age its most frequent incidence is shortly after epiphyseal closure, in late adolescence and young adults.

A fragment of the peripheral osseous epiphysis underlying the articular cartilage undergoes ischemic necrosis. A plane of cleavage separates the dead fragment from the surrounding healthy bone and eventually it may loosen and fall out into the joint space taking along the layer of healthy cartilage which covers it. The cartilage remains viable since it derives its nutrition from the synovial fluid, until the trauma incident to its dislodgement may cause it to degenerate.

Loose joint bodies associated with an epiphyseal defect were probably first described by Alexander Monro[11] and later in 1870 by Sir James Paget,[12] but it was König[13] who described the lesion as an entity in 1888 and gave it the name by which it is known today.

Osteochondritis dissecans is a rather common orthopedic condition. Lavener[14] found 33 cases in 891 roentgenograms of the knee region. This is probably somewhat higher than the general incidence since his material was military service personnel and the disease is more frequent in active young adult males. In most series the peak incidence occurs between the ages of fifteen and twenty-five and one frequently finds the statement that it is rarely seen in children. However, Green and Banks[15] were able to collect 27 cases in patients under fifteen years of age. In reviewing the literature they were able to find reports of only 9 cases in children.

The disease has about the same male predominance as epiphyseal ischemic necrosis, i.e., four to one, though in at least one series the ratio was as high as thirteen to one. In perhaps 10 per cent of cases two or more lesions are found. Multiple lesions have a tendency to be symmetrical. Osteochondritis dissecans is sometimes associated with one or more lesions of epiphyseal ischemic necrosis.

Osteochondritis dissecans may be symptomless and found incidentally on roentgenograms made for other reasons. More often it causes mild to moderately severe pain in the affected joint. The onset may be sudden or insidious. There is usually some limitation of extreme motion and moderate disability. Eventually, there may be muscle weakness and some disuse atrophy. In a few cases the fragment of bone and cartilage which has become loose in the joint has caused locking. In some instances there is swelling and joint effusion. There may be tenderness.

The process usually runs its course over a period of months. The

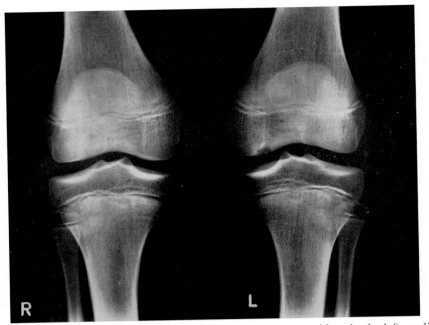

FIG. 166.   Osteochondritis dissecans. A radiolucent defect is evident in the left medial femoral condyle. A tiny fragment of bone is seen within this defect.

defect caused by the separation of the bone and cartilage fragment becomes filled with fibrous scar and the continuity of the articular surface is reestablished though an indentation often remains. If the fragment does not interfere with normal joint motion the patient may become symptomless after a year or more. This is particularly true of cases occurring in children. In adults, pain and disability are apt to persist until surgical intervention.

Ischemic necrosis of a segment of the bony arch which supports the articular cartilage has occurred in most of the weight-supporting bones of the skeleton, but in about 85 per cent of the cases the medial condyle of the femur is involved. No completely satisfactory explanation of this incidence has been offered. Other sites occasionally encountered are the femoral head, the elbow (capitellum), the distal humerus, the head of the humerus and the superior aspect of the astragalus. Involvement of other regions is something of a rarity. In the commonest site, the medial femoral condyle, an area of bone necrosis appears on its lateral border, extending to the margin of the intercondylar fossa adjacent to the posterior cruciate ligament. A circumscribed segment of the arch of bone which supports the articular cartilage dies and then goes on to necrosis. Pressure causes it to collapse so that a depressed area occurs in the overlying articular plate. Just as in an infarct of soft tissue, a zone of hemorrhage occurs about the dead fragment and soon a capsule of granulation tissue is formed. This granulation, bringing with it an increased blood supply, nibbles away the surface of the infarcted dead fragment until a line of separation is established. The lesion now is essentially a sequestrum. The disc of cartilage which overlies the dead fragment usually survives since it does not depend upon the epiphyseal vessels for its nourishment, though as its support gives way it becomes indented to mark the trouble-spot beneath. As a sequestrum, the lesion may persist indefinitely in this state. Sometimes the lysis of the surface of the dead fragment is so extensive that it is completely separated from the surrounding bone, though often the densely collagenized fibrous tissue arising from the granulation may bind it in place. If the loosening process predominates without much scar formation the piece may drop out, taking with it the overlying disc of living cartilage. A vascularized pedicle may persist and tie the loose fragment to its original bed, or the diseased bone tissue and its associated cartilage may be freed to become a loose joint body.

MORBID ANATOMY

The ischemic area of bone is first demarcated by an area of congestion and then a zone of hemorrhage (Fig. 167). If sectioned at

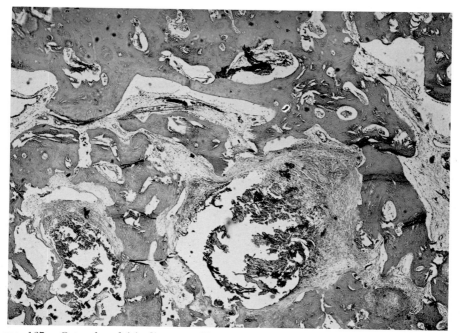

FIG. 167.   Osteochondritis dissecans. Two small areas of hemorrhage surrounded by zones of fibrosis in the bone contiguous to the articular plate. (× 15.)

this time, the bone of the central nidus will be seen to be dead or dying; that is, the lamellae will remain intact but the osteocytes within the lacunae will be lacking or show degenerative change. Next, granulation begins to creep in from the surrounding healthy vessels and soon the hemorrhagic area becomes organized and the dead bone melts away along the advancing granulation surface. Tongues of granulation insinuate themselves along the haversian canals and interspicular spaces bringing sufficient fresh blood and phagocytes to cause bone necrosis. The fate of the lesion now depends upon the degree to which a new vasculature may be supplied. If it is minimal the granulation matures and the crater in the bony epiphysis becomes lined with dense fibrous tissue. If it is more adequate the fragment becomes loosened and eventually detached.

The behavior of the affected cartilage is interesting. Abnormal pressure incident to its lack of support or change in position may cause it to degenerate. If it escapes this fate it may survive even though the fragment becomes completely detached. In this circumstance it usually proliferates to form a complete capsule about the necrotic bone nidus and thus the loose body may become spheroid and actually increase in size.

It cannot be said that the cause of osteochondritis dissecans is known, since the obstructed or interrupted vessels have not actually been demonstrated. The theory of trauma has always been emphasized, and a history of trauma, either acute or chronic, can be obtained in approximately 50 per cent of the cases. It is possible that acute trauma may cause avulsion of an epiphyseal fragment in a few cases in certain sites. However, the most frequently involved areas, such as the medial femoral condyle, are so well protected from acute trauma that it is difficult to accept this as a cause even in those cases in which it appears in the history. Chronic trauma undoubtedly plays a role but its mechanism is almost surely through a thrombosing action upon the vessels. The mechanism of osteochondritis dissecans is almost certainly an ischemic necrosis. Chronic trauma may cause the ischemia by thrombosing the vessels and acute trauma may be the trigger mechanism which dislodges the diseased fragment. It is probable that infection may occasionally cause thrombosis and rarely an embolus may occlude the precise vessel which supplies the area. It is probable, however, that the common sites and the prevalent age incidence are the result of factors conditioned by the development of the normal vasculature pattern. It seems likely that an area on the lateral aspect of the medial femoral condyle is involved in about 85 per cent of the cases because this area normally has a narrow margin of vascular reserve after the epiphysis is ossified.

ANEURYSMAL BONE CYST

Aneurysmal bone cyst is a curious, solitary lesion of bone which has been so named because typically it causes a bulging of the overlying cortex, bearing some semblance to the saccular protrusion of the aortic wall in true aneurysm. The name has caused a good deal of confusion because the lesion happens to be vascular and therefore has been interpreted as an aneurysm of a bone vessel, which it may be, but which implication is not intended by the descriptive name applied.

Ewing, in his first edition (1919) of Neoplastic Diseases, alludes to two lesions in bone which are probably aneurysmal bone cysts, but he classifies them as hemangiomas of bone. In his third edition (1928) he uses the term "malignant bone aneurysm" as a synonym of telangiectatic osteogenic sarcoma and also describes an aneurysmal variant of giant cell tumor which almost certainly is an aneurysmal bone cyst. Until quite recently a number of papers have appeared giving recognizable descriptions of this lesion, but they were always interpreted as vascular variants of other conditions. In 1942, Jaffe and Lichtenstein in their paper on solitary cyst of bone[16] devoted considerable space to the description of two of their cases, each manifesting a large cyst of bone filled with a spongy mass of blood channels. They coined the term "aneurysmal cyst." Eight years later, both had collected sufficient cases to recognize the lesion as an entity and to present their material in separate papers.[17, 18] More recently Dahlin et al.[19] have published a series of 26 cases which were seen at the Mayo Clinic in the period from 1905 to 1952. Most of these cases were misdiagnosed both radiologically and by tissue examination because the features of the lesion had not yet been described. It is obvious that the incidence of this condition is still unknown, but it is probable that it is considerably more common than we have suspected, even in the recent past.

Aneurysmal bone cyst has been found in patients of almost every age over three and under fifty, but about half of them occur in the second decade and most of the rest in the third. Though there has been a female predominance in some series, as more adequate figures are collected it appears that there is no sex predilection. Many of the earlier cases involved the bodies, neural arches and spines of the vertebrae and for a time it appeared that these were the sites most frequently affected, but now it is known that aneurysmal bone cyst probably may involve any bone of the skeleton and that vertebral lesions constitute no more than a quarter of the cases.

Aneurysmal bone cyst usually causes pain. It may be of several weeks' or several months' duration. When a vertebra is affected, severe muscle spasm may be responsible for most of the symptoms or, if there is compression of the cord or nerve roots, the pain may be referred. Though the lesion rarely invades the joint structures, it may occur in the end of a long bone near a joint and thus cause joint pain and disability. Usually before diagnosis is made there is swelling of the area. This has been variously interpreted but the enlargement is actually due to "expansion" of the cortex which overlies the medullary soft tissue mass. The "swelling" is usually accompanied by tenderness. If intervention is delayed, aneurysmal bone cyst may grow to huge proportions. Since it causes lysis of the bone in which it resides and erosion of contiguous bone structures, destruction severe enough to necessitate amputation may eventuate. In the late cases, this disproportionate anatomic distortion makes the diagnosis of malignant bone tumor plausible. In almost every reported series at least one case has been so diagnosed and amputation resorted to. For this reason alone it is mandatory that all orthopedists, radiologists and pathologists learn the diagnostic features of this innocuous lesion.

Aneurysmal bone cyst always begins in cancellous or medullary structures. It may arise at any point in the shaft but it most often affects the ends of the diaphysis, often very close to the epiphyseal line when it involves cylindrical bones. Whether it begins centrally in the medullary tissues and expands further in one direction than another or whether it always begins beneath the compacta is impossible to say, since it cannot be identified on the roentgenograms until the cortex is involved. It apparently has a remarkable lytic propensity because the overlying compacta melts away before it as it expands. The contiguous periosteum is pushed outward and reacts by laying down a thin shell of bone which must be continuously replaced as its inner layers are eroded away. Thus, a bulky structure soon protrudes from the uninvolved cortical surface, pushing soft tissues before it and eroding other bones on contact. It is this appearance and behavior that has given rise to the name aneurysmal bone cyst. When large cylindrical and flat bones are affected the lesion has a saccular, eccentric structure. In shorter or more slender bones the entire circumference is involved and the lesion has a fusiform shape. Aneurysmal bone cyst is a disturbance of the vasculature of marrow tissue. As such it never begins in the cartilaginous epiphysis and rarely, if ever, invades it. After the epiphysis is ossified it may be involved in the process but it is unusual for the lesion to transgress the articular plate and invade the joint cavity. The lesion may grow to a huge size (Fig. 168). Aneurysmal bone cysts over 20 cm. in diameter have been described.

Regardless of size the periosteum manages to maintain a covering

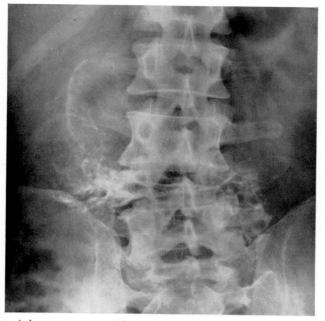

FIG. 168. A huge aneurysmal bone cyst arising from a vertebra. The body has been destroyed and the cyst has ballooned out into the abdominal cavity. A mistaken diagnosis of inoperable malignant tumor was made and the patient was watched until the cyst ruptured and the patient was exsanguinated.

shell of bone but eventually this thin shell fractures and the bloody contents of the lesion extravasate into the soft tissues. Now the lesion becomes much more difficult to recognize because it is essentially a massive hematoma accompanied by the usual reaction of muscle, fat and fibrous tissue to the presence of free blood. The advent of rupture may result in an alarming increase in the rate of growth, inspiring the clinical diagnosis of malignant neoplasm. Excessive lysis may weaken the bone to the point of fracture and erosion of neighboring bones may give the appearance of invasion. Thus, the radiologist is apt to fall into the same trap as the clinician. If the pathologist fails to recognize the lesion for what it is or if the surgeon fails to obtain diagnosable tissue, the condition is almost certain to be misdiagnosed and an amputation may be performed. If a high index of suspicion were maintained and all irregular features of the clinical, radiologic and pathologic aspects carefully considered, this tragedy would occur less often.

ROENTGENOGRAPHIC MANIFESTATIONS

Radiographically an aneurysmal bone cyst presents as a radiolucent area with the density of soft tissue within which are multiple

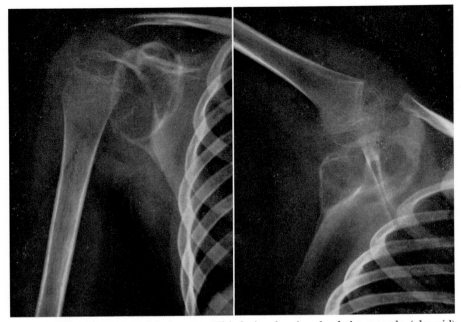

FIG. 169.   Aneurysmal bone cyst. This lesion has involved the scapula (glenoid) of a seven year old white boy. The glenoid is enlarged by the expanding radiolucent lesion. Note the incomplete septa within it, and its scalloped borders. Periosteal new bone defines its extent.

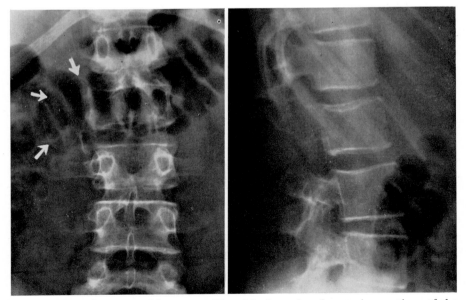

FIG. 170.   Aneurysmal bone cyst. The right lateral and posterior portions of the second lumbar vertebra are involved. There is partial collapse of the lateral portion of the body, the pedicles and lamina are destroyed and the lesion extends well beyond the confines of the vertebra. It is covered by a thin shell of bone (arrows).

fine, often incomplete septa. It is an expanding lesion with sharply demarcated scalloped borders. The lesion erodes bone and after cortical destruction it is covered by a shell of periosteal new bone. At times, rupture and disruption of this thin shell of bone may occur.

The typical aneurysmal bone cyst begins in the cancellous portion of a long bone. It may be centrally or eccentrically located in either the mid-diaphysis or near the end of the shaft. The lesion has been described as parosteal in location[19a] with the bulk of the tumor in the soft tissues and only slight underlying cortical erosion. When a vertebra is involved, it is usually the neural arch that is the site of the lesion.

MORBID ANATOMY

Aneurysmal bone cyst is essentially an aggregate of thick-walled channels carrying streams of blood. Judging from the color of the lesion the blood is probably venous rather than arterial. One important feature to be kept in mind is the fact that the blood is not a stagnant pool but unclotted and in motion, so that there must be a constant supply at one end and a continuous drainage at the other. A second feature is that the tubes which contain this stream of blood are not true vessel walls since they contain no elastic or muscle lamina and in most areas are not even lined with endothelium.

The name aneurysmal bone cyst is misleading in more ways than one since the lesion is not a true cyst. It only appears to be a cyst on the roentgenogram. Actually, it is a sponge-like structure composed of a mass of tangled, interwoven tubes which transport a stream or streams of blood. This excessive blood supply to the area probably accounts for the deossification of normal bone which characterizes the process.

When the surgeon removes a portion of the covering bony shell he usually finds what appears to be a well of blood which bleeds freely and steadily. There is no pulsation. When probed, however, what appears to be a pool is found to be partitioned by tissue walls. Hemorrhage may be exceedingly difficult to control since tangible structures concealed in blood are elusive, retreating into a formless mass as they are approached. The blood spaces are frequently larger in the central portion of the lesion. Sometimes there is considerably more solid matter separating the blood sinuses and then the structure resembles a sponge soaked in blood. When the tissue has been removed and drained, it is found to constitute only a fraction of the mass which filled the exposed cavity. The walls may continue to bleed steadily.

Within the bone the lesion is moderately well circumscribed. If

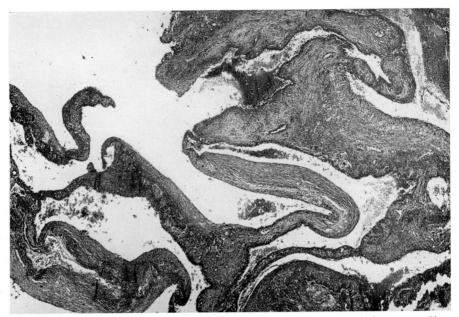

FIG. 171.   Section through the spongy portion of an aneurysmal bone cyst. Since the blood has drained away the sinuses have collapsed but their thick fibrous walls are apparent. (× 30.)

rupture into soft tissue has taken place, the reaction to extravasated blood conceals the margins of the process and makes the selection of representative tissue for biopsy exceedingly difficult. In the area of bone destruction about the periphery of the sinus mass and sometimes within it there are apt to be solid areas of soft tissue. The surgeon is tempted to select these for biopsy. These areas are usually the product of reaction of the injured bone and fibrous tissue rather than the culprit which is causing the injury. Thus, the issue may be confused by the pathologist who must read what he sees rather than what is left behind.

Through the microscope, the aneurysmal bone cyst appears to be a mass of communicating spaces containing fluid blood surrounded and supported by fibrous walls of varying thickness (Fig. 171). There is no organized elastic lamina and if muscle fibers are present they are lost in the collagen of the fibrous tissue which is the main constituent of the walls. Often, slender, smooth spicules of bone are found in the partitions, apparently the product of fibro-osseous metaplasia (Fig. 172). Hemosiderin granules are frequently prominent. Giant cell reaction occurs wherever there has been spillage of blood. In areas, whole fields will have a fibrous matrix and sufficient giant cells to suggest the diagnosis of giant cell tumor or brown tumor of parathyroid adenoma. These fields are usually the solid areas about the periphery of the sinus mass. It is this appearance which accounts for the all too frequent diagnosis of eccentric or subperiosteal giant cell tumor. In an attempt to repair bone defects and infractions there may be a brisk proliferation of new bone and cartilage. The appearance of active osteoblasts or chondroblasts may mislead the pathologist into the diagnosis of osteosarcoma or chondrosarcoma. If the lesion is described by the radiologist as a cyst, and if this is not corrected by the surgeon who fails to obtain sinus material for microscopic study, the pathologist has but one choice of diagnosis, solitary cyst, since the tissue lining a solitary cyst and that surrounding an aneurysmal bone cyst are identical.

There are few clues to the cause and mechanism of aneurysmal bone cyst. It is not a hemangioma nor, indeed, any type of neoplasm since it does not have the microscopic constituents of a true tumor. It has been suggested that an alteration in circulatory dynamics has produced a mass of varicosed venous channels. Against this is the lack of venous wall structure and the bone lysing propensities of the lesion, the latter suggesting that the excess of blood is active rather than passive. Hypothetically, an arteriovenous communication through a plexus of fibrous channels would supply most or all of the criteria found in aneurysmal bone cyst. Congenital arteriovenous fistulas are found in various tissues of the body including bone. They usually

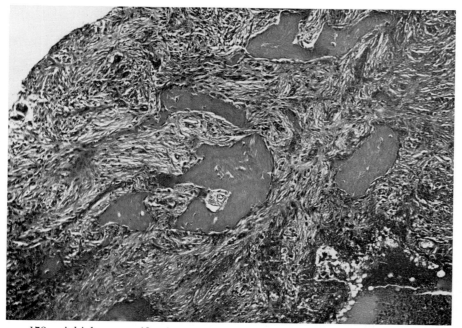

FIG. 172.   A higher magnification through the wall of a sinus of an aneurysmal bone cyst. Spicules of bone are often seen.

result from a failure of complete differentiation of arteries and veins. True congenital aneurysms may form because of a failure of development of the arterial muscle coat. Arteriovenous fistulas are usually associated with varicosities of the associated veins. Against this hypothesis is the frequent occurrence of pulsation in congenital fistula (not reported in aneurysmal bone cyst), birth marks of the skin are frequently associated and though there are no reports of gasometric analysis of the blood in aneurysmal bone cyst, it appears to be no more highly oxygenated than ordinary venous blood.

PROGNOSIS

The destruction of bone in aneurysmal bone cyst appears to be the consequence of an excessive supply of blood to a localized area. Anything which reduces that supply to the normal level should arrest the progress of the disease. This has been found to be true. The lesion may be treated either surgically or by irradiation. The former has usually been used because by the time the diagnosis is made the protruding mass is best handled by excision. It has been shown that even a partial curettement with no attempt to remove all of the vascular tissue has resulted in a cure. There was recurrence in at least one reported case but certainly this is the rare exception.

SOLITARY CYST OF BONE

Solitary cyst (solitary unicameral cyst) is an entity, distinct from other cystic and fibrous lesions of bone, occurring for the most part at the ends of the large cylindrical bones of the extremities in the growing skeleton. It is the only purely cystic lesion of bone.

The term "bone cyst" has been used loosely in the past and still is used, regrettably, in designating a wide variety of bone lesions whose roentgenograms reveal sharply delineated, smooth-walled areas of translucency. A cyst is a collection of gas or fluid enclosed in a capsule. Because the x-ray cannot distinguish between fluid and soft tissue, numerous proliferative lesions which contain no opaque bone salts are casually categorized as "bone cysts." This leads to unnecessary confusion and misunderstanding between the roentgenologist and the pathologist. The clinician is sometimes at a loss to know what either is talking about.

It is true that cystic lesions characteristically occur in a few other bone diseases—parathyroid adenoma (osteitis fibrosa cystica) and less often fibrous dysplasia—but the "cysts" are merely areas of degeneration in proliferative processes and though they contain fluid they should be designated as areas of liquefaction necrosis rather than cysts.

Solitary cysts have been described in the skeleton since the days of Virchow but it was not until the early part of the present century[20] that it was realized that they are an entity apart from osteitis fibrosa cystica and, later, fibrous dysplasia. The more recent account of Jaffe and Lichtenstein[21] adequately summarizes the modern concept of the condition.

Solitary cyst is a disease of the growing skeleton. In the Jaffe-Lichtenstein series of 19 cases, 15 patients were between three and fourteen years of age. One was forty-two. In our own material there are 38 patients, all are under the age of twenty-three years and all but five range between three and seventeen. In almost all series there has been a male preponderance. Of our cases, only 5 of the 38 are in females.

It has been said that solitary cyst occurs only in cylindrical bone and there can be no argument that the large bones of the extremities are the ones most consistently involved. Among our cases two diagnoses of bone cyst were made on lesions in the os calcis and one in a ramus of the pubic bone. Admittedly, neither the microscopy nor roentgenograms of solitary cyst are absolutely specific but when these features are combined with the gross appearance of a fluid-containing bone cyst lined with a thin layer of soft tissue, there is almost no other diagnosis which may be considered. One of the os calcis lesions occurred in a medical student who has been followed after conservative therapy for eight years. It seems highly improbable that the diagnosis is in error.

Lesions in the ends of the femur, the proximal humerus and the proximal tibia will account for approximately nine-tenths of the cases. The incidence is probably in the order named with the proximal femur being the commonest site, despite the preponderant involvement of the upper humerus in some of the earlier series.

Since solitary bone cyst develops very slowly, it rarely, if ever, of itself causes pain. Pain ensues when the overlying cortex is thinned to the point of pathologic fracture. Consequently, though pain is the usual presenting symptom, a roentgenogram will most often reveal a fracture through the wall of an already well established bone cyst. If no fracture lines are apparent it is probable that one or more undemonstrable infractions have involved the periosteal sensory structure.

Because these lesions are symptomless until fracture there has been little opportunity of studying them in the early phase of their development. Occasionally a bone cyst is discovered in x-ray surveys done for another reason. The lesion probably always begins in the spongy bone of the metaphysis, either in contiguity with or near the epiphyseal line. It expands slowly, widening until it occupies the entire diameter of the medullary region and extending through the shaft toward the mid-diaphysis. As it enlarges it first abuts against the surrounding compacta and then slowly erodes it from the inside. As the cortex thins, some appositional bone is laid down on the exterior surface by the periosteum so that the bone becomes expanded, but apparently the stimulus for periosteal bone formation is so gentle that external new bone formation does not keep pace with inner erosion and the expanding wall becomes thinner and thinner until fracture occurs.

Though most lesions are confined to the metaphyseal region and contiguous portion of the shaft, a few very large cysts may expand to involve almost the entire diaphysis. This probably accounts for those rare cysts which are found occupying the mid-third of the shaft; that is, they probably started in the metaphysis and extended to involve that half of the bone, then crossed the mid-point to involve the mid-diaphyseal portion of the remaining half. Since the cysts heal from the metaphyseal pole, the unhealed residuum would eventually come to lie within the middle third of the diaphysis. If this is in fact what happens, this would contradict the most widely accepted theory of pathogenesis, i.e., that of osteogenic defect in the epiphyseal line.

In its typical form the cyst occurs in the end of a large cylindrical bone in the extremity of a patient between the ages of three and seventeen. It may have caused some expansion of the overlying cortex and this "egg-shell" covering often has the slate or bluish discoloration of the blue-domed cysts of the breast. There is almost always a band of normal bone interposed between the cyst and the epiphyseal line.

Because the cyst begins in the metaphysis, possibly immediately contiguous to the epiphyseal line, the band of normal tissue represents the amount of longitudinal bone growth since the establishment of the lesion. As the bone continues to grow, an illusion of drifting of the cyst toward the mid-diaphysis is created. Attempts have been made to judge the age of the lesion by its distance from the epiphyseal line. It has been stated that cysts which appear very near the line are still actively growing and that therapy at this time is more apt to result in a recurrence than if it is in the "latent phase" more deeply situated in the shaft. It is difficult to evaluate this hypothesis but the evidence is probably insufficient to warrant postponement of therapy and risk of further fracture and deformity. A few very large cysts have been observed to impair normal bone growth. When a window is cut in the cyst wall, it is found to contain fluid though it need not be filled. Sometimes incision through the thin, expanded cortex results in a fountain of fluid which may actually spout a centimeter or more because of the intracystic pressure. Usually the fluid is amber though it may be almost clear or have the appearance of pure blood and occasionally it may be clotted. The cyst is lined with a thin layer, often not more than a millimeter in thickness, of red, brown or less often pale membrane. The cyst is unilocular and the wall is usually quite smooth, though it may be traversed by narrow ridges of bone. The lining may be curetted away leaving a more or less complete wall of bone.

ROENTGENOGRAPHIC MANIFESTATIONS

The roentgenographic manifestation of a solitary cyst of bone is a radiolucent defect involving the spongiosa near the end of a long bone. The defect is round or oval and is of the density of soft tissue because it has a wall of soft tissue and contains fluid. The distance between the cyst and the metaphysis varies, probably depending upon the duration of the process. Although expansion of the shaft may occur, the defect is usually no wider than the adjacent metaphysis.

Periosteal new bone is not a feature of this lesion even though the cortex may become quite thin because the migration and erosion of

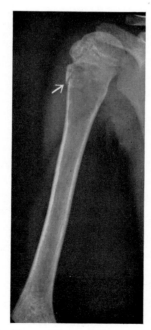

FIG. 173.   Solitary cyst of bone. The radiolucent defect is evident in the proximal humeral diaphysis. Bone separates its superior aspect from the metaphysis. No septa are evident within the lesion. There is a fracture (arrow) through the thinned cortex.

the cyst are so slow. Fracture through the cyst is common. In this instance, the integrity of the cortex over the lesion is lost and deformity may be present. Periosteal new bone is seen as the fracture heals. There is little bone reaction about the cyst, probably because the process is so slow. Its outline is evident by virtue of contrast between bone and the fluid and soft tissue of the cyst.

MICROSCOPY

The microscopic sections only corroborate the clinical and roentgen diagnosis. There are no pathognomonic features about the tissue which is curetted from the bony walls. It usually consists of a more or less definite membrane of moderately young fibrocytes of a rather loose texture intermixed with masses of more deeply staining fibrin (Fig. 174A). The amount of collagen varies considerably. At times it is quite densely collagenized or it may consist almost wholly of quite young granulation. Considerable amounts of granular, yellow-brown pigment are usually in evidence within macrophages and scattered through the intercellular areas. Most of this pigment is hemosiderin and takes the Prussian blue reaction. Its erythrocytic origin is often obvious because of the aggregates of red cells in various stages of degeneration. Pools of recently extravasated blood are sometimes seen. Xanthoid cells whose cytoplasm is swollen and pale with quantities of lipid may occur singly or in small groups. In some areas this material may collect in the intercellular spaces to form masses of fusiform, sharp-pointed crystals. These dissolve in the processing fluid to leave characteristic clefts usually surrounded by collagen. Giant cells occur in varying numbers, their cytoplasm containing lipid, pigment or cell debris (Fig. 174B). They may be clustered about an area of hemorrhage or diffusely scattered throughout the granulation matrix. It is the presence of these cells surrounded by young fibrocytes which has led to the contention that this lesion is a variant of the giant cell tumor of bone. If the material is scant, as it often is, and predominantly composed of this type of tissue, it may be exceedingly difficult to differentiate the cyst wall from the solid masses of giant cell reaction which occur in the metaphyseal region in response to bone injury and hemorrhage, a lesion which is commonly mistaken for benign giant cell tumor. The gross description will usually make the distinction clear because the giant cell reactions are not truly cystic. Bone tissue is usually lacking in the sections but there may be a few irregular fragments of the compacta which have been dislodged by the curette or even some spicules of immature bone from a fracture site or from the subperiosteal region. Osteogenesis is usually not

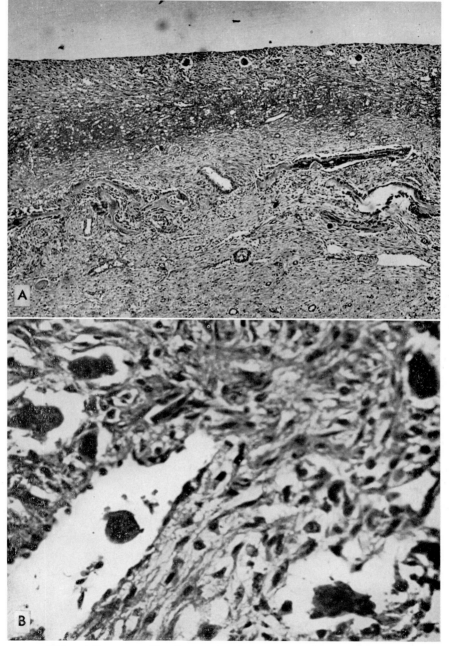

FIG. 174.   *A*, Low magnification (× 40) through the wall of a solitary cyst. There is a fibrous wall containing a few spicules of new bone in its deeper portion. In the superficial layer (above) there is a layer of blood, perhaps the residuum of the original hematoma, and a covering of fibrin. *B*, Higher magnification (× 396) showing a fibroblastic reaction with several giant cells.

prominent enough to suggest the possibility of osteosarcoma. The diagnoses of non-osteogenic fibroma and subperiosteal cortical defect cannot be eliminated on the appearance of the sections alone.

PATHOGENESIS

The pathogenesis of solitary cyst of bone has been the subject of concern of a number of writers. When at last solitary cyst was separated from osteitis fibrosa cystica (parathyroid adenoma) it was reclassified as a variant of giant cell tumor. When rescued from this group it became tempting to speculate on the cause and mechanism of its development. Mikulicz suggested that since the lesion occurred in growing bone it was probably the result of mechanical trauma to an area of bone growth in the epiphyseal line, creating a defect where enchondral bone formation failed to occur resulting in a hiatus which presented as a cyst. Jaffe and Lichtenstein supported this theory and there is much in favor of it, particularly the age group affected. The evidence which appears to contradict this idea is found in those cysts which cross the mid-diaphyseal point. If the cyst is a defect resulting from failure of bone formation in an area of one epiphyseal line, then the defect could involve only the portion of the diaphysis normally formed by that epiphyseal structure. Admittedly, the two epiphyses of a cylindrical bone are not necessarily responsible for an equal amount of the intervening shaft, but in those unusual cases where the cyst has involved two-thirds or more of the diaphysis it is probable that the lesion could not be caused by a defect at one end.

Pommer suggested that the solitary cyst is the result of a hemorrhage into the growing metaphysis. In organization a fibrous wall forms about the extravasated blood which clots and then undergoes liquefaction. The surrounding fibrous capsule acts as a semipermeable membrane and if the specific gravity of the intracystic content is higher than that of the surrounding tissue, water is drawn into the cyst. As the pressure within the wall increases the cyst expands, causing pressure erosion on the surrounding cancellous tissue and then cortex. Eventually, the extra- and intracystic densities are equalized and the process ceases and is now said to be in its latent stage. This theory is attractive for the following reasons. Such expanding cysts are fairly common following subdural hemorrhage. Sections of the bone cyst wall are compatible with the appearance of the capsule about old hemorrhage; there are fibrosis, cholesterol, giant cells, pigment and degenerating red cells. The contained fluid is characteristic of liquefied hematoma. There is sometimes increased pressure within the cyst wall. Sometimes the cyst content is frankly bloody. The age incidence and prevalent sites are harder to explain. It is true that in the growing bone the metaphysis is more vascular and probably less sturdy than after the epiphysis is ossified. It is probably worthy of mention that these areas in the lower extremities may be traumatized by traction when infants are lifted by the feet in changing diapers and in the upper extremities when they are held by the arms in learning to walk.

Against the theory is the apparent fact that patients with hemophilia, in which one expects a high incidence of intramedullary hemorrhage, do not show a high incidence of solitary bone cysts. Also, though the hemorrhages which occur in parathyroid adenoma may produce areas of cystic degeneration, the brown tumors of this disturbance are quite different from solitary bone cyst.

The occasional cyst which occurs in the adult is difficult to explain. Most of them probably represent the residuum of a lesion which developed during childhood or adolescence. The reasons for their quiescence for from several to many years probably vary with each specific case and usually remain unknown.

PROGNOSIS

If the cyst lining is adequately curetted, the lesion almost always heals with replacement by new bone. Recurrence occurs in a small percentage for reasons which are often not apparent. It is said that cysts which undergo pathologic fracture may heal spontaneously. Some of them doubtless do but a favorable result should not be expected in the majority. Very large cysts may cause distortion of bone and inhibit bone growth. Bone cysts do not predispose to neoplasm. Radiotherapy has no proven value in this condition and should not be used.

HYPERTROPHIC OSTEOARTHROPATHY

Generalized hypertrophic osteoarthropathy (pulmonary or secondary hypertrophic osteoarthropathy) is a syndrome triad consisting of clubbing of the fingers and toes, periosteal bone formation of the shafts of the large long bones of the extremities, and a type of osteoarthritis. It is almost always associated with visceral disease, usually situated within the thorax. There is a rarer congenital form of clubbing unaccompanied by periosteal thickening and joint disease which appears to be a separate entity.

Clubbing of the digits was described by the ancients but the syndrome as a triad and its accompanying pulmonary lesions were not described until the last decade of the last century when Marie and Bamberger independently reported the condition. A recent review by Gall, Bennett and Bauer[22] adequately summarizes what is known about the disease and describes the morphologic changes in 7 cases.

Pulmonary neoplasm or longstanding suppurative disease of the lung—bronchiectasis, abscess, empyema or tuberculosis—is usually found to be a precursor of hypertrophic osteoarthropathy. Heart disease, usually of congenital type, was noted frequently in the early reports and so the term "pulmonary osteoarthropathy" was adopted to incorporate the chest pathology. Later it was discovered that primary pulmonary cancer, metastatic tumors to the lung and even benign lesions of the mediastinum and pleura such as lymphadenopathy and fibromas were occasionally associated. At length it was realized that diseases with sites and pathogenesis as widely diversified as those of syphilis, cirrhosis, osteosarcoma, chronic alcoholism and pyelonephritis apparently may cause the condition, so the "pulmonary" portion of the title must be omitted for the sake of accuracy.

The syndrome is much more common in males than females, and though it may occur at any period during adult life it is relatively frequent before the age of forty. During the early phase the complex is usually first manifested by a widening of the ends of the fingers and toes. As this widening progresses the nails curve in both directions, growing down over the ends of the digits to accentuate the typical clubbed appearance. Though clubbing usually occurs first, pain over the shafts of the extremities may lead to an x-ray examination which reveals periosteal thickening in the distal thirds of the diaphyses of the forearms and legs. Stiffness and joint pains are somewhat less common and often later in onset. The pain and periosteal thickening usually spread proximally to involve the remainder of the affected bones and progress to the shaft of the femur and humerus. The symptom complex waxes and wanes with exacerbations and remissions of the primary disease and in a few cases has disappeared when the latter has been cured. Some patients note a worsening of their symptoms during periods of warm and humid weather. Edema of the extremities may be a troublesome complication.

The pathogenesis of hypertrophic osteoarthropathy is unknown though it has been a target for explanation for over a half century. At first it was thought that the suppurative disease within the chest elaborated a toxin which caused the peripheral changes. When cases were discovered without accompanying infection it was proposed that the poor blood supply and stasis in the extremities resulting from cardiac inadequacy caused a proliferative fibrosis at the periphery. Then came the disturbing experimental work of Mendlowitz and Leslie[23] who produced hypertrophic osteoarthropathy in dogs by increasing the peripheral blood flow, and the measurements of Mendlowitz[24] in 35 cases of clubbing (of a variety of causes, excepting the congenital type) in which there was increased arterial pressure and blood flow in the affected digit in all cases with the exception of those with the complete symptom triad of hypertrophic osteoarthropathy. They concluded that secondary clubbing is always caused by an increase in arterial pressure and blood flow in the clubbed member, and that in some cases following clubbing the mean brachial and mean digital pressures equalize so that the digital pressures now appear normal, but the tissue alterations progress to the periosteum and joints and thus produce the triad of hypertrophic osteoarthropathy. If the Mendlowitz hypothesis applies, there is still to be explained why the heterogeneous variety of visceral diseases cause increased peripheral blood flow and indeed why this increased pressure and flow cause the characteristic changes. We must wait for further work before the pathogenesis of hypertrophic osteoarthropathy is clarified.

ROENTGENOGRAPHIC MANIFESTATIONS

The roentgenographic manifestations of hypertrophic osteoarthropathy reflect the changes in the periosteum and cortex which are visible microscopically. Periosteal new bone is laid down about the diaphyses of tubular bones. Early, this new bone may present a smooth outer surface, but later becomes rough and irregular. When severe, the periosteal new bone may blend with and thicken the cortex but a radiolucent line may be apparent between this new cambial bone and the underlying cortex. This line represents the

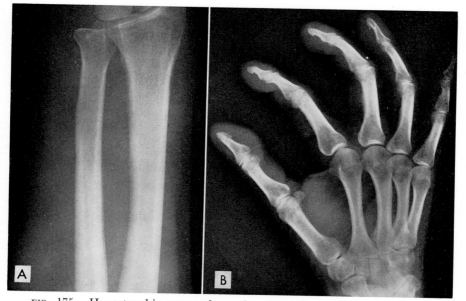

FIG. 175. Hypertrophic osteoarthropathy. Cortical thickening and periosteal new bone is evident in *A*. There is an increase in soft tissue about the distal phalanges, clubbing, without underlying bony alteration (*B*).

fibrous matrix in which the new bone is first formed and in which actual bone marrow appears between the new bone and the cortex. In some areas, perpendicular spicules of bone may be visualized passing through the marrow from cortex to the new cambial bone. Radiographs may reveal the increase in soft tissue about the terminal phalanges of the digits.

MICROSCOPY

Sections made through the clubbed portion of the digit are disappointing. The bulbous enlargement shows little more than hyperemia, edema and a mild infiltration with lymphocytes and plasma cells. The periosteum of the terminal phalanx is usually normal; sometimes the bone is actually atrophic. It appears that the soft tissue enlargement is the result purely of a circulatory disturbance.

The periosteum of the large cylindrical bones, and to a lesser extent the metacarpals and metatarsals and at times the proximal phalanges, shows an interesting alteration. The cambium lays down spicules of bone between it and the cortical surface. At first, the spicules are perpendicular to the cortical surface, unattached to it and embedded in a loose fibrous matrix. As the layer of new bone widens, however, it becomes annealed to the cortex, the spicules become incorporated in lamellae which run parallel to the cortical lamellae and marrow tissue appears. Thus, though the medullary region remains constant the cortex is thickened to as much as twice its normal width. The new bone is quite normal in structure.

The articular structures develop changes which are quite similar to those of osteoarthritis. The changes apparently begin in the synovia with vascular sclerosis and a resultant fibrosis which produces changes like those of a mild villonodular synovitis. The capsule becomes thickened by fibroblastic proliferation. Focal areas of degeneration appear in the articular cartilage and eventually cause roughening and narrowing. A few advanced cases have developed a pannus of granulation like that of rheumatoid arthritis which eventually destroys the cartilage and leads to ankylosis.

PROGNOSIS

Simple clubbing of the digits is a common complication of a wide variety of visceral diseases most of which involve the lung, pleura or mediastinum. Today, bronchiogenic cancer and pleural neoplasms are probably the commonest exciting factors. Some cases of clubbing progress to involve the periosteum of the extremities and the joints, these elements being necessary for the diagnosis of hypertrophic osteoarthropathy. In a few instances, the disease has been so severe that practically all bones, including those of the spine and skull, were involved. Complete disappearance of the osteoarthropic signs and symptoms has occurred in those cases in which the primary disease was completely alleviated. In a few cases the osteoarthropathy has appeared as a forerunner of demonstrable evidence of metastatic disease in the lungs. The ultimate outcome depends upon the underlying visceral disease. Since many cases are caused by malignant tumor the prognosis should be guarded until the condition has been thoroughly studied.

NON-OSTEOGENIC FIBROMA

Non-osteogenic fibroma is a rather common degenerative and proliferative lesion of the medullary and cortical tissues of bone. It occurs most commonly near the ends of the diaphyses of the large long bones, particularly of the lower extremities. It has a predilection for the bones of late childhood, adolescence and early adult life, the great majority of cases occurring between the ages of five and fifteen years. It is frequently multiple. This lesion has been and in some quarters still is called xanthoma or xanthofibroma, and because of the failure of many to recognize it as an entity it is widely confused with solitary cyst, giant cell tumor, fibrous dysplasia, lipid reticuloendotheliosis, chronic osteomyelitis, bone infarct and subperiosteal cortical defect. Despite its common incidence there is surprisingly little written on the subject and most of the older literature is so hopelessly vague and inaccurate because of the lack of a clear concept that it is scarcely worth the reading.

Non-osteogenic fibroma, though badly named, is a definite entity, and with the now available knowledge of its clinical, radiologic and microscopic features the diagnosis rarely should be missed.

Jaffe and Lichtenstein[25] were the first to realize that this lesion has a highly characteristic behavior and appearance which enables one to distentangle it from the unusually large number of similar conditions which masked its recognition as a separate process until 1942. They gave it the name "non-osteogenic fibroma," believing it to be a benign fibrous neoplasm of bone lacking the ability to form osteoid. One wonders why they did not call it simply "fibroma of bone" but since an entity—ossifying fibroma—had already been described, it is possible that they felt the prefixed "non-osteogenic" was warranted to distinguish it. Actually, knowledge of the process which has been garnered since their original paper makes it quite certain that the lesion is entirely non-neoplastic in nature so the term "fibroma" is an unfortunate one, since it has thrown it into the classification of bone tumors where it almost certainly does not belong. If one acccpts the definition of neoplasm, as most oncologists are beginning to, as a hyperplasia of cells which progresses until therapeutic intervention or death of the host, then non-osteogenic fibroma cannot be a true neoplasm, even a benign one, since the natural course of the lesion is one of healing, albeit several years are required. One may justifiably question the grouping of non-osteogenic fibroma with the circulatory disturbances of bone, though Hatcher[26] and some others have apparently reached that conclusion. It is so placed in this monograph to stress the important (from a therapeutic standpoint) point that it is not a neoplasm. Since we freely admit that we do not know its morbid physiology there is no absolutely correct category for its inclusion and we place it here because it is like some other lesions of the group.

Approximately 50 per cent of the lesions diagnosed as non-osteogenic fibroma have given no symptoms and are discovered incidentally in skeletal roentgenograms made for other diseases. For this reason the true incidence of the condition is unknown and difficult to surmise. It is probable that every busy radiologist sees at least a half dozen of these cases each year. Of those cases which show symptoms, the history of trauma can often be obtained just as in a large proportion of all bone diseases. Since the mechanism of the lesion is unknown it cannot be stated whether or not trauma plays a causative role. Pain is the common complaint and it may be of weeks' or even months' duration, suggesting that it usually is not severe. Since the lesion is usually near the end of the diaphysis of a long bone the pain is often interpreted as a type of arthritis. Occasionally enlargement of a bone, particularly if it be a slender bone such as the fibula or the ulna, may be the presenting sign.

The great majority of non-osteogenic fibromas occur during adolescence and the last half of the first decade. Older patients are not entirely spared, however, and in our material a classic lesion developed in the proximal femur of a thirty-two year old woman. Until recently it was thought that non-osteogenic fibroma occurred only in the large cylindrical bones of the extremities but it is now known that they occasionally develop in flat bones. We have made the diagnosis in a lesion of the ilium near the sacrum. Two or more areas may appear in the same bone or in different bones. It may be bilateral.

In its classic form the lesion appears near the end of the shaft a centimeter or more from the unclosed epiphyseal line. Over a period of weeks and months it gradually enlarges, attaining an average size of 3 to 5 cm. In its fully developed state it gives one the impression that it is composed of several confluent areas of deossification, the whole having a bosselated outer "surface." It involves both cancellous and compact bone and appears to begin just deep to the cortical laminae and destroys bone tissue in both directions. It progresses slowly so that the periosteum is enabled to lay down a thin shell of bone over its exterior surface producing cortical expansion, and the cancellous tissue at the inner margin undergoes sclerosis. Eventually, the lesion may extend across the entire diameter of the bone and then it becomes sealed off from the normal medullary tissues above and below by a margin of sclerotic bone and laterally it is covered by a fusiform bulging shell of cortex. If the lesion is followed long enough it will be seen to "drift" toward the mid-diaphysis as enchondral growth pushes the epiphysis away from it. Eventually, it may come to lie well down in the shaft but rarely invades the middle third and probably never reaches the mid-point. In a few cases which have been observed throughout the entire life of the lesion, new bone grows in from the periphery and eventually obliterates the area. The time from the date of diagnosis to that of complete

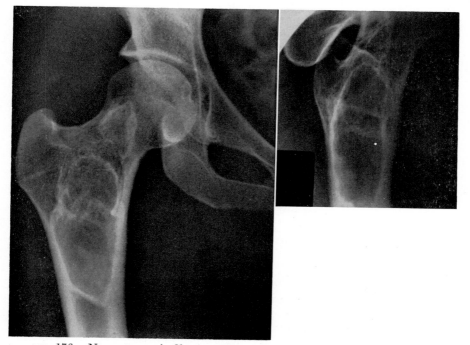

FIG. 176. Non-osteogenic fibroma. The radiolucent defect is lobular in outline with opaque, sclerotic borders. It is sharply limited. There is erosion of the inner aspect of the cortex.

healing in these few cases has been recorded from two to five years. A curetted lesion may appear to heal only to recur later further toward the mid-diaphysis, at a point corresponding to the original site in the younger bone.

Occasionally infractions of the cortical shell or, as in one of our cases, complete fracture may occur. Then the surrounding normal tissues are stimulated to produce callus and the clinical, radiologic and microscopic picture becomes more complex. Pain appears or becomes more severe, the delineating margin changes and unless the biopsy material is chosen from the right area the usual microscopy is replaced by irregular masses of young bone and cartilage in a fibrous matrix.

MICROSCOPY

Non-osteogenic fibroma is essentially an area of cancellous and overlying cortical deossification and replacement by fibroblastic proliferation. It is uncertain whether a true ischemic degenerative process precedes the fibrous hyperplasia or whether a primary and uncontrolled fibrous hyperplasia causes the bone erosion to accommodate its bulk. The expansion of the cortex over many of these lesions suggests the latter explanation. The cause for the fibrous tissue overgrowth is quite unknown. The history of trauma is not constant enough to account for even the majority of the lesions. The results of bacterial culture have been too inconsistent to be impressive. The fact that the process goes on to normal healing appears to exclude a neoplastic nature.

Focal ischemia due to vascular occlusion by trauma or embolism has been suggested as the initiating agent. If the cortical expansion could be accommodated to this reasoning, the other features might conceivably align themselves on a hypothetical basis. It is true that the microscopy of non-osteogenic fibroma is quite different from the lesion which we have come to accept as infarct. But the nidus of dead bone in the latter, with its surrounding zone of fibrous and bone sclerosis, is probably the residuum of an infarcted area which was too large for the ingrowing granulation to resolve completely. If the area of tissue death were small enough to be completely deossified by the granulation growing in from the surrounding normal tissues, it is possible that this process might initiate the fibrosis and other microscopic features which characterize non-osteogenic fibroma. Against this rather fanciful hypothesis is the occasional finding of infarcts no larger than the ordinary non-osteogenic fibroma, and the fact that one is not happy about accrediting the ischemia mechanism as a cause for the progressive enlargement of the lesion and the overlying cortical expansion.

All the microscopic features are consistent with a healed infarct of bone. There is a matrix of rather loosely arranged spindled cells which one has every reason to suppose are fibroblasts and more adult fibrocytes. They are characteristically arranged in rather vague whorls and less prominent trabeculae (Fig. 177). Collagen production is lacking in most areas but at times small fields of collagen may appear. There is no osteoid production. In most lesions at least a few xanthoid cells, large, pale polyhedral cells with abundant, finely granular cytoplasm (Fig. 178A), can be formed. Often these cells are arranged in aggregates or cell islands and occasionally they will dominate the microscopic field. These cells are macrophages, or phagocytizing fibroblasts if a distinction can be made, which have taken up lipid material, largely cholesterol. Higher magnification discloses the presence of coarse pigment granules within the more spindled elements. A Prussian blue reaction identifies this material as hemosiderin. Scattered through most fields one will find giant cells (Fig. 178B). The nuclei are morphogically identical with those of the fibroblasts and they probably represent either a failure of complete division or a tendency of these elements to agglomerate. One gets the impression that these giant cells are somewhat smaller and more spindled than those usually found in the reaction to bone injury. The periphery

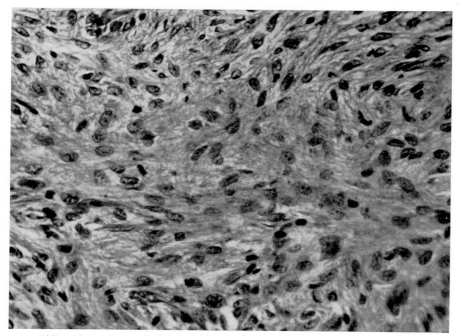

FIG. 177.   Non-osteogenic fibroma. A section through a fibroblastic area. (× 396.)

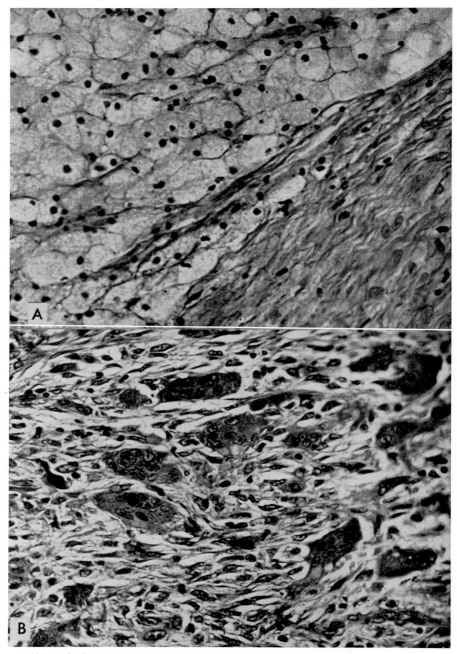

FIG. 178. *A,* An aggregate of xanthoid cells in the left upper half of the picture. (× 396.) *B,* Giant cells are frequently scattered through the matrix. (× 396.)

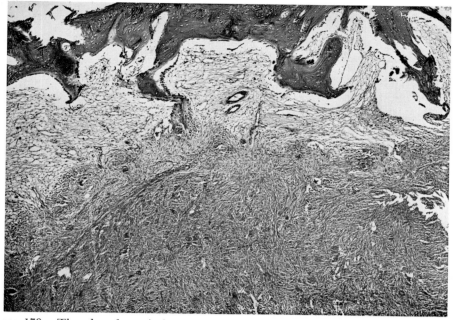

FIG. 179.   The edge of a typical non-osteogenic fibroma. It is surrounded by a thinned layer of cortical bone. ($\times$ 34.)

of the lesion is usually quite sharply delineated and surrounded by a layer of sclerotic bone (Fig. 179).

DIFFERENTIAL DIAGNOSIS

Solitary cyst.   The surgeon should be able to differentiate these two lesions in as much as non-osteogenic fibroma is probably never cystic.

Giant cell tumor probably never occurs before the involved epiphyseal line closes. Non-osteogenic fibroma usually appears before epiphyseal ossification. Giant cell tumor involves the epiphyseal and metaphyseal areas. Non-osteogenic fibroma usually appears farther shaftward. Giant cell tumor is usually more destructive and its microscopic sections reveal a matrix of neoplastic fibroblasts without a whorled and trabeculated pattern.

Fibrous dysplasia.   The diagnosis cannot be made without the presence of at least some bone spicules. Non-osteogenic fibroma does not produce bone.

Lipid reticuloendotheliosis.   Hand-Schüller-Christian disease is a disturbance of the reticulum and its derivatives. Epithelioid cells are prominent and there is usually an eosinophilic infiltration or the presence of other exudative inflammatory cells in response to the presence of the lipid.

Chronic osteomyelitis.   The diagnosis of infectious inflammation is exceedingly risky without the presence of at least some inflammatory exudate.

Bone infarct.   All of the microscopic features of non-osteogenic fibroma might be accounted for on the basis of ischemic necrosis in which complete resolution of dead bone has been accomplished. Since our concept of bone infarct at present includes a nidus of dead bone with surrounding tissue reaction, the lesions are not compatible as we now understand them.

Subperiosteal cortical defect erodes cortical bone from without. Actually, the mechanism and microscopy may be identical though there appears to be less evidence of a whorled pattern and the presence of pigment granules and a greater tendency to form hyalin. Giant and xanthoid cells may appear.

PROGNOSIS

From the evidence currently available, one should expect a non-osteogenic fibroma to disappear in from two to five years from the time it is diagnosed. If it is unusually large, and thereby jeopardizes the strength of the bone, or if infraction causes pain, the most conservative surgical management may be necessary. Diagnostic biopsy is unnecessary except in atypical cases or those which are complicated by other bone disease.

A new name should be devised to more accurately designate the correct character of the lesion. Fibroma is bad if the condition is not a true neoplasm. One should hastily add, however, that it is possible that non-osteogenic fibroma is in reality a tumor, though an uncommon one, and that the lesion which we choose to call subperiosteal cortical defect, a non-neoplastic process, has been so confused with it that we do not have an accurate concept of its behavior. The name "xanthoma" should be abandoned since not all of the lesions contain xanthoid cells, at least not at the outset, and this name implies that a disturbance in lipid metabolism is a major etiologic factor.

SUBPERIOSTEAL CORTICAL DEFECT

Subperiosteal cortical defect is a symptomless rarefaction of cortical bone. To date it has been described only in cylindrical bones and almost exclusively in the large, long bones of the extremities. Though it has been discovered in the skeletons of adults, these lesions appear to represent the persisting residuum of processes which began much earlier. Most subperiosteal cortical defects develop between the ages of twenty-two months and eight years and they rarely, if ever, develop after the age of fifteen years. There is a preponderance in males, rated in some series as high as two to one.

The condition is common. Caffey estimates that it probably occurs in some bone at some time in 20 per cent of all male skeletons and 10 per cent of all female skeletons. It is commonly multiple, sometimes two or more lesions occurring in the same bone, more often a single affected area appearing in each of two or more bones. It may be bilateral and it is sometimes symmetrical.

Despite the considerable incidence of cortical defect, the combined clinical, radiologic and pathologic aspects have not been studied in a sufficient number of cases to insure a thorough and correct concept. Because it is symptomless, it is usually considered of minor importance. When diagnosed by the radiologist it is usually not followed and rarely biopsied. Consequently our factual knowledge at this time depends upon one aspect or another but in no large series has a thorough study of all features, including the microscopy, been reported.

Actually, subperiosteal cortical defect is important. Its nature should be understood by all those dealing with bone disease lest it be overdiagnosed and overtreated. In at least one series a needless amputation has been forthrightly reported. Because this is a common lesion it frequently accompanies more serious bone conditions. Should it accompany a correctly diagnosed malignant tumor, how easy it would be to presume it to be a metastasis and thereby alter therapy.

Kimmelstiel and Rapp were the first to report[27] a series of cases in which the concept of the lesion is one which is limited to the cortex. Later, Caffey[28] reported the clinical and radiologic aspects of a much larger series and applied the name, "cortical defect." We have prefixed "subperiosteal" to more exactly denote the pathology and separate it from other cortical lesions of a variety of causes. In the earlier report of Ponseti and Friedman[29] one cannot be sure that the condition is an entity or that it is confined to the cortex. In the series reported by Sontag and Pyle,[30] cases of what is now known as non-osteogenic fibroma are included with subperiosteal cortical defect. Caffey fails to take cognizance of this in spite of the appearance in the report of such statements as "All of them are situated in the metaphysis or adjacent shaft where they are usually eccentrically placed. The defect often abuts on the cortex or occupies a portion of it," and "In the process of tubulation of the metaphysis the defect may eventually occupy a part of the cortex bone." Also in the illustration of the roentgenogram of their case four, there is shown a lesion of the fibula which in both the anteroposterior and lateral projections extends completely across the diameter of the bone and causes a fusiform expansion of the cortex. Obviously they are describing at least some cases of non-osteogenic fibroma and any conclusions drawn from the report may not be applied to subperiosteal cortical defect.

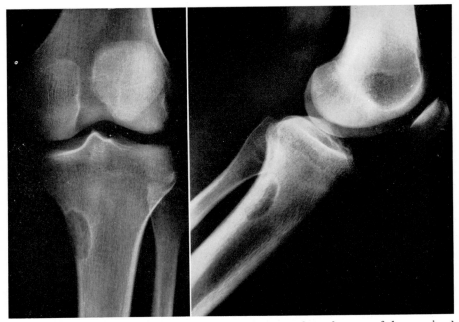

FIG. 180.   Subperiosteal cortical defect. The posterolateral cortex of the proximal tibia is the site of the lesion. The radiolucent defect is surrounded by a sharply defined opaque border. Incidentally, this lesion was observed to heal over a period of several months.

Subperiosteal cortical defect begins most often on the external surface of the medial and posterior cortical walls of the lower end of the femur in children between the ages of three and six years. The second commonest site is the upper end of the tibia where it occurs in the anterior as well as the posterior wall. It is less frequently encountered in the upper end of the humerus and probably occurs occasionally at the ends of all the long bones of the extremities. It always begins near, or perhaps at an epiphyseal line. It enlarges slowly from a spheroid area of demineralization to an ovoid lesion, the greatest diameter in the long axis of the host bone. It grows slowly, requiring months and sometimes years to reach its maximum size. It usually attains a greatest diameter of 3 to 4 cm. and probably never reaches the size of the larger non-osteogenic fibromas. As it grows it may change shape and relative position. Some of the lesions have been seen to drift toward the mid-diaphysis as the growing epiphysis pushes away from it. Others maintain their relative position to the epiphyseal line indicating that they progress in the direction of bone growth and heal in the older portion, thus keeping pace with the normally growing bone. They may heal in a matter of months or persist for a decade or longer but one may expect complete disappearance in from two to five years in most cases.

Certainly the majority of these defects are symptomless. Where pain is a feature, one cannot be sure that it is not due to the trauma which often calls attention to the lesion. Because the involved area is never very large, it rarely leads to fracture.

In those cases which have been adequately studied the defect always begins in the cortical surface directly contiguous to the overlying periosteum. As it enlarges it apparently erodes the bone, producing a dish-like crater. In a few instances a thin subperiosteal shell of bone has roofed the lesion, apparently the product of the related cambium, but there is no evidence to show that the lesion begins within the cortex. As the defect expands the space is filled with a growth of fibrous tissue from the periosteum. No one knows whether the process of deossification is primary and the fibrous proliferation an attempt at healing or whether there is an uncontrolled periosteal fibrous proliferation which erodes bone. There has been a tendency to accept the latter explanation without much justification.

MICROSCOPY

It is almost impossible to obtain a clear concept of the microscopic appearance of subperiosteal cortical defect from the published reports. In the largest series, that of Caffey, no biopsies were taken and the source of the photomicrographs submitted by Jaffe is not absolutely clear. In the series reported by Sontag and Pyle, both non-osteogenic fibroma and subperiosteal cortical defect are included so that one cannot be sure which lesion they are describing. Kimmelstiel and Rapp describe the microscopy of their four cases and include several photomicrographs which are quite different in appearance from those illustrating Caffey's paper. The very limited material of the present authors most closely resembles the descriptions of Kimmelstiel and Rapp.

In our sections the process appears to be a proliferation of fibrous cells from the periosteum which fills the defect produced by a bone erosion (Fig. 181). The appearance of the cells is reminiscent of those which compose the normal fibrous periosteum. Multinucleated giant cells similar to those found in non-osteogenic fibroma are present but xanthoid cells, though present, are less in evidence. There are some foci of hemosiderin granules. The chief distinction between the two lesions, if an over-all distinction can be made, is the presence of hyalin and some intercellular substance resembling osteoid in the subperiosteal cortical defect. The presence of the intercellular products of chondroblasts and osteoblasts, if examination of a large number of cases shows them to be consistent, is of major importance. Numerous studies of non-osteogenic fibroma have shown hyalin and osteoid to be consistently absent. Little more can be said about the microscopy

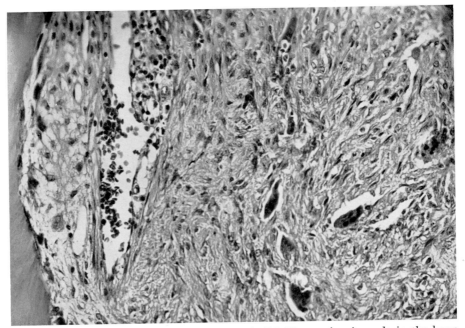

FIG. 181.   Subperiosteal cortical defect. A dish-like erosion is made in the bone seen at the left margin. A fibroblastic reaction with giant cells and xanthoid cells is found between the bone and periosteum. (× 396.)

of this common lesion until a sufficient number of biopsies have been taken to answer our numerous questions.

One can no more than conjecture the pathogenesis of subperiosteal cortical defect. Caffey considers the evidence for trauma and proposes the possibility that muscle pull at points of tendon attachment may initiate the process. After reviewing the evidence for this hypothesis he reminds us that the defects occasionally occur in areas where there are no tendon attachments, that they may be symmetrically bilateral, that two symmetrical lesions may appear and heal synchronously and that a defect may drift away from the point of its origin. These data suggest that the lesion is a variant in normal bone growth.

One is tempted to consider the possibility that non-osteogenic fibroma and subperiosteal cortical defect are one and the same process, the one developing on the inner surface of the cortex and the other on the outer. This may well be, but until we can be more dogmatic about the microscopy of cortical defect and until we can prove with absolute assurance that non-osteogenic fibroma is not a neoplasm, we must consider the two processes as separate entities. There may be some criticism for considering cortical defects under the category of vascular disturbances in bone. This would be quite justifiable but the reasons for placing non-osteogenic fibroma in this category have been given and the two lesions should be considered together, at least for the present.

REFERENCES

BONE INFARCT

1. Kahlstrom, S. C., Phemister, D. B., and Burton, C. C.: Surg., Gynec., and Obst., 68:120, 1939.
2. Kahlstrom, S. C., and Phemister, D. B.: Am. J. Path., 22:947, 1946.
3. Coley, B. L., and Moore, M.: Ann. Surg., 111:1065, 1940.

EPIPHYSEAL ISCHEMIC NECROSIS

4. Emerick, R. W., Corrigan, K. E., Joistad, A. H., and Holly, L. E.: Clinical Orthopaedics, 4:160, 1954.
5. Trueta, J., and Harrison, M. H. M.: J. Bone & Joint Surg., 35B:442, 1953.
6. Legg, A. T.: Boston Med. & Surg. J., 162:202, 1910.
7. Calvé, J.: Rév. de Chir., 42:54, 1910.
8. Perthes, G.: Deutsche Ztschr. f. Chir., 107:111, 1910.
9. Gall, E. A., and Bennett, G. A.: Arch. Path., 33:866, 1942.
10. Zemansky, A. P.: Am. J. Surg., 4:169, 1928.

OSTEOCHONDRITIS DISSECANS

11. Monro, A., Quoted by Phemister, D. B.: J. Bone & Joint Surg., 61:278, 1924.
12. Paget, J.: St. Bartholomew's Hosp. Reports, 6:1, 1870.
13. König, F.: Deutsche Ztschr. f. Chir., 27:90, 1888.
14. Lavener, G.: Am. J. Roentgenol., 57:56, 1947.
15. Green, W. T., and Banks, H. H.: J. Bone & Joint Surg., 35A:26, 1953.

ANEURYSMAL BONE CYST

16. Jaffe, H. L., and Lichtenstein, L.: Arch. Surg., 44:1021, 1942.
17. Lichtenstein, L.: Cancer, 3:279, 1950.
18. Jaffe, H.: Bull. Hosp. Joint Dis., 11:3, 1950.
19. Dahlin, D. C., Besse, B. E., Pugh, D. G., and Ghormley, R. K.: Radiology, 64:56, 1955.
19a. Sherman, R. S., and Soong, K. Y.: Radiology, 68:54, 1957.

SOLITARY CYST OF BONE

20. Bloodgood, J. C.: Ann. Surg., 52:145, 1910.
21. Jaffe, H., and Lichtenstein, L.: Arch. Surg., 44:1004, 1942.

HYPERTROPHIC OSTEOARTHROPATHY

22. Gall, E. A., Bennett, G. A., and Bauer, W.: Am. J. Path., 27:349, 1951.
23. Mendlowitz, M., and Leslie, A.: Am. J. Path., 17:458, 1941.
24. Mendlowitz, M.: J. Clin. Invest., 20:113, 1941.

NON-OSTEOGENIC FIBROMA

25. Jaffe, H. L., and Lichtenstein, L.: Am. J. Path., 18:205, 1942.
26. Hatcher, C. H.: Ann. Surg., 122:1016, 1945.

SUBPERIOSTEAL CORTICAL DEFECT

27. Kimmelstiel, P., and Rapp, I.: Bul. Hosp. Joint Dis., 12:286, 1951.
28. Caffey, J.: Advances in Pediatrics, 7:13, 1955.
29. Ponseti, I. V., and Friedman, B.: J. Bone & Joint Surg., 31A:582, 1949.
30. Sontag, L. W., and Pyle, S. I.: Am. J. Roentgenol., 46:185, 1941.

Metabolic Diseases

OSTEOPOROSIS

The bone mass of the normal skeleton may be reduced to an abnormal status by any of four different mechanisms.

1. Alteration of the blood supply. In complete infarction the osteocytes die but the mineralized matrix remains relatively unchanged until the reparative forces in the surrounding normal tissues are mobilized, a period of several weeks or even months. As granulation is formed about the periphery of the area of dead bone, fresh blood is brought in and the dead bone first becomes necrotic and eventually undergoes lysis as far as the extensions of granulation can reach. The end result depends greatly upon the size of the dead mass. If it is small it may be completely resolved; if large, a nucleus of dead bone surrounded by a zone of sclerotic bone (where vessels have penetrated but the blood supply is subnormal) will persist. The loss of bone mass which follows trauma, infection, and destructive tumors, primary and metastatic, and that due to pressure erosion probably depend to a greater or lesser degree upon alteration of blood supply.

2. Deossification. Excessive parathyroid secretion (parathyroid adenoma, osteitis fibrosa cystica) and Paget's disease are the two best examples of this type of diminished bone mass. Nothing is known of the mechanism of Paget's disease and little more concerning the action of parathormone on bone. The term deossification is used rather than decalcification since the process is a melting away of both mineral and matrix. It is probable that the osteoid fabric never remains after the salts have been leached from normal bone.

3. Inadequate mineralization may account for deficiencies of bone

growth or interfere with the replacement of bone lost by normal wear. Rickets is an example of the former and osteomalacia of the latter. The failure of a normal deposition of mineral may have one of a variety of causes. The mineral intake may be inadequate, or it may not be properly absorbed through the gut wall (vitamin D deficiency) or an adequate mineral supply may be dissipated by abnormal kidney function.

4. The last and most complex mechanism of an eventual diminution in skeletal mass is the failure in the production of an adequate amount of organic bone matrix, osteoid. The result of this failure is known as osteoporosis. This failure may be the result of congenital factors, an inadequate number of osteoblasts or, more likely, osteoblasts with an enzymatic deficiency. Osteogenesis imperfecta is an example of this type of osteoporosis, a disease in which sufficient osteoid for a normal skeleton is never formed. Much more common is the inability to replace the osteoid which is continuously disappearing as a result of everyday wear and tear. Unless specified, it is this mechanism which is meant when the term osteoporosis is used.

Albright[1] defined osteoporosis as "that category of decreased bone mass where the disturbance is the failure of the osteoblasts to lay down bone matrix." Thus, the term osteoporosis has a specific meaning. It should not be used by the radiologist when referring to an area of translucency of unknown etiology nor by the orthopedist to indicate a bone which has lost its normal strength. The mechanism of the development of decreased opacity and loss of strength in osteoporosis is known. It is a failure of osteoid replacement. The cause of this failure cannot always be determined because the physiology of the osteoblast is but poorly understood. However, it is known that there are a number of pertinent factors. In grouping the types of osteoporosis according to these factors we arrive at a classification of the disease.

There must be an adequate number of osteoblasts, which is probably another way of saying that differentiation from the primitive mesenchymal cell mass must be normal. The osteoblasts must be equipped with normal enzymatic systems. They must also be stimulated to action by stress and certain endocrine secretions. They must be provided with the protein and vitamin C building blocks which go into the making of osteoid. Because this rather complex chain must be intact for normal bone matrix production, failure at any point will result in osteoporosis.

The following is an empiric, etiologic classification of osteoporosis:

1. Endocrine
    a. Gonads
        (1) Ovaries—postmenopausal osteoporosis due to inadequate estrogen stimulation.
        (2) Testes—osteoporosis of Fröhlich's syndrome and possibly acromegaly due to inadequate androgen stimulation.
    b. Adrenal Cortex
        (1) Cushing's syndrome—probably due to excessive sugar-active hormone which is antianabolic.
        (2) Adrenal atrophy—senile osteoporosis due to adrenapause of Albright—a deficiency of the anabolic N hormone.
    c. Pituitary
        (1) Cushing's syndrome—probably through the adrenal cortex.
        (2) Acromegaly—possibly through the gonads.
    d. Thyroid
        (1) Osteoporosis of longstanding hyperthyroidism—probably due to excess use of proteins by the accelerated basal metabolic rate.
    e. Pancreas
        (1) Osteoporosis of diabetes mellitus—probably due to excess utilization of protein.
2. Disuse atrophy—Osteoporosis due to loss of stress stimulus.
3. Deficiency—Inadequate intake, absorption or utilization of proteins and vitamin C.
4. Post-traumatic—Osteoporosis secondary to alterations in blood supply due to nerve impulse changes (causalgia).
5. Congenital—Osteoporosis of osteogenesis imperfecta.

Some of these categories probably need further clarification. It has long been known that estrogen, androgen or a combination of the two is necessary for normal osteoblastic activity. The estrogen levels begin to fall soon after menopause and within five to fifteen years may reach a level which is inadequate for stimulation of the osteoblasts. The decrease in androgen and estrogen due to adrenal cortical atrophy of senility is usually considerably later; thus the onset of osteoporosis in males is usually in an older age group.

The osteoporosis of Cushing's syndrome is poorly understood largely because the pathogenesis of the latter has never been satisfactorily explained. Most of the cases show adrenal cortical adenomas, adrenal cortical hyperplasia or adenocarcinomas of the adrenal cortex. Since the osteoporosis of Cushing's syndrome, as well as many other features of the disease, can be induced by the administration of cortisone which is one of the sugar-active hormones, it is assumed that excessive amounts of this steroid cause accelerated glyconeogenesis at the expense of the proteins which are needed by the osteoblasts to form organic matrix.

The osteoporosis of thyrotoxicosis and diabetes mellitus may be due to an overutilization of proteins, in the first as an attempt to balance the increased rate of catabolism and in the second because of its conversion into much needed glycogen. Scurvy is a specific type of osteoporosis. The hemorrhagic factor combined with the inability to form organic matrix makes it a specific entity so that it is never called osteoporosis.

The osteoporosis of disuse is important and interesting. It is well known that without the stress stimulus, the osteoblasts refuse to lay down osteoid. The transitory quality of bone, its continuous dissolution and replacement, is necessary to keep the bone fit for the functional stresses which is must be bear. As pressure trajectories change old laminae dissolve and are replaced by new ones arranged in the new stress lines. If there is no stress, the laminae are not reformed and the bone mass decreases to the status of osteoporosis. A disuse osteoporosis can be noted after only a few weeks of absolute bed rest. If a limb is immobilized in plaster the osteoporosis is more dramatic. As the bone undergoes lysis the minerals are released into the blood stream. The serum calcium and phosphorus rise,[2] presumably because there is insufficient osteoid production to recapture the bone salts, and calcium is spilled into the urine. Urinary calcium excretion may be sufficient to make it necessary to take precautionary measures against nephrocalcinosis and kidney and bladder calculi.

Post-traumatic osteoporosis, sometimes called causalgia or Sudeck's disease, is a curious phenomenon. Following an injury which may be insignificant there is pain, sometimes referred, often swelling and eventually a dramatic decrease in bone substance (Fig. 182). In many instances the osteoporosis appears to be due to an increased blood supply caused by neurogenic insult. In other instances the mechanism is not as obvious and the disuse secondary to pain may play a role.

The most important type of osteoporosis from the standpoint of incidence is that seen in women, usually sixty years or older, a decade or more after the menopause. It is occasionally seen in younger women who have been subjected to an artificial menopause by ovariectomy. The usual complaint is back pain. The onset may be insidious or sudden following injury. The trauma may be disproportionately trivial in relation to the pain. The pain may be referred along the course of involved nerves, particularly down the posterior

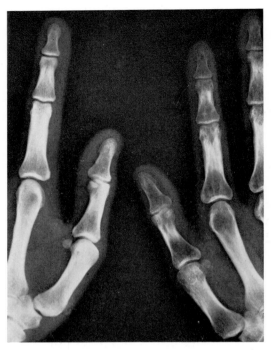

FIG. 182. Causalgia. Deossification of the metacarpals and phalanges of the thumb and index and middle fingers are shown on the right. Normal mineral content is seen on the left. Osteoporosis occurred following a minor injury in the forearm.

aspect of one or both legs. Eventually, the pain may spread to the pelvis, the thorax and the shoulders. If a vertebral body is weakened to the point of collapse there will be a kyphosis and loss of stature. Chemical analysis of the blood reveals nothing abnormal though sometimes there may be an excess of calcium in the urine. Estrogen levels are apt to be low.

ROENTGENOGRAPHIC MANIFESTATIONS

The roentgenographic manifestations of osteoporosis reflect the deficiency of organic matrix and parallel the gross pathologic findings. The cortices are thin and the trabeculae fine and sparse. The skeletal structures are therefore more radiolucent than normal. For the most part all of the skeletal structures are affected except when the cause is a local one such as disuse. In the child diaphyses of the tubular bones may be smaller in diameter than is normal and the zone of provisional calcification may be more apparent in contrast with the adjacent shaft.

Fractures, particularly of the vertebrae and ribs, are not uncom-

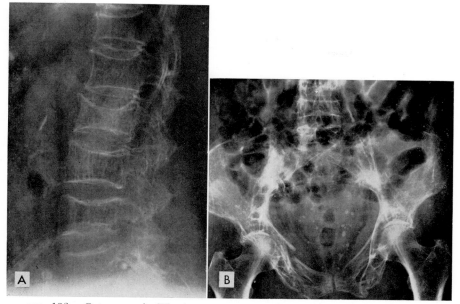

FIG. 183.   Osteoporosis. The bony structures are more radiolucent than normal. There are compression fractures of the lumbar vertebra, *A*, and a fracture of the right pubic bone is evident in *B*. The cortices are thin and only the larger trabeculae are visible.

mon. The vertebral bodies may be collapsed anteriorly with loss of stature and a kyphotic deformity of the spine.

MORBID ANATOMY

When the patient with advanced osteoporosis comes to autopsy the bone changes are quite obvious grossly. The ribs are as fragile and brittle as eggshell. They may be snapped with ease between the thumb and forefinger. When cylindrical bones are carefully examined it will be noted that the silhouette is quite normal except where fracture and infractions have caused distortion. The compacta is greatly thinned, however, because of an enlargement of the medullary area. The thinning takes place from the inside so that the outer surface diameter remains constant. The vertebrae are most markedly involved and one or more may show wedge compression. If a vertebra is dissected and cut vertically in half, it will be seen that the end plates are greatly thinned and cupped inward by the expanding intervertebral cartilaginous plates. The pelvic bones are next severely involved.

When the most important factor causing the osteoporosis is disuse, the skull bones are apt to be spared and the maximum thinning of long bones is found at the ends of the shaft.

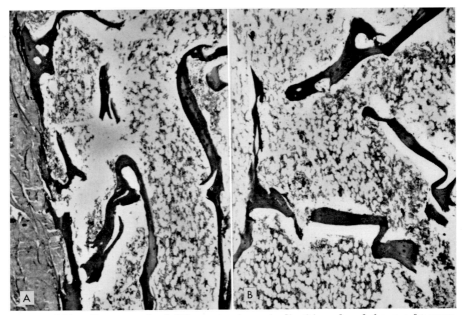

FIG. 184.   Osteoporosis. *A,* The cortex is markedly thinned and shows a fracture. *B,* The ratio of interspicular tissue to bone mass is greatly increased. The spicules are thin, delicate and easily fractured. There is no osteoblastic activity. ($\times$ 15.)

When sectioned the bone tissue appears normal though there is too little of it. The compacta is thin (Fig. 184*A*) and the haversian canals are widened. The trabeculae of the cancellous tissue are thin and often distorted by fracture. The ratio of bone mass to medullary soft tissue is greatly decreased so that the cancellous bone network under low magnification appears as a fine tracery in a matrix of fatty marrow (Fig. 184*B*). Osteoblasts are never numerous and are often entirely lacking.

The cause of the most common variety of osteoporosis, the postmenstrual or senile type, is often complex. The endocrine deficiency is the initiating and often the most important factor. These patients often look older than their age with atrophy of the skin and other features. Frequently, a disuse atrophy complicates the picture. The muscles often show wasting. As these patients approach the sedentary age and as their bone pains appear they take to their rocking chairs and the normal stress stimulus for osteoblastic activity is decreased. Often they become fastidious concerning their diets. As their teeth become less efficient they take more to soft foods and avoid the tough proteins that are necessary for osteoid formation. As they lose interest in food the total caloric intake may be reduced to subadequate levels. Eventually, their diets may include too little calcium or phosphorus or both, and then a superimposed osteomalacia causes a melting away of the remaining skeleton to produce the most extreme weakening and bizarre distortion.

When the etiology of osteoporosis consists of several combined factors it is obvious that no one therapeutic agent will bring about a cure. These patients are usually treated with the deficient endocrine factor, given a high caloric, high protein diet, checked for adequate calcium intake and sufficient vitamin D to insure absorption and put on an exercise schedule. This regimen halts the progress of the disease and usually allays the symptoms but improvement in the roentgenograms is notably slow. It has been stated[3] that as much as half the bone mass of the skeleton may be dissipated in severe osteoporosis. This may amount to a mineral loss up to 3 pounds. Since only about 2 grams of calcium can be retained daily and that only with adequate newly formed organic matrix, to rebuild the skeleton would take two years or longer.

Osteoporosis after the age of fifty is a common condition. It should not surprise one that it is sometimes associated with certain catabolic or deossifying processes such as Paget's disease or parathyroid adenoma. When bone is rapidly broken down and there is no regenerative capacity because of the accompanying osteoporosis, the clinical and roentgenographic pictures are greatly exaggerated. The serum alkaline phosphatase level, which is so characteristically elevated in these two diseases, may be normal because of the lack of osteoblastic activity making accurate diagnosis exceedingly difficult. When osteoporosis becomes combined with osteomalacia in its terminal stages it may be necessary to biopsy the bone to make a diagnosis. Though the clinical picture may be that of advanced osteomalacia, the lack of osteoblastic activity assures the pathologist that at least a part of the process is due to osteoporosis.

Generalized plasma cell myeloma may give the same roentgenologic findings as senile osteoporosis. If the blood and urine chemistry is carefully considered, as it should be in every case of osteoporosis, a mistake in diagnosis will usually be avoided but in some cases a biopsy will be necessary.

OSTEOMALACIA

Osteomalacia is a disease of mature bone occurring in adult life after the epiphyseal ossification centers have closed. The mechanisms of this disease are the same as those of rickets which can occur only in growing bone. The symptomatic differences in the two conditions are due only to the difference in response of the growing and the mature skeleton in a state of chronic calcium or phosphorus or calcium and phosphorus deficiency.

In children, the cause of the disease is almost always a lack of vitamin D in the diet or too little sunlight to synthesize the natural body sources. In adults, the causes are numerous including deficiencies in diet, disturbances in absorption and excessive serum calcium loss. Because full-blown osteomalacia is rare and its causes multiple, the nature of the disease has been poorly understood until relatively recently.

It was not until 1891 that osteomalacia and osteitis fibrosa cystica (parathyroid adenoma) were clearly separated by von Recklinghausen, but he, clinging to the ideas of Virchow, attributed the loss of rigidity of the skeleton to a solvent action of acid in the blood. Cohnheim, in 1889, had a more accurate concept of the disease, but it was not until the publication of McCrudden[4] in 1910 that the mechanism of osteomalacia was accredited to a deficiency of the mineral salts because of either an impoverished supply or an excessive loss.

Even today there is general confusion among clinicians regarding the two conditions, osteomalacia and osteoporosis. Osteomalacia is a disease of mineralization; there is no interference with organic matrix formation. Osteoporosis is a disease of organic matrix formation; mineralization mechanisms would be normal if sufficient matrix could be produced. Both terms have been in the past, and still are, used loosely to mean a softening of the mature skeleton. Such usage is inexact and leads to confusion. Actually, osteomalacia in the older age groups may eventually lead to a combined and superimposed disuse osteoporosis because of pain and deformity. Added to the leaching action of the former is the inhibition of the matrix formation of the latter. Combined, the two diseases produce the most generalized and the most grotesque of the skeletal destruction diseases (Fig. 185).

The causes of the inadequate mineral supplies for skeletal maintenance are numerous. Dietary deficiencies of calcium and phosphorus will cause osteomalacia but are so rare in most civilized populations that the disease practically does not occur from this cause. In remote areas, where the simplest dairy products which abound in these minerals are unavailable, the disease is common.

Vitamin D lack is a much more common etiologic factor, particularly among politically oppressed groups who are forced to live on inadequate rations and are denied sunlight. Deprivation of the actinic rays because of social practices is reported to cause osteomalacia among women of India and the Orient. More common are the fat absorption disturbances which result from chronic disease of the bowel and pancreas. Chronic steatorrhea, sprue, fibrosing pancreatic disease, disturbances in the biliary duct system or even extensive and longstanding ulcerative colitis may result in conditions which inhibit the absorption of the fat-soluble vitamin D. The accompanying excess of fatty acids which may form insoluble soaps with the available calcium and the concomitant diarrhea which moves the intestinal contents too fast for efficient absorption may all add to the difficulties in the transport of adequate calcium and phosphorus from the bowel lumen to the blood stream.

A common type of this condition among women of the lower social strata is known as puerperal osteomalacia. In young women who bear several children in rapid succession and nurse them between confinements, the calcium and phosphorus demand necessitated by the growing fetus and the milk supply for the infant may actually outpace the dietary supply. The skeletal stores are utilized and osteomalacia is the result.

Full-blown osteomalacia practically never occurs in the western hemisphere. Latent or early symptomatic osteomalacia, Milkman's syndrome, is seen occasionally in every active orthopedic clinic. These patients complain of pain, and if a roentgenogram is made early a

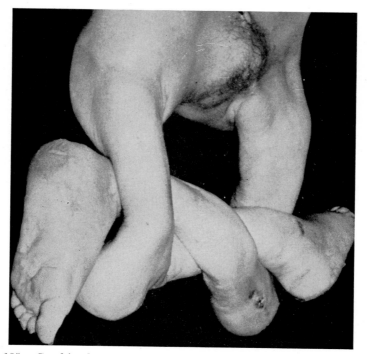

FIG. 185.   Combined osteoporosis and osteomalacia. A postmenopausal woman lived for a prolonged period on a starvation diet. Many factors played a role in the deossification and failure of osteoid maintenance, chief of which were inadequate intake of proteins, vitamins C and A and minerals.

focal area of demineralization in the cortex will be found. These are more often seen in the diaphyses of large cylindrical bones but flat bones, particularly of the pelvis, may also be involved. If periodic roentgenograms are taken over a span of weeks the focal area will be seen to extend slowly across the bone in an irregular ribbon of translucency. These are called Looser zones. They were described long before their significance was appreciated. They are usually multiple, often symmetrical. They have the appearance of fractures without loss of alignment and usually there is no history of trauma. Several such cases were reported in the latter part of the last century and the first three decades of this under a variety of headings. In 1934, Milkman[5] reported a case which he had studied thoroughly. He believed it to be a distinct entity, different from osteomalacia, osteitis fibrosa cystica (parathyroid adenoma) and osteitis deformans (Paget's disease). He called it "multiple, spontaneous idiopathic symmetrical fractures," and since this report the condition has been known as "Milkman's syndrome."

In 1946, Albright and co-workers[6] reported six cases of this condition with carefully controlled mineral balance studies. They concluded that the disease was caused by a chronic, low grade calcium deficiency due to renal tubule dysfunction and classified it as early, symptomatic osteomalacia. Their report has been amply corroborated by numerous workers since and Milkman's syndrome is now considered to be a mild type of osteomalacia. Albright et al. believed that a specific inability resided within the lining cells of the distal convoluted tubules of the kidneys to form an adequate amount of ammonia for urine secretion. There was a resultant withdrawal of the basic ions of the blood, especially calcium, to satisfy this need. The profligate use of calcium in this fashion necessitated a spending of the bone stores, producing symptomatic demineralization. Albright stated that cases of Fanconi syndrome in which it is necessary to excrete abnormal quantities of organic acids may have the same effect.

More recently, Dent[7] has classified four types of congenital, familial renal tubule dysfunction, common to all of which there is an inability to reabsorb phosphates from the glomerular filtrate. Two additional types are not congenital nor familial but acquired, and in addition to the phosphate absorption defect there is an inability to form ammonia. These last two types he considers under the heading of the "Albright-Butler syndrome." Two of the first four types are associated with excessive amino acid excretion and he classifies these as "Fanconi syndrome." But in all cases, he infers, the significant morbid physiology is not the wasting of calcium but the excess drainage of phosphorus. Since inadequate phosphorus supplies are known to cause osteomalacia, his conclusion seems logical. Moreover, if the depleted phosphorus rather than the depleted calcium is the cause of the disease, this may account for the lack of parathyroid hyperplasia which should occur in chronic hypocalcemia but which has not been reported in clear-cut cases of osteomalacia of this type. This mechanism also suggests that since extravagant parathyroid hyperplasia apparently does not occur in renal tubular bone disease but does in renal glomerular bone disease (renal rickets), a high serum phosphorus level which occurs in the latter but not in the former may be an activating factor in the parathyroid hyperfunction and enlargement.

As the disease progresses from Milkman's syndrome into florid osteomalacia the fractures increase in number and severity. Eventually, malalignment takes place and then it will be noted that the entire skeleton is beginning to show deossification. Why certain focal areas (the regions of partial and finally complete fracture) are selected in early involvement is unknown. The Looser zones are usually, though not always, found at points of stress. Even in stress areas it is difficult to understand why a circumscribed portion of the bone under-

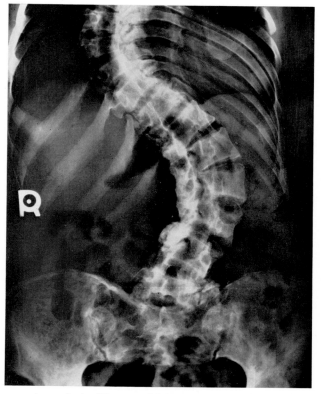

FIG. 186.   Severe osteomalacia. The vertebral column has suffered deossification until it can no longer bear the normal stresses to which it is exposed.

goes demineralization and replacement with fibrous tissue while the adjoining region remains relatively normal.

As the skeleton softens, weight-bearing inflicts greater deformity. The long bones, particularly of the lower extremity, bend and twist. The pelvis becomes flattened laterally causing the pubic bones to protrude anteriorly. The vertebral column wilts like a warm candle (Fig. 186). Eventually, the directions of stress are so altered that the articular cartilage surfaces no longer serve their normal purpose and degenerative change induces a traumatic osteoarthritis. Pain from arthritis and fracture and disability due to deformity completely inactivate the patient. Then, disuse osteoporosis sets in and the progress of the disease is hastened to a state of helplessness and eventual death.

ROENTGENOGRAPHIC MANIFESTATIONS

The roentgenographic manifestations of osteomalacia may be difficult to differentiate from those of osteoporosis, since in both the skeletal structures are more radiolucent than is normal. Early in the course of osteomalacia only a coarse trabecular pattern associated with focal areas of radiolucency (Looser zones) may be evident. The

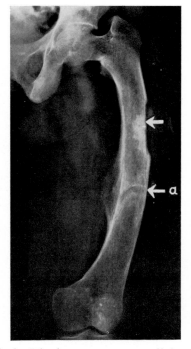

FIG. 187.   Osteomalacia. The bones are more radiolucent than normal, but the trabecular pattern is coarse. Bowing of the femur is present and a Looser zone is evident in the mid-shaft (a). The defect in the cortex (arrow) marks the site of a biopsy.

cortices then become less opaque and thinner. Deformities of the long bones, pelvis and spine follow as a result of softening of the bones. In the final stages, osteoporosis as a result of disuse complicates the picture so that severe and marked radiolucency of the skeletal structures is evident.

The coarse trabecular pattern is a consequence of inadequate mineralization of secondary trabeculae; the larger primary trabeculae are well seen in contrast with the unossified osteoid and soft tissues of the marrow. Radiolucent streaks in the cortex, representing unossified osteoid, precede thinning of this compact bone. In contrast with the brittle bones of osteoporosis, the unossified osteoid in osteomalacia permits deformities such as extensive bowing and bending.

Looser zones are radiolucent by virtue of their composition of osteoid and fibrous tissue. They often occur early in the course of the disease before the generalized skeletal manifestations of osteomalacia are apparent radiographically. These focal areas of radiolucency may be seen in other diseases, e.g., Paget's disease and fibrous dysplasia, but when evident in bones that appear otherwise normal radiographically, they strongly suggest the presence of osteomalacia.

MICROSCOPY

Sections made through areas of osteomalacia have much the appearance of rickets without the participation of cartilage. Sections

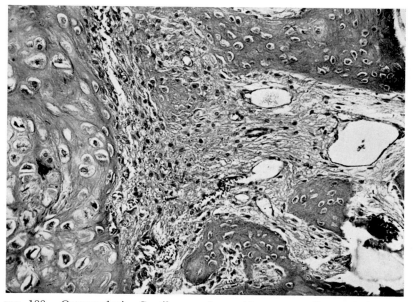

FIG. 188.   Osteomalacia. Cartilage and osteoid are normally produced but the latter is not mineralized to produce normal rigidity. The section reveals scrambled islands of cartilage between which there are masses of unmineralized osteoid. ($\times$ 150.)

through the Looser zones have shown a transverse stratum of bone destruction with replacement by a rather loose feltwork of fibrous and osteoid tissue. Mineral salts are completely lacking. As the disease advances the entire skeleton melts away. At the ends of the long bones the spicules of the spongiosa become thinner and thinner. Wide seams of osteoid are laid down to ensheath them and the interstices are filled with collagenizing fibrous tissue (Fig. 188). Osteoblasts and osteoclasts are abundant. There is less hemorrhage than in osteitis fibrosa cystica (parathyroid adenoma) and, therefore, giant cells are not so prevalent. The cortices become more and more attenuated by enlargement of the haversian canals until they come to resemble spongiosa. There is less osteoid proliferation in these areas except at the sites of infraction and frank fractures. Here the disarray of osteoid masses reminds one of callus formation.

PROGNOSIS

The bone lesions of osteomalacia are much more insidious in their development than those of parathyroid adenoma. An early distinction between the two processes is important because of the completely different therapy. The cause of the bone softening must be ascertained. Dietary deficiencies are easy to supplant. Intestinal disease may require replacement or even surgical treatment. The method of alleviation of puerperal osteomalacia is obvious. Cases of Milkman's syndrome due to renal tubular insufficiency are usually treated by making available an alkaline salt to substitute for the calcium ions being used, massive doses of vitamin D to stimulate tubular phosphate reabsorption and a high calcium and phosphorus diet. Results depend largely upon the cause and available means to eradicate it. Most cases diagnosed early respond completely.

PAGET'S DISEASE

Paget's disease, named osteitis deformans by Sir James Paget[8] in 1877, is a disease of bones in which repeated episodes of osteolysis closely followed by excessive attempts at repair result in a weakened, deformed skeleton of increased bone mass. In its advanced and symptomatic stage it is rarely seen before the age of 40 though at least one case has been reported as early as eighteen years. The writer has seen one case strongly suspected of being Paget's disease in a woman aged 28.

Since the roentgenogram is reasonably characteristic in the majority of cases, considerable numbers of asymptomatic, monostotic or solitary focus Paget's disease may be discovered on skeletal survey studies carried out for other reasons. Many of these lesions never will manifest themselves symptomatically, others will progress into clinically obvious Paget's disease. In its florid state most of the bones of the skeleton may be involved with crippling or complete invalidism, and numerous and severe complications, most often involving the cardio-vascular system, may lead to a fatal termination.

Paget's disease is usually slowly progressive over a period of months and years. It starts as a small focus and gradually spreads to involve large areas of both cylindrical and flat bones. At first there is a demineralizing process which causes skeletal radiolucency and a coarsening of the trabeculations. But as it progresses areas of density appear which may eventually overshadow in opacity the surrounding normal bone. Even though the bone mass ultimately may be increased, the repair is not normal in lamellar stress lines so that pathologic fracture is a common occurrence. These fractures often heal poorly with excessive, poorly distributed callus. In long bones the ends are usually involved first but the process may spread to involve the entire bone.

Several reports have emphasized the greatest incidence in the bones subjected to the greatest stress. Thus in Schmorl's reported studies[9] on autopsied cases, the sacrum was the most common site of the disease and the related structures, upper femur, lower spine and pelvic bones were almost as often affected. The skull, too, is frequently involved for a reason which is harder to name. The over-all incidence of the disease probably approaches the level of 3 per cent, but if all instances of radiologically presumed cases were included the figure would be somewhat higher.

When the focus is solitary and in but one bone, the condition may remain silent indefinitely. As the lesion progresses it may cause pain and a sensation of stiffness. Eventually this may be severe enough to bring the patient to his physician or, if the bone is sufficiently weakened, minor trauma may cause fracture. If a skeletal survey is done at this time other smaller and probably younger lesions are often found.

When large areas of numerous bones are affected the deformity and symptoms are quite characteristic. There is a slowly progressive deossification which appears to begin along the inner cortical surfaces. As it continues, the substance of the bone disappears. It becomes weakened and distorted under pressure. Collapse of the anterior portions of the vertebral bodies causes a typical kyphosis of the thoracic spine which thrusts the head forward and downward. The femora bend outward to produce bowing and this deformity is accentuated by an outward and forward bowing of the tibias. These various curvatures cause shortening of the stature. Softening of the femoral necks results in coxa vara. The bones of the feet are usually spared but when involved there is collapse of the arches and plantar elongation. The feet appear to enlarge, requiring bigger shoes.

Flat bones are involved as often as cylindrical bones. Softening of the sacrum and the iliac bones, together with the coxa vara, causes a waddling gait. The ribs and sternum also may be involved in severe cases. There is a lateral flattening of the thorax with increase in the anteroposterior diameter. This deformity together with the kyphosis interferes with the lifting of the ribs in normal respiration. This feature may play at least a part in the respiratory difficulty which these patients experience. Poor ventilation may add to the increased work load of the right heart. The forward curvature of the spine causes the belly to protrude.

The weakening of the normal bone structure is doubtless due in large measure to the progressive deossification process. But, some time in the course of the disease, probably when the deossification is fairly well advanced, an attempt at repair sets in. There are no data available which prove unquestionably that the bone destructive process is transitory and cyclic with interspersed periods of repair. One gets the impression on examination of the bones in advanced Paget's disease with a hand lens that irregular areas are destroyed throughout the entire thickness of the cortex, and that around the fragments that remain a poorly constructed and disoriented substitute is laid down. The resulting cortex is thicker than the original but it is coarser, less dense and obviously not as strong, since fractures continue to occur during this stage.

Some time during this period the cambium of the periosteum begins to form coarse primitive bone which is often arranged in spicules more or less vertical to the outer cortical surface. When long bones bend from weakening, infractions occur along the convex surface and the periosteum lays down new bone on the opposite side to strengthen the member. The periosteal osteogenesis, whether it occurs in cylindrical or flat bones, is additive in effect, causing widening of the bone as a whole without decreasing the medullary volume. If the medullary area is decreased, and it sometimes is (Fig. 189), the narrowing is due to the replacement of the original cortex which is now thicker and more porous than normal. Thus, the cranial capacity and the marrow space are never greatly intruded upon by the increasing bone mass, though the latter may be invaded by fibrous proliferation at the expense of hematopoietic tissue.

A concept of the Paget's process may be gained by examining the sawed edges of the calvarium by means of a hand lens. In the normal bones of the calvarium one sees an inner and outer table of dense cortical bone which together approximately equal in thickness the middle layer of more porous bone. The calvarium in Pagent's disease shows an outer layer of relatively dense bone which is more porous and often thicker than the combined three layers of the normal (Fig. 190). The dural surface is quite smooth and normal in appearance. What was previously the outer table is extremely rough and jagged. Applied to this "surface" there is a much thicker layer of very porous bone which apparently has been laid down by the periosteum. It is so coarse that it has much the appearance of pumice. The outer surface is irregularly scarred and pitted. Occasionally, a thin layer of more dense bone may be found immediately beneath the periosteum.

Attempting to reconstruct the process which results in the final appearance, there is first destruction of the normal cortex in widely disseminated but finely patchy areas, then there is replacement about the irregular fragments that remain by osteoblastic proliferation within the remaining cortex, and some time during the process an addition of a very poor and primitive type of bone on the outer surface by periosteal activity.

Anemia has been reported in Paget's disease and it may be severe.

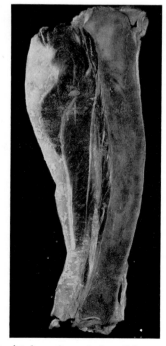

FIG. 189.   Paget's disease. Sagittal section of the tibia reveals anterior bowing and replacement of the cancellous tissue with compact bone.

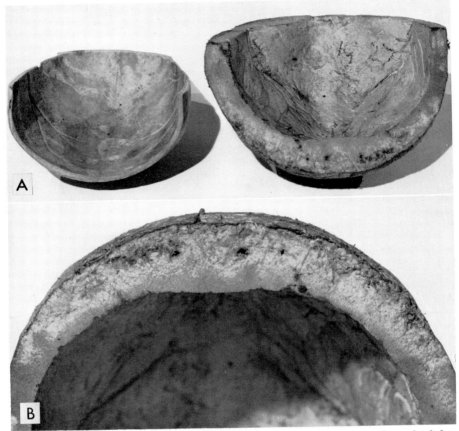

FIG. 190. Paget's disease. *A,* A Paget's calvarium on the right and on the left a normal specimen. The cranial cavities are about equal in volume but the bone thickness is enormously increased in the Paget's skull. *B,* Higher magnification of a Paget's calvarium. Note that the inner table is fairly normal. Apposed to this is a thick layer of coarse bone. The outer surface is rough and pitted.

However, it is certainly not common and if one examines the normal hematopoietic areas one wonders why a greater incidence is not found, since there is usually a considerable amount of fibrosis in these regions. The reason may lie in the fact that during the decades when Paget's is found, only a relatively small proportion of the medullary space is utilized for hematopoiesis. The remainder is filled with fat. But this fat may shift back to hematopoietic tissue if the demand arises, so the compensatory reserve is usually adequate to make up for the fibrosis.

Where periosteal bone formation impinges upon the foramina of emerging cranial and spinal nerves, pressure may interfere with nerve function. Impaired vision and deafness have been ascribed to this cause. The squeezing of other cranial and spinal nerves may result in both motor and sensory disturbances.

The weight of the brain and the enlarged skull may cause the softened bones at the base to flatten. The plane of the foramen magnum becomes inclined dorsally and the odontoid process is thrust up into the posterior fossa. Thus, the brain stem must bend over the odontoid and ventral margin of the foramen magnum,[10] the olivary processes sink into the cervical canal, and tension is made on nerve roots.

The mechanism of the pigmented corneal degeneration and the choroidal atrophy and pigmentation which has been reported in Paget's disease is not clear unless they are etiologically associated with pressure atrophy of the optic nerves. Since a large number of patients with Paget's disease eventually develop hypertension, this may be responsible in part.

A few cases of mental degradation have been reported with the far advanced disease. Since Paget's and arteriosclerotic cerebral disease occur in the same age group, the association may be coincidental though there are a few reports of alteration in the capacity of the brain box.

Cardiovascular disease is listed as the most common cause of death in advanced, generalized Paget's disease. There are several factors each of which probably play a role. The cervicothoracic kyphosis and the impaired motion of the ribs result in a limited ventilatory capacity. This in turn may increase cardiac output, right-sided hypertrophy and eventual right heart failure.[11] The incidence of hypertension, arteriosclerosis and valvular disease is reported to be higher in generalized Paget's disease than in the average population of comparable age. These complications may be related to the observation that the cardiac output in Paget's disease is considerably elevated.[12] It has been known from almost the first observations of the disease that the affected part is warmer than the normal. Surgeons have noted that during the active stage the tissues bleed abnormally, and microscopists have frequently mentioned the unusual vascularity of the fibrous proliferation that forms a matrix for the abnormal bone. It has been supposed either that there are multiple small arteriovenous aneurysms or that the large vascular sinuses in some way create their effect. If such is the fact, the increased cardiac output might be so explained, and it is conceivable that the arteriosclerosis, the valvular and coronary calcification and eventually even the hypertension might be related, but the actual mechanisms of these complications are still unexplained.

One would expect the serum calcium level to be elevated in generalized Paget's disease in the destructive phase. Yet this is rarely true, and perhaps any elevation which occurs may be the result of disuse atrophy in those patients who are incapacitated by the disease. A hypothetical explanation may be offered. In the natural course of the disease new osteoid is laid down and mineralized in the wake of the destructive process. This new bone formation may utilize most of the mineral that is liberated except when a lack of the stress stimulus causes slowing down or failure of osteoblastic activity. Excessive quantities of alkaline phosphatase are found in the serum. In active, severe, generalized Paget's disease the levels may be quite high. When one sees the flamboyant display of osteoblastic activity which is occasionally encountered in Paget's one is not surprised. The serum phosphorus level remains normal.

ROENTGENOGRAPHIC MANIFESTATIONS

The roentgenographic manifestations of Paget's disease reflect osteolysis and excessive repair, alone or in combination. Thus areas of radiolucency and opacity result. The trabecular pattern is prominent and coarse. The smaller trabeculae are not evident, but the larger ones in the line of weight-bearing increase in size. Particularly do the bones of the pelvis show this alteration in trabecular pattern. The long bones may be thick and opaque but pseudofractures and bowing belie the apparent strength of the bones.

The destructive or osteolytic phase is often most characteristic on radiographs of the skull. The radiolucent defect slowly enlarges and is in sharp contrast with the normal surrounding bone. The cortex, particularly the external cortex, becomes indistinct and hazy in outline. The term osteoporosis circumscripta has been applied to this de-

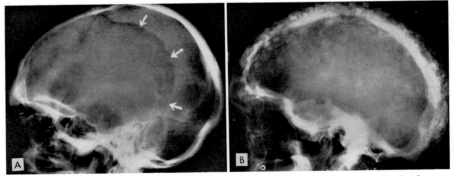

FIG. 191.   Paget's disease. *A*, Osteoporosis circumscripta is apparent in the fronto-parietal region. The margin of this area of radiolucency is well defined posteriorly (arrows) by normal bone. Marked thickening of the cranial bones is evident in *B*. The inner aspect of these bones is well defined. Deformity at the base of the skull is the result of softening of the bone in this region.

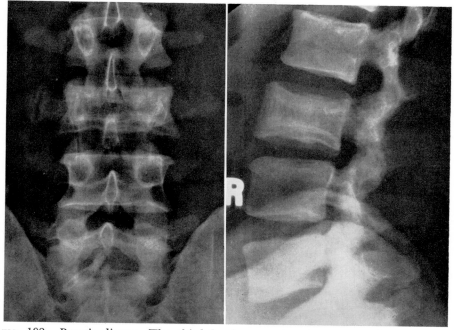

FIG. 192. Paget's disease. The third lumbar vertebra is compressed. Horizontal opaque lines parallel the superior and inferior surfaces of the body.

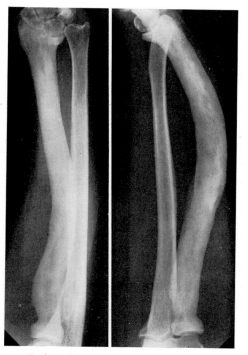

FIG. 193. Paget's disease. Deformity of the entire radius with bowing is apparent. The bone is thickened and opaque, and the medullary canal obliterated.

mineralization. As the disease progresses, areas of opacity appear within the radiolucent region and then excessive new bone becomes evident with thickening of the cranial bones. The radiograph shows coarsely granular cranial bones reflecting areas of osteolysis and excessive new bone formation.

The involved tubular bones increase in size. Most of the new bone is produced by the periosteum so that the cortex is thickened with no encroachment on the medullary canal. At times, however, the canal may be narrowed by the excessive repair. Often, osteolysis and new bone formation are seen in combination resulting in radiolucency and opacity of a most bizarre nature. Immobilization of affected bones appears to accentuate the osteolytic phase.

Coarse trabeculations in affected vertebral bodies are common. These tend to be horizontal and accentuate the margins of the body. Compression fractures are not uncommon which result in narrowing of the vertebral body anteriorly. Almost homogeneous opacity of a vertebral body may be evident without fracture or coarse trabeculae.

MICROSCOPY

The mosaic pattern described by Schmorl remains the hallmark of the full-blown, mature Paget's picture. When an osteone is formed, that is, a haversian canal with its complement of ensheathing lamellae,

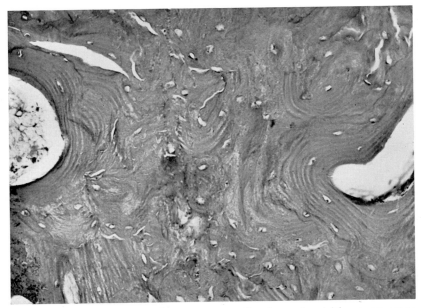

FIG. 194.   Paget's disease. Irregular osteones are fitted together without respect to the haversian pattern. This produces the mosaic appearance. (× 170.)

the external surface of the outermost layer acquires a peculiar staining quality. It takes the hematoxylin stain more avidly than related tissue areas so that when the osteone is cut in cross section it is seen to be delineated by a heavy blue line called the cement line. Thus the province of one osteone can be distinguished from that of its neighbor.

In Paget's disease portions of osteones are irregularly gnawed away. To this rough and erratic surface new osteoid is applied by the repairing osteoblasts. But the new bone is never annealed to the old as are the lamellae of an osteone and consequently, when cross sectioned, a crazy quilt pattern of areas of all sizes and shapes is outlined by the cement lines that are formed (Fig. 194). This does indeed look like a mosaic done by an artist who had forgotten his objective. These irregular areas have been called breccie.

When these irregular breccie dominate the microscopic section there can be little doubt of the diagnosis. However, Paget's disease does not show the mosaic pattern in all phases and any condition in which there is irregular bone destruction and immediate osteoid apposition may mimic this picture to some degree. Then the histologic diagnosis becomes more difficult.

Much of the new osteoid is laid down by osteoblastic activity and it is not unusual to see the entire length of an irregular fragment of bone solidly surfaced by these cells. In other areas a fibroblastic proliferation dominates the picture, and in the midst of such a field

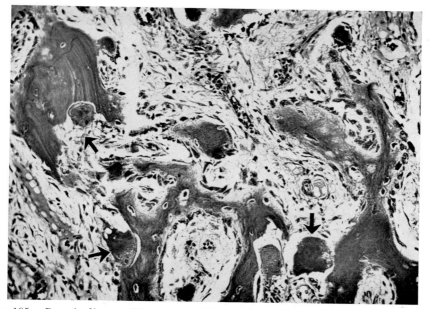

FIG. 195.   Paget's disease. There is a brisk osteoblastic activity in a fibrous matrix. Abnormal numbers of osteoclasts (arrows) are usual. ($\times$ 150.)

one may find a coarse-fibered osteoid and obvious fibro-osseous meta-plasia. In the phase of deossification large numbers of osteoclasts are often encountered (Fig. 195). Sometimes one finds them nestled against a spicule the opposite surface of which is being built up by osteoblasts. Eventually, both osteoblasts and osteoclasts disappear leaving a sponge-work of massive spicules demonstrating the mosaic pattern. The fibrous matrix eventually may be converted to fat.

It is true that the feltwork of fibrous tissue that forms the back-ground for the irregular bone spicules may show numerous, large, thin-walled vascular sinuses along with evidence of blood extravasation and an incidental sprinkling of exudative inflammatory cells. If numerous arteriovenous sinuses exist, however, ordinary technique does not show them. Moreover, it is difficult to account for the changes visualized by microscopy on the basis of an increased blood supply. It is true that bone appears to demineralize when exposed to abnormal quantities of arterial blood, but the bizarre changes seen in Paget's disease do not then materialize. It is probably best to admit that the cause and mechanism of Paget's disease are still unknown. If increased vascu-larity plays a role, then we must await a better demonstration of this phenomenon.

PROGNOSIS

It is exceedingly difficult to predict the behavior of Paget's disease. As mentioned earlier in this chapter, it is almost certain that some monostotic lesions will remain asymptomatic throughout life. Others progress and a small percentage will become generalized, cardiovascular and respiratory complications will develop and the patient will almost certainly die in a state of heart failure, but the course of the disease may run for many years.

One of the most interesting complications of the condition is the superimposition of malignant mesenchymal tumor, usually in an area previously affected by the Paget's. The sarcoma may be osteo-sarcoma or fibrosarcoma, and in the material of the author a chondrosarcoma developed (Fig. 196). Though these cancers run approximately the same course that they do in younger patients, they are much more apt to occur in the bones of the pelvis and other flat bone sites that would be unusual in the younger age group.

There has been considerable controversy concerning the inci-dence of this tragic complication. Jaffe[13] states that the figure may be set at about 4 per cent of all symptomatic Paget's disease. In the author's material a very high percentage of osteosarcomas and fibrosarcomas in patients over 45 has occurred in the pelvic and

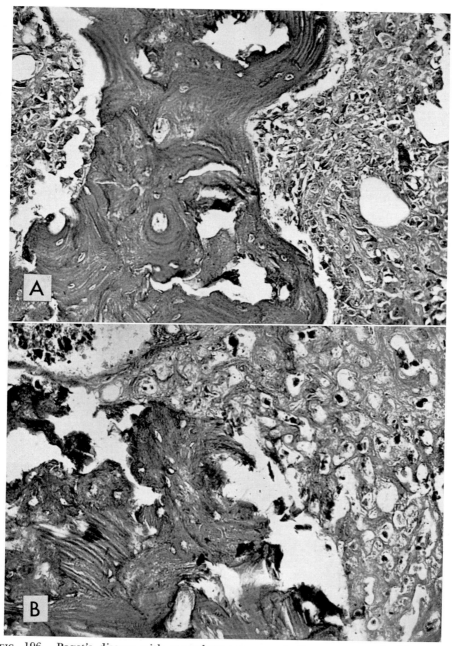

FIG. 196. Paget's disease with secondary sarcoma. *A*, Osteosarcoma. *B*, Chondrosarcoma. (× 186.)

other flat bones, and a considerable number of these have shown microscopic or x-ray evidence or both of concomitant areas of Paget's disease. Some authors have made the statement that approximately one third of the osseous and fibrous cancers of the older age group are superimposed on Paget's disease. It is possible that if multiple samples were taken from various levels an even higher coincidence could be shown.

SLIPPED EPIPHYSIS

Slipped epiphysis, epiphysiolisthesis, epiphysiolysis or epiphyseal coxa vara is a condition in which there is a separation of the epiphysis from the metaphyseal diaphysis along the lattice line. This separation may or may not progress to a displacement of the epiphysis in relation to the diaphysis in a manner which suggests a sideway slipping. Though several epiphyses have been reported to demonstrate this curious behavior, the condition is relatively so much more frequent in the superior femoral epiphysis that when the site is not specifically designated one assumes the lesion to be in this region. In areas other than the capital femoral epiphysis the so-called "slipped epiphysis" is probably always due to acute trauma.

Slipped epiphysis was described nearly a century ago but the pathology of the early cases was unknown and the condition was confused with a number of other diseases of the hip of a variety of etiologies. Monk's report, in 1886, was probably the first non-traumatic case the identity of which is unmistakable. Sprengel correctly demonstrated the pathology in 1898, and in the same year Poland reported a thorough search of the literature. The best modern reviews of the subject are those of Key[14] and the later report of Howorth.[15]

Slipped epiphysis is not a rare condition. The busy orthopedist is apt to encounter two or three cases each year. The lesion is more common in males, the proportion varying in different series from four to one to a "slight preponderance." When it occurs in females the onset is usually one or two years earlier than in males. The disease begins and runs its active course during adolescence, between the ages of 10 and 18. This age incidence is so common that the process is sometimes called epiphyseal coxa vara of adolescence. Slipped epiphysis probably never begins after the closure of the superior femoral epiphysis.

The preponderance of these adolescent patients in whom no frank and significant history of trauma can be obtained are heavier than average; indeed, a considerable proportion are frank cases of Fröhlich's adiposogenital dystrophy. The association is so common that should one encounter persistent hip pain of recent onset and inability to properly abduct and externally rotate the thigh in a child after puberty who is fat and manifests an underdevelopment of the genitals, the diagnosis of slipped epiphysis must be assumed until disproven.

The disease runs its active and healing course in from one to three years. It is bilateral in about 15 per cent of the cases. It begins with a widening of the epiphyseal line of the capital femoral epiphysis. It is apparent that the epiphysis is now loose upon the proximal end of the neck. If there be no unusual strain or trauma it may remain here, held in place apparently by the ensheathing periosteum and perichondrium. Eventually, the epiphysis begins to shift downward and backward, usually with some clockwise rotation. The periosteal-perichondrial covering is first stretched and twisted and then torn. As the head slides downward and backward the posterior-inferior margin of the end of the neck penetrates into the substance of the epiphysis and the anterosuperior margin is bared. This change in relationship of the femur with the pelvis causes some outward rotation, a slight degree of flexion and a small amount of shortening.

The onset of the disease is usually accompanied by pain which may be minimal or quite severe. There is usually a limp which at first is due to the pain, but after the disappearance of the pain, which usually persists for several months, the disability remains, presumably owing to alteration in the mechanics of the joint. When examined, the leg is found to be externally rotated, slightly adducted and a little shortened. The trochanter is slightly elevated and prominent. There may be a minimal atrophy of the thigh. There is frequently a permanent flexion of 15 degrees or more and flexion limitation to about 80 or 90 degrees. Abduction and internal rotation are also limited.

Without intervention the epiphysis remains in its abnormal position and eventually becomes fixed there by fibrous tissue and callus formation. This permanent fixation is accomplished in two or three years. The process has usually become static by the time of normal epiphyseal closure. The limp and disability may in a few cases completely disappear, may persist unchanged or become progressively worse as atrophy of the acetabulum and neck and new bone formation take place in response to changed trajectory lines. Later on, an osteoarthritis is apt to set in because of the altered weight-bearing surfaces.

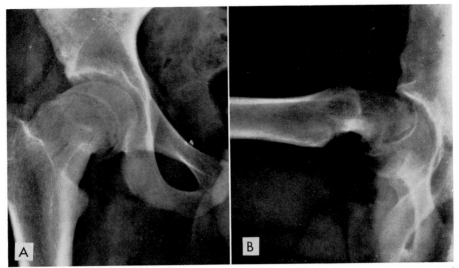

FIG. 197. Slipped epiphysis. The deformity of the femoral neck and the femoral capital epiphysis is evident on both the anterior-posterior (*A*) and lateral (*B*) projections. The widened epiphyseal line is best seen on the lateral projection. New bone is most evident at the posterior-inferior aspect of the femoral neck adjacent to the epiphyseal line.

ROENTGENOGRAPHIC MANIFESTATIONS

The roentgenographic manifestations of slipped femoral capital epiphysis depend on the degree of displacement of the femoral head. If the examination is made early in the course of the process only widening of the epiphyseal line is apparent. Minimal displacement of the epiphysis may not be appreciated in the A-P projection because the displacement is downward and posterior, but it will be apparent on the lateral projection. When the displacement is more severe, the abnormality will be appreciated on both projections.

Because the process is a slowly progressive one, adaptive changes take place in the neck of the femur. New bone is formed at the posterior-inferior aspect of the neck and at the exposed anterior-superior margin. Anterior bowing of the neck is common as a result of which the neck appears short and broad on films exposed in the A-P projection. The femoral head maintains its relation with the acetabulum; it is the femoral neck which is actually displaced. Changes in the joint in untreated patients are manifest early by narrowing of the joint space.

Traumatic slipped femoral capital epiphysis may be differentiated from the spontaneously occurring lesion by virtue of displacement without associated new bone formation and without adaptive changes in the neck of the femur.

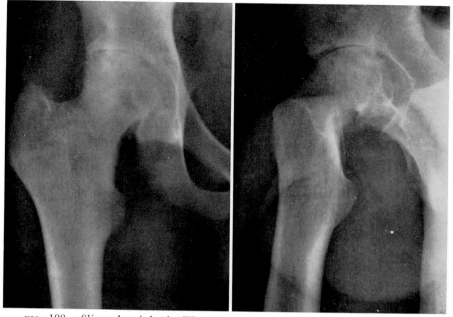

FIG. 198. Slipped epiphysis. The epiphyseal line has closed. The residual deformity of the proximal femur is apparent as well as is the marked narrowing of the joint space. This was an untreated case and the joint abnormality reflects abnormal mechanical factors secondary to the deformity of the femur.

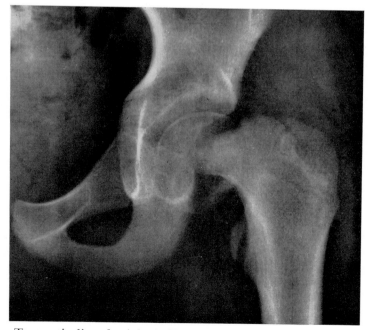

FIG. 199. Traumatic slipped epiphysis. Note the lack of new bone formation adjacent to the epiphyseal line. There is no deformity of the femoral neck.

PATHOLOGIC MORPHOLOGY

The gross appearance of slipped epiphysis depends, of course, upon the degree of displacement of the femoral head. Cases may now be diagnosed in the pre-slipped stage so that there is little alteration of the gross anatomy when the surgeon approaches the region. Or the epiphysis may slide downward and backward until a considerable portion of its subchondral surface becomes applied to the posterior-inferior surface of the neck. In the non-traumatic cases the progression is usually slow and there is considerable reparative tissue proliferation by the time the lesion is fully developed. The denuded portion of the end of the femoral neck becomes covered with a thick layer of densely collagenized fibrous tissue. In the interstices between the convex outer surface of the cortex of the neck and the subchondral surface of the epiphysis there is a proliferation of fibrous scar tissue and callus with irregular masses of cartilage and later bone. When the epiphysis comes at last to rest, the stress lines of cortical and cancellous bone are altered to the local topography by absorption and reformation of bone lamellae. Corresponding changes take place within the acetabular cup to accommodate the new position of the articular surface.

The microscopy of slipped epiphysis in sections taken at various periods of the process fails to give a clue as to the etiology of the disease. Nothing is found on microscopic examination that cannot be accounted for on the basis of traumatic loosening and eventual displacement of the epiphysis. The early changes all take place along the line of separation. The cartilage cells of and on both sides of the line of provisional calcification become deranged and distorted by pressure. The degenerative changes in this region are probably secondary to the disturbance in the normal vasculature. The osseous nucleus of the epiphysis remains intact until impingement by the neck or altered stress lines cause changes. The granulation which first appears, then the fibrosis and callus formation and eventually the active osteogenesis are all normal responses to bone injury. If there is interruption of the epiphyseal arteries in consequence of the epiphyseal migration, an epiphyseal ischemic necrosis may result with eventual collapse of the osseous nucleus and flattening of the articular cartilage.

PATHOGENESIS

The mechanisms of slipped epiphysis are now quite clear thanks to periodic roentgenograms taken during the course of the process and a correlation with the gross and microscopic pathology. The cause of the disease is still unknown. In the earliest accounts it was thought to be a type of tuberculosis and later of rickets. Today, we can be definite in stating that neither infection nor a bone salt deficiency is associated with the typical case of slipped epiphysis. Other causes which have been proposed and warmly supported, at least for a time, are arthritis, osteomalacia, chondrodystrophy and nutritional disturbances. In our present state of knowledge there is nothing to support any of these contentions. It is well known that acute trauma may dislodge the epiphysis from the femoral head but most cases fail to give a history of a single episode of frank trauma commensurate with the lesion, and besides a single episode of trauma does not account for such other features as the age incidence in adolescence, a tendency for bilateral involvement, the male preponderance and the characteristic obese body type. Yet the closest scrutiny of the lesion both grossly and microscopically fails to reveal evidence for a cause other than trauma.

All or most of the features which characterize slipped epiphysis are satisfied in the hypothesis that excessive strain in a conditioned structure may produce the lesion. The excessive strain may be accredited to the abnormal weight found in a large number of the subjects. The conditioning may be the result of the normal changes which take place at the site about the time of puberty. If one sections any actively growing long bone longitudinally one finds the weakest point in the cortex immediately beneath the line of provisional calcification. At this level only the cancellous bone is well formed; the cortex is paper thin because there has not been sufficient time for the deposition of intramembranous bone by the periosteum. The periosteum and perichondrium probably play an important role in holding the epiphysis fast to the shaft. The junction of the head and neck of the femur is one of the several points of great stress in the skeleton. The last hurdle in the chronic trauma or strain hypothesis is the consistent occurrence of slipped epiphysis during adolescence. One might ask why it does not occur with equal frequency during the first decade. Key contends that, until osseous union of the epiphysis with the shaft, the surrounding periosteum is much thicker and more dense than it is after epiphyseal closure, and that in the years immediately preceding closure it atrophies to assume the post-closure thickness. If this be true, then excessive strain due to overweight or unusual activity or frank trauma at a stress point (the femoral epiphyseal line), at a time when the normal cortical thickness has not been attained and the supportive periosteum is weakened, might result in a lesion or lesions with all the clinical and pathologic features of the disease, slipped epiphysis. Such, at present, appears to be the most logical explanation.

Because the normal sequence of changes is related to bone growth and because obesity is related to glandular or nutritional disturbances, the disease is classified as and discussed with the metabolic diseases of the skeleton.

Bone Changes of Pituitary Dysfunction

GIANTISM

The somatotropic hormone (STH) is a potent factor in the growth of all mesenchymal tissues including cartilage, bone, periosteum, perichondrium and fibrous tissue. It has recently been isolated from the eosinophilic cells of the anterior lobe of the pituitary gland. Its actions and mechanisms are as yet not entirely understood, but experimentally at least it speeds somatic growth and perhaps prolongs the growth period. In certain instances of excessive growth during childhood and adolescence, tumor-like nodules of hyperplasia or a diffuse proliferation of the eosinophilic cells of the pituitary has been noted. This condition has been called pituitary giantism or gigantism.

As early as 1886, Marie called attention to abnormal stature in relation to the function of the pituitary gland but it was not until 1910 that Cushing hypothesized that it was the specific secretion of the eosinophilic cells that caused the remarkable overgrowth of the skeleton and soft tissues.

Giantism, which seems a better term than gigantism, is presumably caused by abnormally rapid growth during the normal growth period and often prolongation of the growth period. It is known that, in the experimental animal, somatotropic hormone will reestablish active enchondral bone growth after the enchondral plate has ossified, provided a residuum of hyalin cartilage remains. Since the articular cartilage at the ends of long bones and at the boundaries of joints and synostoses provides this residuum, new bone growth may take place wherever articular cartilage is found. It has not been shown conclusively that somatotropic hormone specifically delays systemic epiphyseal closure. It is known that gonadotropic hormones play a very important role in the establishment of the date of epiphyseal ossification, and that, in virilism due to excessive androgen stimulation, dwarfism may result from premature closure and cessation of linear growth. Since in some cases of giantism and often in acromegaly there appears to be inadequate gonadotropin secretion, it may be that the prolonged growth period in the former is due to delayed closure caused by hypogonadism.

Pituitary giantism is not a common condition. It has been defined

as enchondral growth in excess of 6 feet 8 inches. This type of abnormal growth has resulted in statures which have exceeded 8 feet. It is
relatively much more common in males than females.

Since, by definition, giantism is excessive growth of bone,
cartilage and fibrous tissue during the period of normal growth, often
with some prolongation of this period, the active phase of giantism
occurs during adolescence. The same process after the secondary
epiphyseal centers have closed also results in excessive growth of bone,
cartilage and fibrous tissue, but since the epiphyseal centers have been
ossified, bone growth is different because it arises from the articular
plate[16] rather than the enchondral plate and so the pattern of growth
is quite distinctive. This condition is known as acromegaly.

Giantism presents a variety of patterns depending upon the stage
of body development at which the condition begins. It should be kept
in mind that the somatotropic hormone stimulates growth mainly and
perhaps only in mesenchymal derivatives. Thus, bone, cartilage and
fibrous tissue are the principal tissues affected, but if the stimulus is
applied early in their normal growth period the result will be simply
an exaggeration of the normal. Both length and mass of the skeleton
are increased and concomitantly there is a proportionate growth in
fibrous supportive tissue. The result is a huge but symmetric and well
proportioned figure. There is some evidence to support the hypothesis
that epidermal derivatives merely provide the necessary physiologic
functions that support the mesenchyme. If this be true, it would explain the increased and balanced visceral size which accompanies
mesenchymal growth. Since growth and maturation of the organic
structure takes place earlier in the brain than in other parts of the
body, this organ is not involved in giantism or acromegaly.

In summary, if the effects of excessive STH secretion begin before puberty, growth will be balanced in all areas and the result will
be simply an exaggeration of the normal. But, periodically throughout
adolescence, certain epiphyseal centers close and after closure enchondral bone formation is not nearly so rapid nor is it normal in type.
Consequently unbalanced growth takes place and the eventual product
will reflect the result of normal and abnormal bone growth. If the
stimulus is applied after closure of all epiphyseal centers the picture,
acromegaly, is quite different from giantism. If the stimulus continues throughout adolescence and into adult life the result is acromegaly superimposed on giantism.

The cause of abnormal skeletal growth in giantism is an excessive production of somatotropic hormone by the eosinophilic cells
of the anterior lobe of the pituitary. Since this excess is due usually

to an increase in the number of these cells, their other secretory products, thyrotropic hormone (TSH), glycotropic hormone and lactogenic hormone, are increased also. The cellular increase may be focal and well delineated—eosinophilic adenoma; diffuse—pituitary hyperplasia; or, as in a very few cases, giantism may be accompanied and presumably caused by an adenocarcinoma of the anterior pituitary lobe. In another few cases the pituitaries have been reported normal. There may be a functional increase without cellular hyperplasia.

The signs and symptoms of giantism fall into four groups: (1) Those due to excessive STH. (2) Those due to stimulation by other hormones elaborated by the eosinophilic cells. (3) Those due to the imbalance created by abnormal eosinophilic cell secretion and a deficiency of basophilic cell secretion because of basophilic cell destruction by the eosinophilic cell hyperplasia. (4) Those due to the space-taking character of the lesion in the anterior pituitary lobe.

The excessive growth resulting from the elaboration of abnormal amounts of STH involves all mesenchymal derivatives. The skeleton is large but so is the musculature. The viscera enlarge to accommodate the massive frame. This is especially true of the heart and kidneys. The latter show increased renal glomerular infiltration rate and proximal tubule activity.[17] Distorted growth takes place after the epiphyseal center closes so that in late adolescence the victim begins to take on the character of acromegaly superimposed on giantism. The increased height and weight sometimes leads to a thoracic kyphosis and to atrophic disturbances in the soft tissues of the feet.

Besides STH the eosinophilic cells also secrete thyroid-stimulating hormone (TSH), glycotropic hormone and lactogenic hormone. In the second group of symptoms one may find exopthalmos (excessive TSH is associated with, if not the cause of exopthalmos), hyperthyroidism and sometimes diabetes mellitus. The last may be explained on the basis of the antagonistic action of the glycotropic hormone to hexokinase, an enzyme which is necessary for the normal conversion of glucose to glycogen.

The third group of symptoms is due to the suppression of function or the pressure atrophy of the basophilic cells. Since these cells are supposed to produce adrenal cortical stimulating hormone (ACTH) and other hormones (follicle-stimulating, FSH, luteinizing, LH, and luteotropic, LTH, hormones) one may find sterility in females and osteoporosis in both males and females. The osteoporosis, which is seen more often in acromegaly than giantism, is presumably the result of excessive sugar-active hormone from the adrenal cortex which is stimulated by ACTH.

The fourth group of symptoms arise from the pressure effects of an enlarging, space-taking lesion within the cranial cavity. In most cases of giantism one finds a focal area of eosinophilic cell hyperplasia, termed eosinophilic adenoma. In some cases there may be several such adenomas or the hyperplasia may involve the entire anterior lobe. In a few cases no hyperplasia has been found. Whether minute nodules of eosinophilic cells were missed or whether there was a hyperactivity without increase in cell number is not known. In a very few cases an adenocarcinoma of the anterior lobe has been reported in giantism or acromegaly. The amount of increase in intracranial pressure depends, of course, upon the size of the lesion. Since adenomas are usually small and slowly growing, there may be no pressure symptoms or symptoms may not occur until many years after the somatic signs appear. Then erosion of the sella takes place. Headache is a frequent complaint. Extrasellar expansion of the lesion may result in pressure on the optic tract at the chiasm producing bilateral temporal hemianopsia.

Pituitary giantism must be differentiated from eunuchoid giantism. In cases of failure of proper descent and maturation of the testes or in males castrated before puberty, there is excessive growth of mesenchymal tissues. This phenomenon is comparable presumably to capon development in fowls. The body type is characteristic in eunuchoid giantism and growth never reaches the proportions of pituitary giantism. In the eunuchoid type the patient is always male, the lower half of the body exhibits greater growth than the upper half, there is failure of development of the external genitalia and the epiphyseal lines remain unossified for a prolonged period. This prolongation of the growth period is presumably responsible for the excessive size attained in areas which grow predominantly by enchondral ossification.

MORBID ANATOMY

There has been a great paucity of material available for study in giantism. The patients rarely die before adult life when acromegaly supervenes and too little attention has been directed to the epiphyseal growth centers. Bone is increased in both length and thickness. Excessive chondroblastic growth maintains the epiphyses in proportion. Perichondrium and periosteum apparently share in the accelerated and prolonged growth activity. Most reports agree that the sites of enchondral ossification show no cytologic evidence of growth disturbance.

PROGNOSIS

When giantism develops early in youth and persists throughout adolescence, the prognosis for normal life span is poor. The patients may die of their intracranial lesion or polyglandular dysfunction may lead to other conditions such as diabetes or hyperthyroidism. The patient usually develops sterility and often becomes impotent. Eventually a condition of hypopituitarism may intervene, presumably due to destruction or exhaustion of the hypophysis. There is weakness and loss of weight similar to that seen in Simmonds' disease. Most patients fail to reach middle age, and treatment—surgical eradication or irradiation of the adenoma and endocrine replacement therapy—may be beneficial but rarely curative.

ACROMEGALY

Acromegaly is the condition which results from excessive growth of mesenchymal tissues during adult life. It is caused by an abnormal secretion of the somatotropic growth hormone from the eosinophilic cells of the anterior pituitary. This increased secretion may be the product of an eosinophilic cell hyperplasia, one or more focal areas called adenomas or a diffuse multiplication throughout the lobe. In some instances it may be due to excessive secretion of a normal number of cells. A few cases have been reported accompanying adenocarcinoma of the anterior pituitary lobe.

Acromegaly may begin at any time during adult life or it may be superimposed on giantism which has developed during adolescence. The features which characterize acromegaly are the result of abnormal growth of cartilage, bone and fibrous tissues after the normal growth period has ended. Since the normal sites of enchondral bone growth, the epiphyseal lines, have been ossified, bone is formed from remaining cartilage deposits, the articular plates[16] and from fibrous tissue, the periosteum. The first is enchondral in type and the second is intramembranous. Enchondral bone formation from the deep layers of the articular cartilage is slow and abnormal, leading to skeletal distortions which characterize the disease. Excessive intramembranous bone formation from the periosteum causes abnormal thickening of the cortices without proportionate longitudinal growth. At points where the cartilage completely disappears in the course of closure of ossification centers no growth occurs, and so the over-all picture is one of disharmonious skeletal enlargement.

Where considerable amounts of fibrous tissue are normally concentrated, growth at these points results in a curious type of enlargement. This accounts for the tufting of the fingers and toes which resembles hypertrophic osteoarthropathy and the bizarre thickening of the lips. There is a generalized thickening and sagging of the skin.

Where cartilage is not directly associated with bone, the chondroblastic hyperplasia increases the cartilage mass but does not go on to enchondral bone formation. This type of growth accounts for the enlargement of the nose.

Periosteal intramembranous bone growth not only causes generalized cortical thickening but it is accentuated at certain points. In the frontal area a supraciliary ridge is produced, and from the external occipital plate there grows a torus sometimes of considerable magnitude. The mandible is increased in length by enchondral growth from the cartilage remaining at the condyle, and its length is accentuated to grotesque proportions by the apposition of bone to the outer lamina of the anterior surface of the mandibular body. The huge jaw with failure of dental occlusion is one of the most characteristic features of the disease. The walls of the sinuses and mastoid become greatly thickened and the air spaces are enlarged. Despite this growth of bone in the cranial and facial areas there is no enlargement of the cranial cavity. This is probably due to the complete ossification of the centers of cranial growth before the onset of the disease.

Longitudinal growth of long bones is never proportional to the increase in thickness. Since reactivation of chondroblastic activity takes place at all sites of residual cartilage, the areas with the greatest number of articular cartilages will exhibit the greatest increase in length. This is found in the disproportionate growth of the hands and feet where each of the digits has four units with seven articular cartilages.

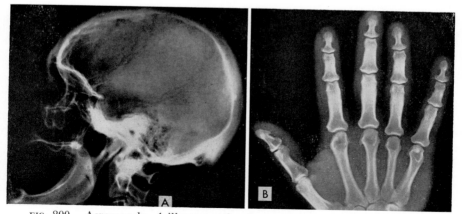

FIG. 200.   Acromegaly. *A* illustrates the changes in the mandible and the skull. The mandible is elongated, the frontal and maxillary sinuses prominent and the sella turcica enlarged and eroded. The hand (*B*) shows wide phalanges with thick cortices and enlargement of the tufts of the distal phalanges.

The ribs are increased in diameter by periosteal apposition of bone and in length by enchondral bone formation at the costosternal junction. This increase in length anteriorly causes the characteristic chest deformity with an abnormal anteroposterior diameter.

The vertebrae enlarge by apposition of bone to the lateral and anterior surfaces of the body. This new bone is intramembranous in origin and forms a collar of cortical bone surrounding the vertebra on three sides.

Thus the well advanced acromegalic acquires a typical facies and habitus. There is enlargement of the face due to the disproportionate growth of the masticatory skeleton. The mandible is widened and greatly lengthened. The lips are thick and prominent. The nose is large. There may be a prominent supraciliary ridge and an occipital torus. The skin is thick and coarse. The anteroposterior diameter of the chest is increased; there is often a thoracic kyphosis. The hands and feet are enlarged both in length and breadth with tufting of the distal ends of the digits.

Even more commonly than in giantism there is apt to be evidence of dysfunction in other endocrine glands, diabetes, exopthalmos and hyperthyroidism being most common. Males may exhibit testicular atrophy and loss of libido. Amenorrhea and sterility may develop in females.

As in giantism the prognosis is not very cheerful. The pituitary lesion may be removed surgically or an attempt may be made to reduce the eosinophilic cell secretion by irradiation. In either case the resulting endocrine disturbance is not easy to control.

PITUITARY DWARFISM

Failure of the mesenchymal derivatives to attain a size within the limits of the normal variation results in dwarfism. The commonest variety of dwarfism is seen in achondroplasia, a congenital, hereditary condition of unknown mechanism. Failure of normal bone and cartilage growth in osteogenesis imperfecta and osteopetrosis may in the rare, severe cases result in statures of subnormal proportions. Inability to mineralize the organic matrix of bone because of insufficient calcium or phosphorus or both at the osteoid site may be encountered in advanced cases of renal rickets and vitamin D refractory rickets. A deficiency in hormonal stimulation may result in slow or impaired growth and such cases are typified by cretinism and pituitary dwarfism.

The eosinophilic cells of the anterior lobe of the pituitary secrete the somatotropic hormone, STH. When there is insufficient hormonal stimulus there is inadequate growth of fibrous tissue, cartilage and bone. Since it is obvious that the failure in hormonal stimulation must apply before growth has taken place, the active phase of pituitary dwarfism always occurs in childhood or early adolescence.

The deficiency in STH may be due to a congenital lack of eosinophilic cells or to destruction. When the deficiency is congenital, most cases exhibit deficiencies of other pituitary hormones in a balanced ratio. The result is not only a failure of growth in stature but a complete and synchronized lack of somatic development. The body may remain diminutive but well proportioned. There is a concomitant failure of maturation and sex development. This rare type has been called, appropriately, the Peter Pan type of dwarfism. Destruction of the normal eosinophilic cell complement is usually caused by tumors or tumor-like (lipid reticuloendotheliosis) processes. Here the destruction is usually selective and unbalanced and bizarre combinations of signs and symptoms including dwarfism emerge. These can be accurately diagnosed only by thorough and meticulous endocrine, roentgenographic and chemical analyses. As such they are scarcely to be considered orthopedic problems.

Bone Changes of Thyroid Dysfunction

HYPOTHYROIDISM

A hormone elaborated by the thyroid gland plays an important role in the normal growth of the mesenchymal frame of the body. It may or may not be identical with the hormone that is concerned with iodine metabolism and the regulation of the metabolic processes within the cell. It is uncertain whether this hormone controls skeletal growth directly or whether its effect is achieved through its influence on the pituitary. It has been shown that when the thyroid is completely removed, the eosinophilic cells of the anterior pituitary lobe gradually become greatly reduced in number. It has been hypothesized, therefore, that the thyroid hormone stimulates the transformation of eosinophilic cells from the neutral chromophobe cell reserve. Since the eosinophilic cells produce the somatotropic hormone which regulates mesenchymal growth and maturation, this may be the mechanism by which the thyroid affects cartilage and bone formation. In support of this hypothesis is the report that somatotropic hormone will prevent dwarfism in athyroid patients but does not control myxedema and mental retardation. This finding might be countered with the explanation that myxedema is not the direct result of hypothyroidism but is due to an excess secretion of thyrotropic hormone (or a very similar and closely associated hormone) from the pituitary gland in hypothyroidism. Still to be explained is the finding of increased intramembranous bone formation (judged by increased cortical thickness) in hypothyroid patients. Pituitary somatotropic hormone is supposed to control both enchondral and intramembranous bone formation.

In order that skeletal growth may be retarded, the thyroid deficiency must be severe and occur early. Myxedema is the condition of hypothyroidism characterized by a curious increase in water-binding capacity of the fibrous collagen. The meaning of the term is enlarged to include the low basal metabolic rate and the mental lethargy that occur in this condition. When dwarfism and retardation of mental growth are a part of the picture, the disease is called cretinism. It is obvious that cretinism can occur only during the growth period, usually beginning in infancy or early childhood. Myxedema may occur in either childhood or adult life.

Cretinism or thyroid dwarfism is usually caused by a congenital lack of thyroid formation. It may be produced by complete or nearly complete removal of the thyroid gland in early childhood. The body appears immature for the chronologic age. Skeletal growth does not catch up with fetal cranial growth so the head appears abnormally large and the extremities short. The disturbance in collagen function manifests itself early. There is apparently an increase in its water-binding capacity so that it swells and takes on a myxomatous appearance. The excess water is not free as in ordinary edema so that it cannot be drained by incision or removed through the kidneys by reducing the sodium content. There appears to be a colloidal bond between the collagen protein and the fluid. Since the water cannot be displaced by pressure, pitting does not take place. This swelling of all the collagenous structures accounts for many of the signs and symptoms of the condition.

The skin is dry and scaly. It and the subcutaneous tissue are much thicker than normal, giving the myxedematous appearance. The eyelids and tongue are greatly enlarged, causing disturbance in function. Mental growth is seriously retarded; at times the patient attains an intellect no greater than that of a three to four year old child. There may be failure of development of secondary sex characteristics with hypogonadism.

Skeletal growth is greatly inhibited. The fault appears to be in the conversion of cartilage to bone, i.e., in enchondral bone formation. Intramembranous bone formation progresses at a normal rate so that eventually the cylindrical bones become disproportionately wide for their subnormal length. The mechanism of inhibited enchondral bone growth is not understood. The osseous nuclei within the cartilaginous epiphyses are late in appearing, so that in mapping the cretin skeleton it appears to be much younger than its chronologic age. Multiple centers may develop instead of a single osseous nucleus and later merge to form an irregular area of opacity. There is probably decreased chondroblastic multiplication in the enchondral plate since the mature cells at the foot of the epiphyseal columns are not actively dissipated, and if new, young cells were added at a normal rate in the depths of the plate the latter would soon become abnormally thick. This does not occur in cretinism. Chondroblastic proliferation cannot be the sole disturbance, however, since there appears to be a slowing of mature chondrocyte utilization to produce the calcified cartilaginous lattice which is necessary for the initial deposition of osteoid. Indeed, a dome or end plate of osteoid which becomes normally mineralized to bone is laid over the cartilage surface, sealing it away from the metaphyseal tissues. Thus, it appears that there is no fault in collagen, hyalin or osteoid formation nor in mineralization of osteoid. Since hyalin is very similar to collagen in chemical constituency one is led to wonder if the same disturbance in water metabolism occurs here. And, if it does, if this affects the formation of the hyalin lattice for enchondral bone formation.

There is delay in eruption of the deciduous teeth and irregular and delayed shedding which eventually leads to impaction of permanent dentition. The teeth, however, appear to be normally formed, suggesting that there is no disturbance in normal matrix formation or mineralization. Dental difficulties probably stem from the failure of normal growth of the jaw.

The cretin fails to grow in height. Since apparently fibrous and intramembranous osseous growth is not disturbed, they appear heavier than normal. Not only is there delay in appearance of the osseous epiphyseal centers but there is delay of ossification of the enchondral plate. All enchondral bone growth is inhibited, resulting in dwarfism. The bones which enlarge predominantly by enchondral growth, particularly those of the extremities, are the ones most dramatically affected. The fontanels, frontal sutures and the synchondroses at the base of the skull remain unossified for prolonged periods. The vertebral discs appear to be thickened. This is probably relative since the bodies fail to achieve normal stature.

The serum cholesterol is usually elevated in cretinism and there is a hyperlipemia. As one would expect in decreased thyroid function, the protein-bound iodine is low. The diagnosis should not be difficult since other types of dwarfism—pituitary dwarfism and renal rickets—are not complicated by the changes of myxedema.

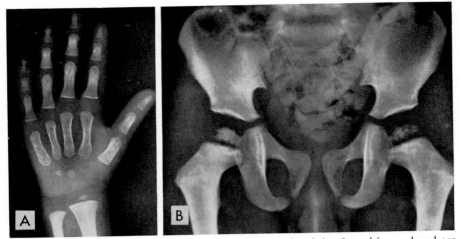

FIG. 201.   Hypothyroidism. Hand and wrist and pelvis of a white male whose chronologic age is 4 years, 3 months. The bone age as reflected by the wrist (A) approximates 15 months. There are no phalangeal epiphyseal centers and the number and development of those in the wrist is deficient. The femoral capital epiphyseal centers (B) are irregular in outline and show punctate areas of ossification.

ROENTGENOGRAPHIC CHANGES ASSOCIATED WITH DYSFUNCTION OF THE THYROID

The roentgenographic manifestations of hypothyroidism are related to the severity and duration of the condition and are present only in growing bones. The appearance of centers of ossification is delayed. When the centers do appear, they tend to be smaller than normal and are often irregular in outline and spotty in their ossification. The cortices may be thick at the expense of the medullary canal and irregularities of the epiphyseal line may mimic rickets. The tubular bones are shorter than normal. The retarded bone age may be ascertained by comparison of the radiographic appearance of the hands, wrists and knees with available standards.

REFERENCES

OSTEOPOROSIS

1. Albright, F.: Ann. Int. Med., 27:6, 1947
2. Deitrick, J. E., Whedon, G. D., and Shorr, E.: Am. J. Med., 4:3, 1948.
3. Stein, I., Stein, R. O., and Bellar, M. L.: Living Bone in Health and Disease. J. B. Lippincott Co., Philadelphia, 1955.

OSTEOMALACIA

4. McCrudden, F. M.: Arch. Int. Med., 5:596, 1910.
5. Milkman, L. A.: Am. J. Roentgenol., 32:622, 1934.
6. Albright, F., Burnett, C. H., Parson, W., Reifenstein, E. C., and Roos, A.: Medicine, 25:399, 1946.
7. Dent, C. E.: J. Bone & Joint Surg., 34B:266, 1952.

PAGET'S DISEASE

8. Paget, J.: Tr. Roy. Med. and Chir. Soc. London, *60*:37, 1877.
9. Schmorl, G.: Virchows Arch. f. path. anat., *283*:694, 1932.
10. Wycis, H. T.: J. Neurosurg., *1*:299, 1944.
11. Sornberger, C. F., and Smedal, M. I.: Circulation, *6*:711, 1952.
12. Edholm, O. G., Howard, S., and MacMichael, J.: Clin. Sc., *5*:249, 1945.
13. Jaffe, H. L.: Arch. Path., *15*:83, 1933.

SLIPPED EPIPHYSIS

14. Key, J. A.: J. Bone & Joint Surg., *8*:53, 1926.
15. Howorth, M. B.: J. Bone & Joint Surg., *31A*:734, 1949.

BONE CHANGES OF PITUITARY DYSFUNCTION

16. Weinmann, J. P., and Sicher, H.: Bone and Bones, 2nd Ed. C. V. Mosby Co., St. Louis, 1955.
17. Gershberg, H., Heinemann, H., and Stumpf, H.: J. Clin. Endocrinol., *17*:377, 1957.

14

Disturbances of Parathyroid Function

Hyperparathyroidism

PARATHYROID ADENOMA

Circumscribed hyperplasia of the secretory cells of one, rarely more than one, parathyroid gland is known as parathyroid adenoma. If these abnormal cells secrete an excessive amount of parathyroid hormone, and our knowledge is limited to those which do, then this excess acts upon the skeleton and the kidneys to produce a condition called osteitis fibrosa cystica generalisata or von Recklinghausen's disease of bone. Because certain types of kidney disease may cause secondary parathyroid hyperplasia (renal rickets) and because the term osteitis fibrosa disseminata refers to a completely different condition (fibrous dysplasia), and osteitis fibrosa cystica localisata still another, and because von Recklinghausen's neurofibromatosis may affect bones but has no relation to von Recklinghausen's disease of bone, it seems best to side-step this semantic nightmare and refer to the condition which is caused by adenomatous parathyroid hypersecretion as parathyroid adenoma. There is a distressing tendency to report cases of parathyroid adenoma under the title of "primary hyperparathyroidism," thus leaving the reader in a state of uncertainty whether the case is parathyroid adenoma or idiopathic primary hyperplasia.

Before discussing this disease, it would be well to review what is known and what is assumed concerning the parathyroid glands and their secretion.

These endocrine structures vary considerably in number, in size and in position. Any operative procedure calculated to accomplish their removal should take these variations into consideration. Usually the glands are four in number, the superior pair lying one behind the upper pole of each thyroid lobe, the inferior pair just below and behind the lower poles of the thyroid within the fibrous supportive tissue of the neck. One or more glands may be situated in the thyroid capsule, within the substance of the thyroid gland, at some distance from the thyroid or even in the mediastinum. These structures are usually moderately flattened anteroposteriorly, light tan in color, and have an average measurement of 5 by 3 by 3 mm. When sectioned and examined through the microscope they are found to consist of fields of polyhedral gland cells (chief cells) with very little tendency to acinus formation. Among them one often finds aggregates of larger cells the cytoplasm of which stains poorly or not at all (clear cells). It is supposed by most that this variation in morphology is due to differences in secretory activity in the same cell type. Mature fat cells are dispersed through the gland. At about puberty, large cells whose cytoplasm stains pink with eosin appear and increase in numbers with age (oxyphil cells). The relationship of these cells to the chief cells is unknown (Fig. 202).

A substance supposed to be the secretion of the chief and clear cells was extracted by Collip in 1925. It is known as parathormone. A relationship between the physiology of the parathyroid glands and the skeleton was realized shortly after their discovery by Sandström in 1880, and Askanazy reported a parathyroid tumor and concomitant bone disease in 1904. Erdheim expressed the opinion in 1907 that the parathyroid enlargement represented a compensatory hyperplasia. MacCallum and Voegtlin[1] reported the relationship of parathyroid insufficiency and tetany in 1909. It was not until 1926, however, that proof of the relationship of excessive parathyroid activity and demineralizing disease of bone was reported by Mandl who, believing with Erdheim that parathyroid hyperplasia was the result rather than the cause of osteitis fibrosa cystica, transplanted glands into such a patient. When the condition became worse he removed the transplanted glands, and dissecting the neck region found a parathyroid

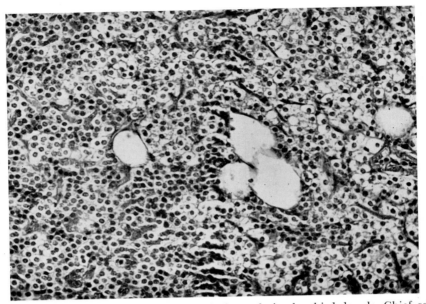

FIG. 202.   Normal parathyroid gland of a male in the third decade. Chief cells predominate. On the right there is some clear cell transition. Oxyphil cells are located in the left lower corner but are difficult to discern in a black and white photograph. (× 215.)

adenoma which on removal caused reversal of the disease. Until 1891 the condition in the skeleton produced by parathyroid adenoma was widely confused with osteomalacia and certain other demineralizing diseases. In that year von Recklinghausen separated and described an entity which he called osteitis fibrosa cystica and which has since come to bear his name.

Today it is known that a focal hyperplasia of a parathyroid gland —adenoma—by secreting excessive amounts of parathormone will cause a demineralization of the skeleton, focal areas of bone destruction, brown tumors, a lowering of the serum phosphorus level, increase in serum calcium which eventually produces metastatic and dystrophic soft tissue calcification, kidney stones and often kidney insufficiency. The mechanism of the action of the hormone upon the bones and the kidneys is still unknown, but there is no subject in the experimental literature which has been the topic of a more polemic discussion.

The matter is exceedingly complex because both calcium and phosphorus are involved, because the controlling mechanism of parathyroid secretion is not known, because kidney dysfunction can be both the cause and the result of high serum mineral levels and because the physiology of ossification is not completely understood.

It has been postulated that parathormone increases the solubility of calcium and phosphorus in blood and thus dissolves out the bone salts, that it stimulates osteoclasts to destroy normal bone, that it causes a phosphorus diuresis by inhibiting phosphorus reabsorption of the renal tubules, thus lowering serum phosphorus which is replenished by drawing phosphorus (and calcium) from bone resulting in an elevated calcium level, and that it acts directly upon the organic matrix of bone to release its mineral. In 1950 it was shown by Chang[2] and later corroborated that parathyroid transplants in contiguity with bone will cause local deossification. Until further concrete evidence is forthcoming, this mechanism of bone demineralization must be accepted as a cause of the increase in serum calcium. This does not rule out the phosphorus diuresis hypothesis, which may still apply. It is still unproven that parathormone acts upon the renal tubules to cause increased calcium reabsorption from the glomerular filtrate and this hypothesis is not necessary to satisfy the known facts concerning parathyroid adenoma. The increase in the calcium level in parathyroid adenoma appears to be proportionate to the rate and severity of deossification. At a critical level, the serum calcium spills over the kidney threshold to cause hypercalciuria. The increase in urinary mineral content leads to the formation of kidney stones. If the stones obstruct the urinary passages, altered pressure plus infection may lead to overwhelming kidney damage and kidney insufficiency. The excess calcium in the serum is deposited first in collagenous tissues which have been damaged to become calcifiable—dystrophic calcification—and finally into normal tissues—metastatic calcification. Eventually it may produce nephrocalcinosis (Fig. 203) and this may lead to impaired kidney function.

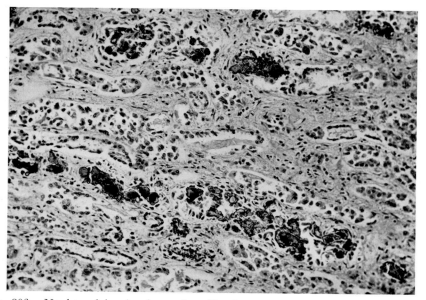

FIG. 203.   Nephrocalcinosis of parathyroid adenoma. The tubule lining cells and their supportive stroma are infiltrated with crystalline calcium salts. ($\times$ 125.)

The low serum phosphorus level is now generally believed to be the result of the action of parathormone upon the distal convoluted renal tubules. Here it apparently inhibits the reabsorption of phosphates from the glomerular filtrate, thus causing a phosphorus diuresis.

The tetany which has frequently been reported occurring immediately following the removal of a parathyroid adenoma is probably best explained on the basis of involutional atrophy of the uninvolved glands because of the reciprocal action of the high parathormone levels. This same type of atrophy has been described in other endocrine glands which are the seat of a functioning adenoma and in instances consequent to overenthusiastic endocrine therapy. Apparently the normal stimulus for secretion is inhibited by the excessive hormone and the unaffected glands undergo a disuse atrophy. After a period in which the low calcium levels must be controlled by therapy, the glands become reactivated and a normal balance is reestablished.

Parathyroid adenoma is approximately twice as common in women as men. The incidence is highest in the middle years, but may occur in children and the aged. There is usually no gross evidence of the offending parathyroid mass. In all but two of the 19 cases reported by Castleman and Mallory,[3] the adenoma involved but one gland. In the other two, two glands revealed adenomatous proliferation.

It is now known that functioning parathyroid adenoma manifests itself clinically in many ways and that the bone changes usually represent an advanced stage of the disease. The symptoms may be divided into three groups: first, those caused by the high serum calcium levels, second, those due to bone demineralization and finally, those which arise from deposits of calcium salts in the soft tissues.

The disease usually begins insidiously with lethargy, loss of muscle tone and weakness. Since the calcium ion acts as an "insulator" for nerve impulses, it may be assumed that motor impulses do not elicit a normal response. Visceral non-striated muscles are affected as well as skeletal muscles and soon there is anorexia and constipation, followed by nausea and often vomiting. In a few patients with prolonged elevated serum calcium levels, a deranged psyche may be noted.

As the skeleton is weakened by actual thinning, stress may cause bone pain. This is often misdiagnosed as arthritis, though it is probably due to infractions. In perhaps a quarter of these patients, focal areas resembling bone tumors may develop (Fig. 204). These are usually seen at the ends of cylindrical bones. They represent brown tumors. The teeth may become loosened owing to loss of the lamina dura. Eventually, fracture due to an insignificant trauma will occur and this focuses the attention of the physician on the disturbance in bone maintenance. Roentgenographic and chemical studies may then reveal the true nature of the disease.

Calcium salts may be deposited in many areas and types of tissues in the body. The most common related symptoms are those due to nephrolithiasis. Some authors have estimated that as many as 5 per cent of all kidney stones are due to parathyroid hyperactivity. It is true that all cases manifesting renal colic should be investigated for this possibility. Other signs of kidney involvement are polyuria and polydipsia. Eventually evidence of kidney insufficiency may appear. The blood urea nitrogen, creatinin and chlorides rise and there is a fall in carbon dioxide combining power. The patient develops a chronic uremia and a certain proportion will succumb.

The diagnosis is usually made, or at least verified, by laboratory examination. The serum calcium should be above 12 mg. per 100 ml. and has been reported as high as 18. The phosphorus level is less constantly low, but averages 2.5 mg. per 100 ml. The serum protein should be estimated at the same time since in hypoproteinemia a high ionizable calcium level may be masked by the low protein-bound calcium content. Since in osteitis fibrosa cystica there is an attempt on the part of the osteoblasts to repair the destruction in the skeleton, the alkaline phosphatase levels are consistently elevated. During the active phase of bone demineralization abnormal amounts of calcium should be found in the urine.

Actually, parathyroid adenoma is an uncommon disease. It is

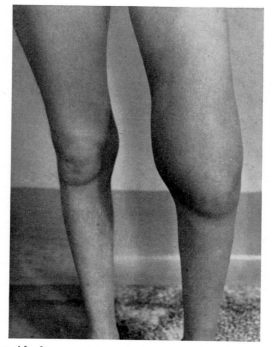

FIG. 204.   Parathyroid adenoma. A large brown tumor in the lower end of the femur. Other bones showed similar masses.

important less from the standpoint of its incidence than from the fact that there are several demineralizing bone and kidney insufficiency conditions which are commonly mistaken for it. One might hazard the guess that most tentative diagnoses of parathyroid adenoma are ultimately proved to be wrong. This only emphasizes the importance of understanding the condition thoroughly.

ROENTGENOGRAPHIC MANIFESTATIONS

The roentgenographic manifestations of hyperparathyroidism are characterized by demineralization of the skeleton and localized areas of bone destruction—brown tumors. These alterations may not be de-

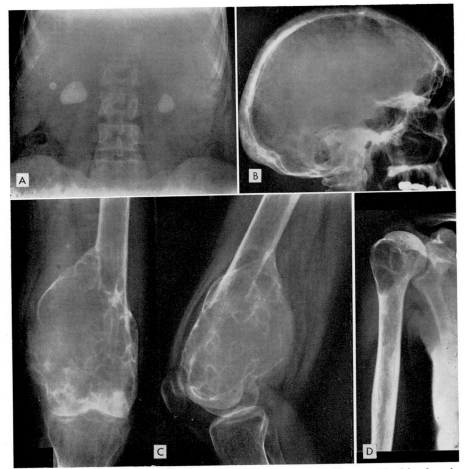

FIG. 205. Hyperparathyroidism. Extensive change in a 25 year old white female secondary to a parathyroid adenoma. Large renal calculi are present (A) as well as bony alterations. The cranial bones (B) show diffuse granular radiolucency. The large cyst-like lesion in the distal femur (C) represents focal demineralization and proliferating fibrous tissue. A similar lesion is present in the proximal humerus (D).

tected until late in the course of the disease. Certain areas, however, may show evidence of demineralization when the skeleton in general appears normal. These are the lamina dura, the phalanges and the cranial bones. When mineral salts are removed from bone, the finer trabeculae disappear and the larger ones become smaller. The cortex becomes thin and spongy bone is evident in areas that normally are composed of compact bone. Thus, the medullary canal widens. Subperiosteal demineralization is also evident; this is an important radiographic manifestation.

The lamina dura represents cortex about the tooth sockets and is evident as a dense, opaque line about each socket. Disappearance of this cortex is a result of subperiosteal demineralization. The phalanges also exhibit such change so that the external surface of the cortex is indistinct and lacy in appearance. The outer table or cortex of cranial bones becomes indistinct and the diploic bone between the inner and outer cortices becomes coarse and granular with loss of trabecular detail.

Localized destructive areas of brown tumors are most often seen in tubular bones and are of the density of soft tissue of which they are composed. Their margins may be indistinct. As they expand bone,

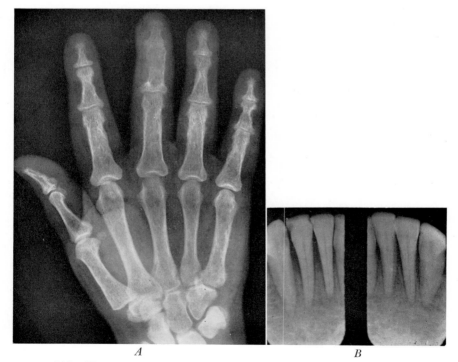

A   *B*

FIG. 206. Hyperparathyroidism. Extensive subperiosteal resorption of bone is evident in the phalanges (*A*). The cortex is thin and lacy in outline. A radiolucent cyst-like lesion is present in the middle phalanx of the third digit. *B*, The lamina dura about the teeth is absent.

a thin shell of periosteal new bone surrounds and marginates them. These lesions may be multilocular in appearance and may become extremely large or may be evident as small radiolucent cyst-like areas.

In growing bones, attempt at repair is evident at the metaphyses and result in large amounts of poorly ossified osteoid. The radiographic appearance is that of osteomalacia or rickets. Secondary hyperparathyroidism results in a radiographic appearance akin to rickets associated with demineralization that is generalized and particularly subperiosteal.

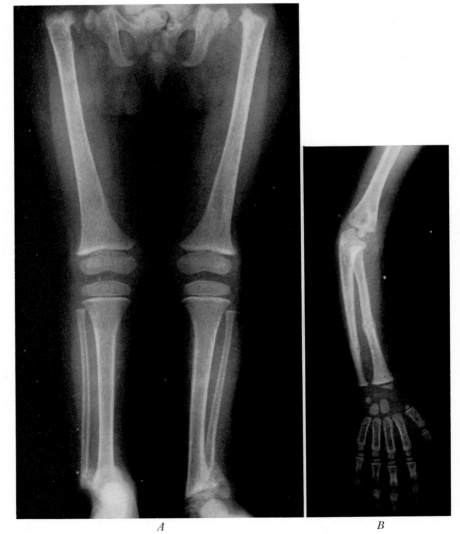

A   B

FIG. 207.   Hyperparathyroidism secondary to renal abnormality has resulted in skeletal demineralization and fractures of the proximal femurs and distal tibias and fibulas (A). The lamina dura were absent and subperiosteal resorption of bone evident in the phalanges (B).

MICROSCOPY

The name osteitis fibrosa cystica was doubtless used for this disease because of the prominence of the proliferating fibroblastic tissue which characterizes the sections. This fibrous tissue replaces the bone which disappears under the influence of abnormal amounts of parathormone and fills in the intervals between the remaining bone spicules (Fig. 208). There is nothing unique about the appearance of this fibrous tissue but the cause for its growth is not understood. The weakening of the rigid bone structure leads to multiple infractions and these in turn cause hemorrhages. Wherever there is extravasation of blood into mesenchymal tissues fibrous proliferation is stimulated. There is ample evidence of old blood pigment in the lesions, and aggregates of giant cells which accumulate especially about areas of hemorrhage are one of the hallmarks of the disease. It is unknown whether this fibrous reaction is the direct response to hemorrhage or whether other factors as yet unknown play a role.

There is an actual decrease in bone mass, seen in both the spicules and the compacta. Since there is a constant attempt at repair, the lamellation of new bone over old results in prominent cement lines. Since the pattern of destruction and replacement is not so confused

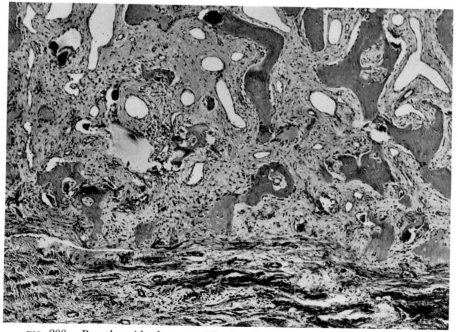

FIG. 208. Parathyroid adenoma. Fibroblastic proliferation between the thinned bone spicules is usual. There is almost complete deossification of the cortex in this area. Note the numerous osteoclasts.

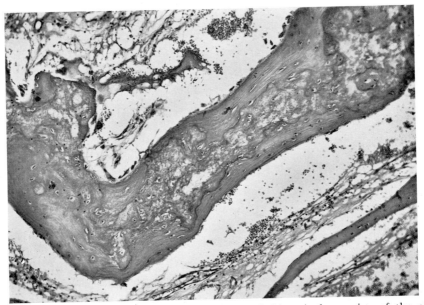

FIG. 209.   Parathyroid adenoma. The core of this spicule consists of the old, original bone. On both sides there are wide seams of newly formed osteoid which smooth out the irregularities of abnormal deossification. Along the upper seam there is osteoblastic activity. (× 102.)

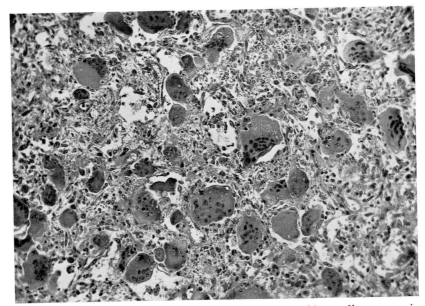

FIG. 210.   Parathyroid adenoma. Section of a brown tumor. Giant cells are prominent. They lie in a fibrous matrix which lacks the characteristics of neoplasia. (× 125.)

as that in Paget's disease, the mosaic is rarely seen so prominently. Within the diaphysis new bone formation is never prominent[4] but in the metaphyses, particularly in growing bone, wide seams of recently formed osteoid are usually encountered (Fig. 209). Along the surfaces of these seams one often finds a row of active osteoblasts. It is this osteoblastic activity which produces the increase in serum alkaline phosphatase. The presence of considerable amounts of osteoid may present a picture similar to that of rickets or osteomalacia. In sections of the metaphysis it may be impossible to distinguish these conditions though as a rule ostoid production is not as florid or as irregular in parathyroid adenoma as it is in rickets and osteomalacia.

The sections through the brown tumor areas present a highly characteristic appearance. Here again, there is evidence of old hemorrhage with considerable amounts of hemosiderin. The matrix consists of a proliferation of fibroblasts. In it are thickly dispersed hundreds of giant cells (Fig. 210). The combination of giant cells and a fibrous matrix presents the problem of differentiation from giant cell tumor of bone. This is not always possible. Indeed, it is the opinion of the writer that a certain percentage of the lesions diagnosed as "giant cell tumor" are, in fact, focal giant cell response to medullary hemorrhage. In general, the stromal cell nuclei of bona fide giant cell tumors are younger, and therefore contain more chromatin, more closely packed and less uniform in size and outline. The giant cells of giant cell tumor are apt to be somewhat smaller and to contain fewer nuclei, the nuclei show more chromatin and morphologic irregularity and they are less apt to be peripherally arranged. In brown tumor the giant cells are usually clearly separated from the stromal matrix by a space whereas in giant cell tumor they often merge with the stromal

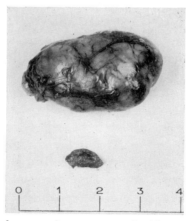

FIG. 211.   Parathyroid adenoma above compared with a normal parathyroid gland.
The scale is in centimeters.

cells. The amount of hemorrhage may also be a helpful distinguishing feature.

The importance of differentiating a brown tumor from giant cell tumor can hardly be overemphasized from the standpoint of the pathologist, since, in the past, numerous patients have undergone surgical treatment for the former, a procedure which can hardly be construed as beneficial to the patient with parathyroid adenoma.

Microscopic diagnosis on parathyroid tissue alone also presents its problems. Usually the adenoma is composed largely of chief cells, but clear cell forms, transitional types and combinations of all of these are not unusual. Moreover, in adenoma, there is a tendency for the cells to form acini which often contain a colloid-like material, thus making difficult the distinction from thyroid tissue (Fig. 212). At times a margin of compressed but otherwise normal parathyroid tissue may be encountered at the periphery of a parathyroid adenoma. This, when present, will distinguish the adenoma from secondary hyperplasia in which the entire gland is involved. In secondary parathyroid hyperplasia, the cells are chief cells or mixed chief and clear cells. It is thus impossible on the basis of parathyroid sections alone to differentiate the two. In primary hyperplasia, the proliferation is of the clear cell type and, at this moment at least, this picture is considered pathognomonic of this condition.

Throughout this discussion the parathyroid lesion of osteitis fibrosa cystica has been referred to as "parathyroid adenoma." The subject should not be closed without mentioning that most oncologists no longer consider it a true neoplasm. It is a focal hyperplasia of functional cells which mature and secrete very much as normal cells. It is their increase in number and their failure to respond to the stimulating and checking influences that govern normal cells that result in the excessive amounts of parathormone. The reason for this breaking away from normal control is not known since the parathyroids are apparently not affected by the secretions of other ductless glands. Such functioning "adenomas" also occur in the thyroid, adrenal cortex, pituitary and pancreas. In these, however, a complex hormone balance is involved which may be responsible for their behavior.

The factors which govern the secretory activity of the normal parathyroid gland are not certainly known. Some are of the opinion that a high serum phosphorus level is the stimulating agent but most writers now concur with Albright that the initiating factor is a critical low serum calcium content. Most of the facts known about the clinical aberrations of this gland are consistent with this idea, though in those cases of hyperplasia which are known to be secondary (renal rickets) there is always an elevated serum phosphorus. The secretory activity

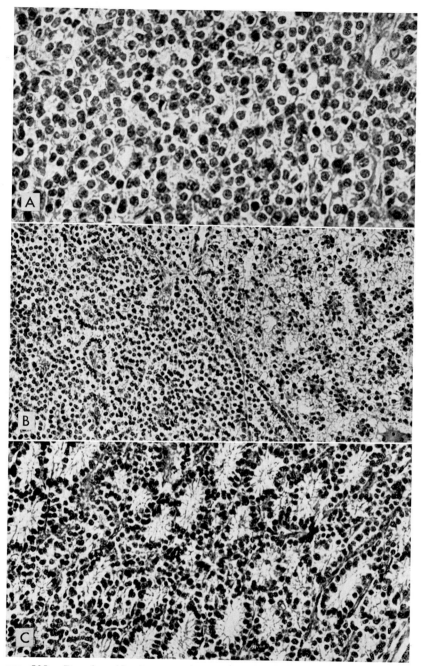

FIG. 212. Parathyroid adenoma. *A,* The entire field is composed of chief cells. (× 350.) *B,* The left half of the illustration is composed of chief cells, the right half of clear cells. (× 170.) *C,* The adenoma cells may have an acinar arangement. All three sections were taken from the same gland. (× 200.)

of most ductless glands is checked by a high level of their secretory product. For the present, at least, this may be assumed to be true of the parathyroid gland.

True tumors of the parathyroid have been reported but these are exceedingly rare and, since their cells are usually non-functional, these lesions do not pertain to this subject.

This subject has been presented primarily as a disturbance in parathyroid function rather than as an entity of skeletal disease. Since the manifestations in bone are only signs of this disturbance and frequently late ones, this approach appears to be a logical one. Furthermore, since the therapy is directed toward the gland rather than the bones, it is the parathyroid adenoma which should be emphasized. Its surgical removal should completely cure the disease.

SECONDARY PARATHYROID HYPERPLASIA

(Renal Rickets)

Secondary parathyroid hyperplasia (secondary hyperparathyroidism) is a chronic disease of the kidneys in which there is a dissipation of the serum calcium and an elevation of phosphorus, one or the other or the combination resulting in a stimulation of parathyroid hyperactivity. The low serum calcium level makes it impossible to mineralize newly formed osteoid of growing bone, and the presumable excess of parathormone causes deossification of bone which has been normally mineralized. The result in relation to the skeleton is that of a combination of rickets and hyperparathyroidism. Because of the symptoms of renal insufficiency plus those of bone destruction the disease is generally known as "renal rickets."

The association of renal and skeletal disease was first called to the attention of the profession by Lucas in 1883.[5] During the next thirty years numerous such cases were reported, but it was not until the physiology of the parathyroid glands was carefully mapped that our present concept of the skeletal disturbance on the basis of parathyroid hyperplasia was presented. Even today, all the steps in the complex mechanisms of the disease have not acquired the security of factual proof, but from analysis of experimental data and of the morbid physiology of other types of renal disease and of parathyroid adenoma we are able to assume much that has hitherto been complete mystery.

The type of parathyroid hyperplasia known as "renal rickets" is by definition a disease of growing bone and, therefore, occurs only in children. Its counterpart in the mature skeleton is frequently called "renal osteomalacia" and, in a sense, differs from the childhood form just as vitamin D deficiency rickets differs from other types of osteomalacia. Dent suggests that the terms "glomerular rickets" and "glomerular osteomalacia" be used to distinguish the type secondary to total kidney disease from "tubular rickets and osteomalacia" due to a congenital disturbance of resorption ability of the renal tubules.

The disease is almost always seen in childhood. The earlier it occurs, the more profound the bone changes are apt to be. The background is usually a congenital disturbance in kidney development. Polycystic disease or hypogenesis is common, or there may be alteration in the pressure of the calyces due to congenital ureteral stricture or valves of the urethra. The congenital malformation is usually overlaid by a chronic pyelonephritis so that there is a gradual but progressive limitation of renal efficiency. Thus, a chronic uremic state is induced. It is unusual for renal rickets to be caused by a pure glomerulonephritis though this is the usual cause of renal osteomalacia.

The signs of impaired kidney function are usually present if searched for. Albuminuria and polyuria are commonly found and there is an inability to concentrate the urine normally. There is usually a reduction in the power to excrete phenolsulfonphthalein and an increase in the blood non-protein nitrogen, chlorides and uric acid levels. The history of longstanding kidney disease before the onset of skeletal symptoms is usually the most helpful diagnostic criterion. The association of kidney disease with bone demineralization does not necessarily mean secondary parathyroid hyperplasia since in parathyroid adenoma there may be eventual renal insufficiency due to nephrocalcinosis.

The stimulation of the parathyroid glands to excessive secretory activity is probably the result of a long continued low serum calcium content. The exact cause of the low calcium level is not known. It may be due to the incompetence of the renal tubules to synthesize ammonia with a resulting substitution of the serum base ions of which calcium is one of the most important. The serum calcium may be thus expended along with other ions such as sodium and potassium. In chronic nephritis the damaged glomerular filter results in retention of phosphates. It has been presumed by some that under normal conditions there is physiologic saturation of the serum with the calcium and phosphorus ions and that the addition of one above this saturation level necessitates a fall in the other. It has been shown by other workers that an increase in one of the components elevates the solubility product and causes a precipitation of calcium phosphate which is deposited in the tissues and in motile blood phagocytes. There being a superabundance of phosphorus ions, this level is not materially affected but the available calcium stores are thus depleted. The usual serum calcium level in renal rickets is normal or slightly depressed; the phosphorus may be normal but is often elevated. The changes in ion levels are almost never as dramatic as those in parathyroid adenoma and idiopathic spontaneous parathyroid hyperplasia. The most important distinguishing feature is the high calcium level in the primary parathyroid diseases and the low level in that secondary to renal disease.

Metastatic calcification is not nearly as common in secondary parathyroid hyperplasia as it is in the primary parathyroid disturbances. But nephrocalcinosis may occur and even widespread calcific deposits possibly due to the increased solubility product related to excess phosphorus. When the kidney disease supervenes in parathyroid adenoma the serum calcium level may fall. Then the combination of kidney insufficiency, metastatic calcification, parathyroid hyperplasia and skeletal deossification makes it almost impossible to ascertain the correct nature of the disease unless there is a clear history of renal disease before the appearance of bone disease. It may be of significance, however, that the bone changes develop more slowly, are more chronic in nature and less severe in renal hyperparathyroidism with the exception of those cases which begin very early in life.

The bone changes in renal rickets depend upon the severity of the kidney disease, its duration and the stage of skeletal development at which it began. If the nephritis results in a profound uremia early, the patient succumbs before osseous changes occur. If the kidney insufficiency is moderate, beginning early but sparing the child for several years, the skeletal changes may become very severe by the time he reaches seven to ten years. In this type, dwarfism is usually the outstanding feature and the skeleton may show all the changes of advanced rickets, since there are insufficient calcium ions to produce enough calcium salts to mineralize the osteoid of growing bone. The more rapidly the skeleton grows, the greater is the mineral lack and the more severe the bone changes will be. In addition to the changes which are characteristic of rickets, one may find fractures with faulty healing such as those encountered in parathyroid adenoma.

If the disease is later in onset, dwarfism does not occur. Here the clinical findings are largely those of chronic renal disease and skeletal deformity such as that found in parathyroid adenoma. The normally formed skeleton becomes less rigid owing to demineralization and stress causes abnormal bending.

MICROSCOPY

Examination of the kidneys reveals maldeveloped or shrunken and fibrotic organs. The appearance is usually that of the end stage of pyelonephritis often accompanied by a hydronephrosis. Microscopic sections will show extensive disease in both the glomeruli and the tubules (Fig. 213). Often there are fine deposits of fine calcium salts in the supportive tissue of the tubules and even in the glomerular tufts.

When the parathyroid glands are dissected, all or the majority will usually be found to be enlarged. Through the microscope the entire parenchyma is seen to be involved in a cellular hyperplasia. At times, this hyperplasia is entirely of chief cells but usually some of the cells are somewhat enlarged and moderately clear (Fig. 214). Scattered single or aggregates of oxyphil and fat cells may be encountered. If the entire gland is composed of clear cells arranged along a fibrillar septum with a basal arrangement of the nuclei, the case is surely one of idiopathic spontaneous hyperplasia and not of renal rickets. The difficulty for the pathologist comes in attempting to differentiate the glands of parathyroid adenoma and those of secondary hyperplasia on microscopy alone. In the majority of cases

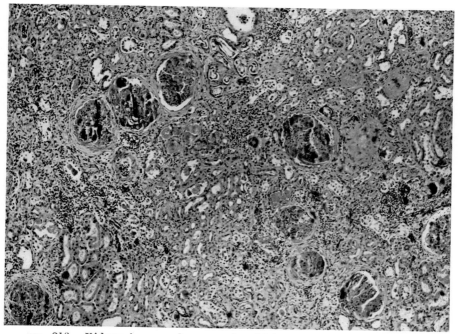

FIG. 213.   Kidney in secondary parathyroid hyperplasia (renal rickets). Both glomeruli and tubules show post-inflammatory scarring and calcium deposition. (× 25.)

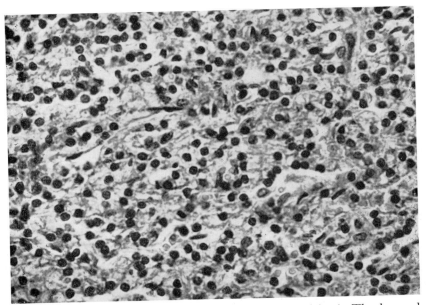

FIG. 214.   Secondary parathyroid hyperplasia (renal rickets). The hyperplasia is predominantly of the chief cell type. One can make out some tendency to clear cell transition. ($\times$ 455.)

this cannot be done, since in both the components may be mixed and variable. If a rim of normal parathyroid tissue can be found this is a strong factor for parathyroid adenoma, since in secondary hyperplasia the entire organ is usually involved.

If sections are made through the epiphyseal plate and the metaphysis of a long bone in secondary parathyroid hyperplasia (renal rickets) the changes of vitamin D rickets may be found, since here too there is inadequate calcium to form sufficient calcium salts for mineralization (Fig. 215). The provisional line of calcification may be incomplete or irregular. Failure of hyalin bar mineralization may allow the mature cartilage cells to persist. They are pushed downward to form islands within the metaphysis. Since there is no disturbance in osteoid production, in growing bone this material is formed just as in true rickets though usually it is not as abundant. Because of the failure in provisional calcification and the persistence of chondrocytes a normal hyalin lattice is not formed so that the osteoid is laid down in irregular masses or as seams along old bone spicules and abnormal cartilage islands. On comparing this section with one of true rickets a distinction cannot be made.

Sections through areas of intramembranous bone formation show less characteristic changes. Masses of fibrous hyperplasia replacing the disappearing cortex are the most obvious finding. Osteoclasts are abundant and there may be some narrow seams of new osteoid.

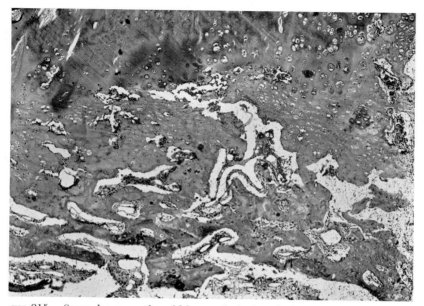

FIG 215.   Secondary parathyroid hyperplasia (renal rickets). The epiphyseal line (above) shows a lack of scaffolding. The metaphysis contains large amounts of unmineralized osteoid. ($\times$ 25.)

PROGNOSIS

The prognosis in well developed renal rickets is eventually poor. The disturbances of bone growth and deossification can be arrested by raising the serum calcium level with high calcium and low phosphorus diet and by giving adequate vitamin D. Special attention should be directed to the primary difficulty, the kidney disease. Renal insufficiency profound enough to cause bone disturbance will almost certainly result in fatal uremia but the patient may be carried along a number of years, sometimes well into adult life, until this ultimate event.

RENAL OSTEOMALACIA

Osteomalacia due to calcium loss–phosphorus retention glomerulonephritis, preferably known as renal osteomalacia, is actually a combination of calcium loss osteomalacia and secondary parathyroid hyperplasia. By definition, the disease can occur only after the epiphyseal ossification centers are closed so that bone growth is not affected.

The disease is considerably less common than renal rickets since the most common cause of the type of renal malfunction which results in disturbances of bone growth and maintenance is congenital mal-formation. In rare instances, however, a chronic glomerulonephritis may be severe enough to cause a longstanding low-grade uremia yet spare the life of the patient for a number of years. With sufficient time the resulting calcium-phosphorus imbalance induces secondary parathyroid hyperplasia and the bone changes are reflections of excessive parathormone activity.

The symptoms are primarily those of chronic renal insufficiency on which are superimposed the bone symptoms of osteomalacia.

MICROSCOPY

The microscopic features of hyperparathyroidism are bone destruction, fibrous replacement, hemorrhage and brown tumors. Those of osteomalacia are bone lysis and replacement with considerable amounts of osteoid which remains unmineralized. There have been too few cases to date to allow a critical comparison of the material from cases of renal osteomalacia with that from true osteomalacia and osteitis fibrosa cystica. Until such comparisons have been made, it is impossible to say whether renal osteomalacia can be differentiated on the basis of bone tissue examination.

IDIOPATHIC (PRIMARY) PARATHYROID HYPERPLASIA

In 1935, Castleman and Mallory[6] reported the results of their study of 25 parathyroid glands removed from patients with demineralizing skeletal disease. In 19 cases they were able to make the diagnosis of parathyroid adenoma, a single gland being involved in 17 and two glands in two cases. In another case, there was ample evidence that the hyperplasia in three of the four glands involved was secondary to longstanding kidney disease. In the remaining five cases the cellular morphology and pattern was strikingly similar, an appearance which was quite different from the other 20 cases. All of these five patients had kidney stones. In none was there clinical evidence of preceding, chronic renal disease. In three of the cases all four glands were involved, in one, three of the four, and in the fifth the only two glands found were enlarged.

Thus, it appears that three classes of hyperparathyroidism must be recognized: (1) parathyroid adenoma, (2) secondary parathyroid hyperplasia due to renal disease and (3) idiopathic parathyroid hyperplasia.

In the years since this report numerous cases of this third class have been found, most of them presenting symptoms of nephro-lithiasis but showing little evidence of the severe skeletal disturbance which characterizes parathyroid adenoma. The condition is now commonly called "primary hyperparathyroidism."

If the hyperplasia of these glands is truly "primary," then of necessity it must be of neoplastic nature. This would suggest that the parathyroid glands are not autonomous in relation to other ductless glands but that normal secretion is part of endocrine balance, and that "primary" hyperplasia is the result of breaking away from the normal control just as the multiple nodules of the thyroid establish independent activity. Since the serum chemistry appears to be the same as that in parathyroid adenoma and since preceding renal disease is not found in these cases, there is much to be said for this hypothesis.

On the other hand, the multicentric foci and the diffuse involvement of all or most of the parathyroid tissue have led some to insist that this is a secondary hyperplasia of unknown cause. To avoid a term which suggests the mechanism, it is probably best to refer to the condition as idiopathic parathyroid hyperplasia.

An insufficient number of these cases has been studied to give a clear picture of the clinical, roentgenologic and pathologic aspects. Most cases are initially admitted to the urologic service because their most prominent symptoms are those of kidney stones. An analysis of the serum phosphorus is found to be below 3 mg. per 100 ml. and the calcium level is above 12.5 mg. A skeletal x-ray survey may or may not reveal deossification though it may be assumed that the bone stores of calcium are being utilized in order to maintain the high serum level. To date, no means of separating this entity from parathyroid adenoma has been suggested other than microscopic examination of the parathyroid glands.

MICROSCOPY

Sections of the parathyroids reveal such a unique picture that even the novice should recognize the condition (Fig. 216). The entire architecture of the normal chief, clear, oxyphil and fat cells is replaced by monotonous sheets of large cells with distinct limiting membranes and cytoplasm that is almost devoid of opacity. This appearance has led to the term clear cell or wasserhelle hyperplasia. The nuclei are comparable to those of normal chief cells but in these cells appear relatively small. The cells are grouped by thin, linear strands that traverse the section and the nuclei are placed in the portion of the cell in contiguity with its septum.

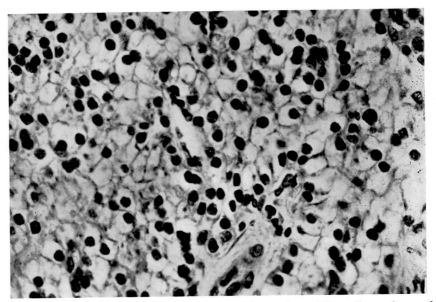

FIG. 216.   Primary (clear cell) parathyroid hyperplasia. The cells are large, the cytoplasm clear, the nuclei darkly staining and arranged along linear trabeculae. (× 412.)

In secondary hyperplasia the entire gland may be composed of chief cells but usually there is an intermixture of other normal elements and in some fields the appearance may be that of clear cell hyperplasia. Such is also the case in parathyroid adenoma and these two conditions cannot as a rule be differentiated on cytologic grounds alone. Unless the sections are composed entirely of clear cells, the diagnosis of idiopathic (primary) hyperplasia should be questioned.

Several cases of idiopathic hyperplasia have been treated by removal of all or the major portion of the hyperplastic gland tissue. In those that have been reported, the serum calcium and phosphorus levels have reverted to normal within a few days. If the diagnosis of hyperparathyroidism is reasonably certain, if the serum phosphorus is low and the calcium high and if primary chronic renal disease and fat absorption disturbance can be ruled out, surgical exploration of the neck should be undertaken. If an enlarged parathyroid is found, it should be removed and immediately sectioned by frozen technique. If it is composed of chief cells or a variety of transitional types the condition is probably one of parathyroid adenoma and nothing further need be done. If the sections reveal a clear cell hyperplasia the remaining glands must be dissected and removed. If the preponderance of the abnormal tissue is excised, the calcium and phosphorus levels should revert to normal and the disease should be arrested.

Hypoparathyroidism

CHRONIC HYPOPARATHYROIDISM

The exact action, the sites and mechanisms of the secretory product or products of the parathyroid glands is not known. Whereas it has been assumed that a single hormone was elaborated, recently some evidence has been presented to indicate that there are more than one.[7, 8] Since the glands are composed of more than one morphologic type of cell, this seems a reasonable hypothesis. Most writers agree that the parathyroid hormone has at least two actions. It lowers the serum phosphorus level by inhibiting reabsorption of phosphates through the renal tubules, thus causing phosphorus excretion in the urine. It probably acts directly upon the organic matrix of bone, freeing calcium salts which are then washed into the blood. These two actions may be accomplished by the same hormone or they may be caused by two different hormones, and no one can be sure that the glands have only these two activities.

On the assumption that the above two activities are valid, we might expect in hypoparathyroidism a failure of phosphorus excretion in the urine and an inability to move stored calcium from bone to replenish a falling serum level. The serum phosphorus level, therefore, should be high and the serum calcium low in cases in which the parathyroid glands have been removed. This is precisely what is found in cases in which the glands have been removed accidentally in thyroidectomy, called secondary hypoparathyroidism. It occurs also in cases in which no known damage to parathyroid function can be found and this is known as idiopathic hypoparathyroidism. In a few of these cases investigation has shown the apparent lack of the glands or their replacement by fat. This type has been called spontaneous hypoparathyroidism. In other cases, the glands are histologically normal or hyperplastic. This type is known as pseudohypoparathyroidism.

The commonest type of deficient parathyroid function is secondary hypoparathyroidism in which the glands have been removed at surgery. The second commonest type is spontaneous hypoparathyroidism of which about 60 cases have been reported.[9] The least common type in the literature, totaling something less than 20 cases, is pseudohypoparathyroidism.[10]

Regardless of the type, the signs and symptoms of hypoparathyroidism are much the same. Since the report of MacCallum and Voegtlin[11] in 1909, it has been known that a deficiency in parathormone secretion results in tetany. The serum calcium level falls and the phosphorus content rises. The muscle spasms which occur, in the larynx (laryngospasm), the wrists and ankles (carpopedal spasm) and in severe cases of the entire skeletal musculature (convulsions), are widely accepted as being caused by a deficiency of calcium ions in the peripheral nerves, sympathetic ganglia, the myoneural end plates and perhaps the intracerebral pathways where nerve excitability is increased. When the patient gives a history of thyroidectomy with onset of tetany soon after, these symptoms are readily recognized and controlled with proper therapy. When no such history is obtainable a diagnosis of epilepsy may be made, and because in longstanding, chronic idiopathic hypoparathyroidism there may be dwarfism, skeletal changes and metastatic calcification the cases may be confused with orthopedic diseases.

The first case of idiopathic spontaneous hypoparathyroidism was reported by Albright and Ellsworth in 1929. Since that time a considerable number of adequately studied cases have accumulated. The diagnosis is made in patients who have muscle cramps, spasms or convulsions. The serum calcium is low and the phosphorus high. The alkaline phosphatase may be elevated. Many patients suffer from opacities of the lenses. The Chvostek and Trousseau tests are positive, the latter being the manifestation of ischemia in the presence of hypocalcemia. There are often multiple defects in the ectodermal structures including scant scalp and body hair, dryness and coarseness of the skin, flecking and cracking of the nails, and poor development and early loss of the teeth. Symmetrical areas of calcification occur in the cerebral basal ganglia and in a few cases symptoms of Parkinsonism have developed. In several cases, mental deterioration has occurred along with headache and papilledema. These signs have led to the mis-diagnosis of an expanding intracranial lesion. They are thought to be due to an accompanying cerebral edema. Monilia infection of the skin, nails and mucous membranes has been reported in a number of cases.

An increase in the density and width of the cortices of the long cylindrical bones and less frequently the calvarium has occurred in some patients. This is not a constant finding and, indeed, some patients have shown generalized osteoporosis and in others the skeletal roentgenographic survey is normal. The Ellsworth-Howard test depends upon a rise in urine phosphates following the injection of parathormone. It has been shown that, performed as originally outlined, this test may be misleading particularly if parathormone has been used therapeutically. However, if the above signs and symptoms are present and if renal disease and a fat absorption defect can be ruled out, the patient is suffering from idiopathic hypoparathyroidism. Most cases respond fairly well to sustained therapy with dihydrotachysterol, showing a gradual rise in serum calcium and fall in phosphorus levels.

In 1942, Albright, Burnett, Smith and Parson reported three cases[12] of idiopathic hypoparathyroidism which did not respond to parathormone injection and considered them cases of pseudohypoparathyroidism. They believed that in these cases the parathyroid glands were normal but that the target organs were non-responsive. They felt that these cases were examples of what they called the "Seabright bantam" syndrome. The Seabright bantam cock bears the plumage of the hen because, it was thought, the target organ, in this case the feather follicles, were unresponsive to gonad secretion. It has since been shown that upon castration this particular animal does become responsive to male hormone stimulation so the term "Seabright bantam syndrome" has become meaningless. However, numerous cases of hypoparathyroidism which are refractive to parathormone stimulation have been reported. In addition, the patients are apt to be dwarfed with heavy stature, round faced and show a curious deformity of the hands and calcified or ossified nodules in the soft tissues about the joints. The deformity of the hands, and less often the feet, is due to a failure of normal growth and an early closure of the epiphyseal growth centers of the first, fourth and fifth metacarpals and

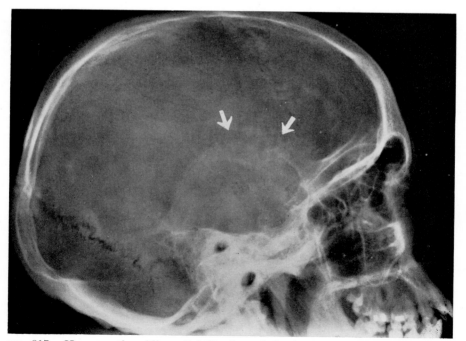

FIG. 217.   Hypoparathyroidism. Calcification of the basal ganglia is evident. The bones of the skull are normal in thickness.

metatarsals. Thus, the index finger is apt to be longer than the others. MacGregor and Whitehead point out that dwarfism and the moon face are unsafe criteria, but that if there is hypoparathyroidism in the absence of fat absorption defect and renal disease and if the patient fails to achieve a normal serum calcium level within one week of treatment with at least 200 U.S.P. units daily of parathormone the case is one of bona fide pseudohypoparathyroidism.

It has also been noted that these cases respond poorly to dihydrotachysterol and there is a high incidence of familial occurrence.

MICROSCOPY

In the few cases which have been studied by microscopic section the glands have revealed a normal cellular picture or a moderate chief cell hyperplasia.

REFERENCES

PARATHYROID ADENOMA

1. MacCallum, W. A., and Voegtlin, C.: J. Exper. Med., *11*:118, 1909.
2. Chang, H.: Anat. Rec., *106*:266, 1950.
3. Castleman, B., and Mallory, T. B.: A. J. Path., *11*:1, 1935.
4. Jaffe, H. L.: Arch. Path., *16*:63, 1933.

SECONDARY PARATHYROID HYPERPLASIA

5. Lucas, R. C.: Lancet, *1*:993, 1883

IDIOPATHIC PARATHYROID HYPERPLASIA

6. Castleman, B., and Mallory, T. B.: Am. J. Path., *11*:1, 1935.

HYPOPARATHYROIDISM

7. L'Heureux, M., Tepperman, H., and Wilhelmi, A.: J. Biol. Chem., *168*:167, 1947.
8. Stewart, G., and Bowen, H.: Endocrinology, *51*:80, 1952.
9. Robinson, P. K., Carmichael, E. A., and Cumings, J. N.: Quart. J. Med., *23* (92) : 383, 1954.
10. MacGregor, M. E., and Whitehead, T. P.: Arch. Dis. Childhood, *29*:398, 1954.
11. MacCallum, W. G., and Voegtlin, C.: J. Exper. Med., *11*:118, 1909.
12. Albright, F., Burnett, C. H., Smith, P. H., and Parson, W.: Endocrinology, *30*: 922, 1942.

Infectious Diseases of Bone

ACUTE AND CHRONIC SUPPURATIVE OSTEOMYELITIS

Bone is no less vulnerable to the ravages of animate, biologic agents than are soft tissues. Because, under normal circumstances, bone is never exposed to the external environment, these agents must reach their site of colonization by the blood or lymphatic stream, usually the former, except in compound fracture or iatrogenic infection due to surgical manipulation. It is probable that transient episodes of asymptomatic bacteremia are common. Because the organism is usually non-pathogenic or of very low virulence or because the host resistance is high, these agents are killed before they have the opportunity of establishing growth and tissue damage. If the host resistance is low or the resistance of a focal area has been impaired, a virulent organism may find a situation suitable to its reproduction and a site of infection becomes established. Suppurative osteomyelitis has a high incidence in the debilitated and in bone regions which have suffered trauma. It is probable that minor trauma causes a minute hemorrhage which lowers the resistance of a focus. If there happens to be a bacteremia and the organisms are carried to this exact area, they are able to multiply because bactericidal factors are inhibited.

Bone which suffers from the lowered oxygen tension of sickle cell disease is prone to develop one or more foci of osteomyelitis.[1] It is peculiar that in these instances organisms of the Salmonella group have been most often reported. These infections are more apt to involve the shaft than the metaphyseal region and children appear to develop this type of osteomyelitis more often than adults.

In perhaps a third of the cases a primary focus of infection can be found. Furuncles, subcutaneous abscesses and paronychiae are the usual sources of the organisms which contaminate the blood stream. Visceral or serosal pus collections may supply the infectious agent and produce the debility which predisposes to secondary bone involvement. Other diseases such as lobar pneumonia and typhoid fever may be responsible for the bone focus during the stage of systemic infection.

The Staphylococcus aureus accounts for the great majority, perhaps as many as 90 per cent of the cases of suppurative osteomyelitis. A member of the streptococcus group is involved in about half of the remainder and a small percentage are caused by Escherichia coli, Salmonella typhosa and Neisseria gonorrhoeae.

Suppurative osteomyelitis occurs most often in children under twelve years though it may occur, of course, at any age in situations conducive to its development. It is from two to four times more common in boys than girls, the reason usually offered to explain this preponderance being the greater occurrence of trauma in the former. The disease usually affects the large cylindrical bones of the extremities, the femur, the tibia, the humerus and the radius being involved in the order named.

Suppurative osteomyelitis may involve any part of any bone but the great majority of the primary foci are found in the metaphyses and usually at the end of most rapid growth. Thus the knee region, lower end of the femur and upper end of the tibia are most commonly involved, just as in tumors. This predilection is difficult to explain though there apparently is an association with areas having the richest blood supply. In adults the shaft may be affected as often as the metaphysis.

The onset is usually sudden though occasionally it is insidious. Pain, which is usually deep and often intense, ushers in the bone involvement. Tenderness is focal and usually exquisite. Soon there is swelling of the soft tissues over the area of bone involved and heat and redness appear. The systemic signs and symptoms are those of infection wherever it occurs. There is fever, malaise and anorexia, a sharp rise in the leukocyte count and a marked shortening of the sedimentation time.

The infection probably always starts in the soft medullary tissues. In the early stages there is hyperemia, change in capillary permeability and edema. Granulocytic leukocytes soon infiltrate the area in most types of infection. These are destroyed by the bacteria or their products and liberate a proteolytic enzyme. Tissue necrosis ensues and the bacteria, the lytic products of necrosis, the pus cells and debris are mingled to form a focus of suppuration.

The fate of this lesion now depends upon many factors including, of course, the virulence of the organism and the resistance of the host. But much also depends upon the portion of the bone involved and the integrity of the blood supply to the area.

In the metaphyseal area the compacta is very thin and the infection finds ready access to the subperiosteal tissue of this region. It pushes up the periosteum and travels along the external cortical surface. Spread in this fashion may be quite rapid in growing bone where the periosteum is only loosely attached. Advancing along the venous and lymphatic channels of the spongiosa the infection permeates the cancellous metaphysis (Fig. 218) and works its way toward the mid-

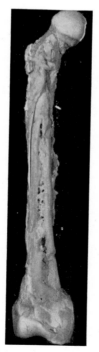

FIG. 218.   Suppurative osteomyelitis. The infection has extended through the length of the shaft. A "troughing" operation was done for drainage.

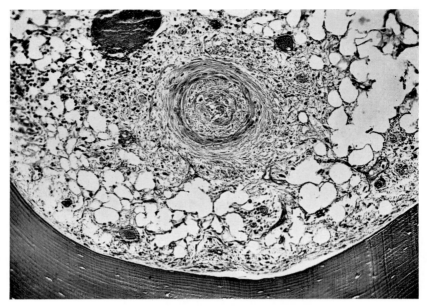

FIG. 219.   Osteomyelitis. Cross section through a small cylindrical bone. Portion of compacta at bottom. The fatty marrow shows an infiltration with inflammatory cells. A medullary vessel is completely thrombosed. It is the alteration of blood supply, decreased by thrombosis and increased by granulation, that produces the characteristic changes of the disease. ($\times$ 109.)

diaphysis. Thus the cortical cylinder becomes bathed in pus on both sides.

The initial hyperemia results in bone absorption which may be sufficient to register on the roentgenograms within one week. The inflammatory reaction causes thrombosis of vessels producing irregular areas of bone ischemia (Fig. 219). As the infection is controlled or contained there is production of excess osteoid which becomes mineralized, revealed as irregular areas of increased density on the roentgenogram. As the infection travels along the tortuous channels of the spongiosa and through the haversian canals, granulation is formed in the wake of the advancing acute process. With the increased blood supply carried by the numerous budding capillaries of the granulation there again is lysis of bone. The haversian canals are increased in diameter causing the compacta to become porous.

Vascular thrombosis induces varying degrees of ischemia. Where the blood supply is decreased below normal but is still sufficient to maintain the life of the bone tissue, the osteoblasts respond by laying down excessive amounts of osteoid. Where nutrients are diminished beyond the point of viability the osteocytes die and after a few days appear as pyknotic masses or disappear entirely, leaving the lacunae empty. Now the bone is dead and as such it is inert. Until the circulation is reestablished it remains exactly as it was at the time of cell death. What happens to this piece of dead bone depends greatly upon its size. If it is small, fingers of granulation from the contiguous living tissue will bring in a fresh blood supply which causes its lysis. Eventually, it will be completely removed and replaced first by granulation, then by fiberbone and eventually by mature, lamellated bone. If it is a large piece, the granulation will extend into its substance as far as its vessels will support it. The periphery of the dead bone becomes canalized and eventually lysed and surrounded by a zone of granulation. The central residuum remains as a static mass. This piece of bone is known as a sequestrum (Fig. 220). The sequestrum remains intact until it is revascularized or surgically removed.

The sequestrum may be composed of a mass of cancellous bone, an area of compacta or a combination of the two. It will vary in size from a minute fragment to the entire shaft. In cancellous bone it is identical with a bone infarct except that it is complicated by infection. If the process is in spongiosa the surrounding zone of granulation collagenizes, calcifies and then is converted into a shell of living bone which encapsulates the dead fragment. If the sequestrum is com-

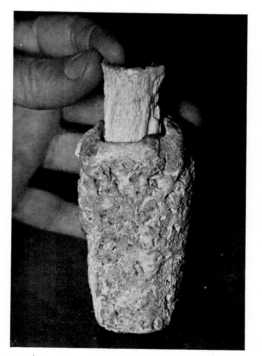

FIG. 220. Suppurative osteomyelitis. There are two separate cylinders of bone. The inside cylinder (the sequestrum) represents the residuum of the original bone. The outside cylinder (the involucrum) represents new bone laid down by the elevated periosteum.

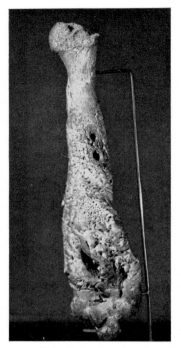

FIG. 221. Suppurative osteomyelitis. Infection has traveled the full length of the shaft and penetrated the cortex at numerous points to produce sinuses.

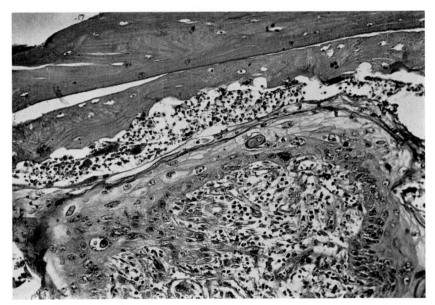

FIG. 222. Chronic suppurative osteomyelitis. The squamous cell carcinoma seen in the lower half of the picture arose in a chronic sinus and penetrated into the bone. ($\times$ 117.)

posed of compacta, a surrounding shell is produced by the overlying periosteum. In either case this ensheathing layer of bone is called an involucrum. The involucrum may be intact or incomplete depending upon the stage of the incarcerated infection. Usually it is punctured with numerous channels through which pus may escape from inside. The nature of the lesion now tends to wall off pockets of infection which may lie dormant for long periods and then undergo exacerbations of activity. Thus chronic sinuses are formed (Fig. 221) which eventually reach the surface and drain. They suppurate until the infection becomes static and then the channels are plugged with granulation and remain closed until the pressure of the pus within builds up to the point of reopening the sinuses or establishing new ones. Thus the process may continue over a period of many years or until the bone becomes so riddled and useless that amputation is imperative. In a small percentage the sinus tract opening onto the skin becomes lined by stratified squamous epithelium growing down from the surface. Constant inflammation of these lining cells may induce cancerous change. The resulting neoplasm behaves in all respects like a squamous cell carcinoma (Fig. 222).

ROENTGENOGRAPHIC MANIFESTATIONS

The roentgenographic manifestations of suppurative osteomyelitis are related to destruction of bone, to the formation of new bone as a reaction to infection and to the presence of devitalized bone. Radiographic examination will reveal no abnormalities early in the course of the process and changes will not be apparent until there is microscopic evidence of bone destruction or of new bone formation. The early administration of antibacterial agents will further modify the radiographic manifestations, so that with mild infections there may be no radiographic evidence of the disease or with more severe infection there may be a marked delay in the radiographic manifestations of the process. Since osseous changes are dependent upon destruction of bone or new bone formation, the first evidence of an underlying osteomyelitis may be the presence of a soft tissue swelling adjacent to the affected bone.

In the untreated case, small irregular areas of radiolucency are evident in the spongiosa, usually in the metaphyseal end of the bone. These represent areas in which trabeculae have been resorbed as a result of local hyperemia and necrosis. The spread of infection through the cortex causes elevation of the periosteum with resultant production of a thin, visible layer of bone. Extension of infection through

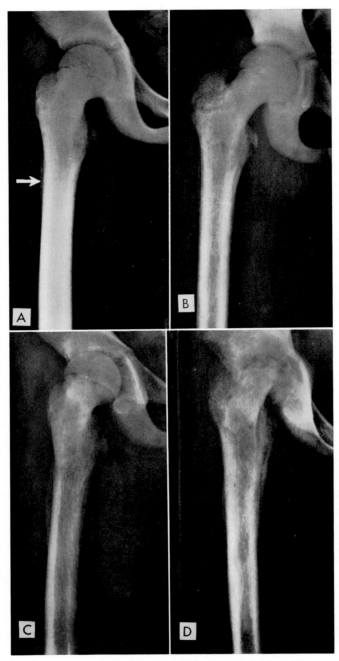

FIG. 223.   Acute suppurative osteomyelitis. The initial radiograph (*A*) shows only minimal periosteal reaction along the lateral aspect of the proximal femur (arrow). Ten days later (*B*) periosteal reaction is more marked and small irregular radiolucent areas are evident within the cortex and spongiosa. The joint space is narrowed. Two months later (*C*) marked bone destruction and narrowing of the joint space are evident. Eight months after the onset (*D*) there is gross destruction of the joint and proximal femur and marked new bone about the femur.

the tissues of the medullary canal results in the extension of osseous destruction and the presence of more and larger areas of radiolucency.

Thrombosis of vessels by the inflammatory process causes ischemia and death of bone. Spicules of devitalized bone appear quite opaque in contrast to the surrounding granulation tissue and demineralized bone. This is accentuated by the fact that they cannot respond to hyperemia as does the surrounding bone. These spicules of dead bone (sequestra), which may be cortical or medullary in location, vary in size, are usually smooth in outline and are surrounded by a radiolucent area of granulation tissue, which in turn is surrounded by an area of reactive living bone (involucrum). Multiple openings are present in large involucra and it is through these cloaca that drainage of debris occurs, often to the skin surface.

Infection may penetrate the epiphyseal line and cause disturbances of growth. If the joint is involved, rapid destruction of the articular cartilage follows initial swelling of the joint space. This is followed by narrowing of the joint space and ankylosis.

After the initial roentgenographic manifestations of osteomyelitis appear, roentgenographic examination is invaluable in delineating the extent and chronicity of involvement and the presence or occurrence of subsequent disturbances in bone growth.

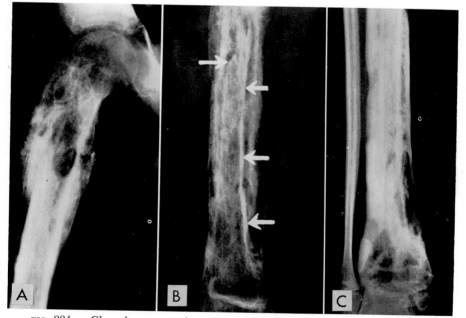

FIG. 224.   Chronic suppurative osteomyelitis. Examples of chronic suppurative osteomyelitis are illustrated. In *B* the cortex (arrows) is a sequestrum, opaque and smooth in outline. A large involucrum surrounds it, in which there are multiple cloaca. The ankle joint has been destroyed in *C*.

MICROSCOPIC FEATURES

The microscopic appearance of suppurative osteomyelitis depends upon the stage of the process at which the tissue is taken. Early the section is dominated by fields of polymorphonuclear leukocytes, living and dead with areas of liquefaction necrosis and cell detritus (Fig. 225). Later the exudate is composed largely of lymphocytes, macrophages and plasma cells. Eventually a fibrotic marrow becomes the predominating feature and it may be necessary to search through numerous fields to find exudative cells (Fig. 226). Spicules of quite normal appearing bone may be found in which the lacunae are empty. If no lacunar osteocytes can be demonstrated in entire fields, the bone is quite probably dead. The compacta often shows enlargement of the haversian canals. Some of these are empty, others are filled with granulation and still others with fibrous connective tissue. Regeneration of new bone will be found in those areas where the infection has been controlled and the debris removed by macrophage activity. The novice may have difficulty in differentiating exudate in cancellous bone from normal marrow. This mistake is not as ridiculous as it may sound since the components of an exudate, polymorphonuclear granulocytes, plasma cells, lymphocytes and red cells, may all be found in normal

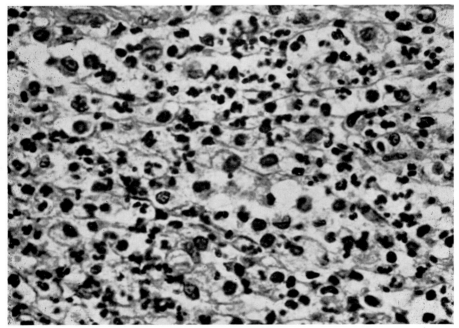

FIG. 225.   Suppurative osteomyelitis. There is necrosis with a rich infiltrate with exudative inflammatory cells. Note the numerous polymorphonuclear leukocytes. (× 534.)

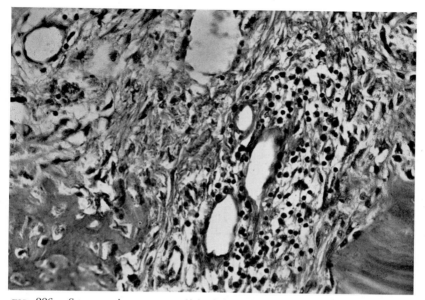

FIG. 226.   Suppurative osteomyelitis. There is a piece of new bone in the left lower corner and of old bone in the right lower corner. Between the two there is fibrosis with a perivascular infiltration with lymphocytes. (× 247.)

bone marrow. But marrow always has a distinctive fat cell pattern—large, circular, clear spaces evenly distributed throughout the cell aggregates. Exudate never contains these evenly dispersed fat cells.

Long continued infection in the subepiphyseal region, though it rarely violates the enchondral plate, may inhibit enchondral bone growth so that a long bone may fail to achieve normal stature. In some instances the excessive blood supply to the growth area consequent to nearby infection may speed growth so that the cylindrical bone becomes longer than its opposite member. Longstanding suppurative disease of medullary tissues predisposes to secondary amyloidosis, most often occurring in the spleen, kidneys and liver. The mechanisms of amyloid formation are not well understood but apparently the function of the globulin-forming tissues is perverted, so that instead of producing specific antibody gamma globulin they produce an abnormal globulin which is somehow incorporated into the chemical constituency of amyloid.

BRODIE'S ABSCESS

In certain cases a suppurative osteomyelitis may be established but the host may be able to control the infection and its spread to large areas of cancellous tissue and the subperiosteal region does not occur. Instead, the central area of suppuration and necrosis becomes

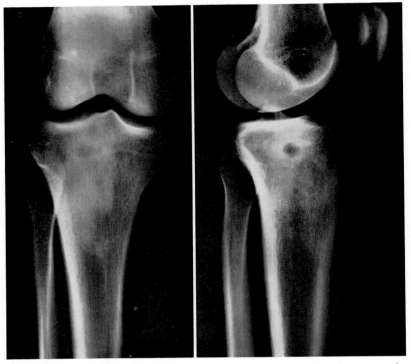

FIG. 227. Brodie's abscess. A localized area of osteomyelitis is present in the proximal tibia. There is a radiolucent lesion surrounded by opaque reactive bone. Culture of the material obtained from the lesion at surgery revealed Staphylococcus aureus

incarcerated by a wall of granulation which collagenizes to form a fibrous capsule. Thus a focal abscess of bone develops and becomes static. The offending organisms are killed and the pus is usually found to be sterile. Since auto-drainage is impossible the abscess remains until surgical intervention.

Brodie's abscess represents an aborted acute suppurative osteomyelitis. Early symptoms of the latter may disappear entirely or there may remain a focal area of bone pain and tenderness. In those cases which have yielded positive bacterial culture the same organisms have been found as in cases of diffuse suppurative osteomyelitis. It is probable that the mechanisms of development are the same.

PROGNOSIS

Suppurative osteomyelitis is no longer the dreaded disease of the past. Antibiotic therapy has completely changed the mortality and the morbidity. Treated early and efficiently the infection may be expected to yield with the same consistency as like processes in soft tissues. The principal difficulty is in making a firm diagnosis before extensive bone destruction has occurred. Because clinically and radiologically the differential diagnosis often includes Ewing's tumor, a biopsy and culture should be resorted to if necessary. Recently numerous cases have appeared which seem to be attenuated infections caused by the antibiotic used. These may run a smoldering course which make diagnosis exceedingly difficult since the cultures may be consistently negative. Usually the biopsy showing a fibrotic marrow with scattered aggregates of lymphocytes and plasma cells will supply the last piece of information necessary for accurate diagnosis.

Rarely a non-pathogenic organism or one of extremely low virulence will gain access to bone. A very low-grade infection is established which may progress so slowly that osteomyelitis is not suspected. Such lesions are sometimes seen in the vertebrae months or even longer after a spinal puncture and it is assumed that the organism has been introduced by a non-sterile needle. The very best bacteriologic work may be required to culture the organism and some cases have been known to continue for years before the cause is determined.

Non-suppurative Osteomyelitis

TUBERCULOSIS OF BONE

Tuberculous osteomyelitis used to be one of the most important problems of orthopedic practice. With but rare exception it is secondary to a tuberculous infection elsewhere in the body, usually in the lungs. With the advent of a much more efficacious therapy of this disease both the incidence and morbidity have decreased.

Tuberculous osteomyelitis may occur at any age but the great preponderance of cases affect the prepubertal child. The vertebral bodies are the most common sites of involvement, after this the upper end of the femur and the ends of cylindrical bones near large joints. In most instances there is a related tuberculous arthritis and it is impossible to state whether the infection begins within the joint or the cancellous tissue of the metaphysis. The close physiologic relationship between the subchondral cancellous tissue of the metaphysis and the soft tissues which constitute the joint has been pointed out in several instances. In rheumatoid arthritis, if biopsy material is taken from the metaphysis contiguous to the affected joint an exudative reaction similar to that of the soft tissues will be found. A like condition pertains in villonodular synovitis. Apparently the lymphatic channels of the joint capsule serve as the pathways by which processes in one area gain access to the other. It is not remarkable that tuberculosis often involves both sites. It is remarkable that tumors and suppurative arthritis so rarely do the same.

The pathology of tuberculous osteomyelitis may be classified for the sake of discussion into four groups: (1) tuberculosis of the spine; (2) combined tuberculous arthritis and osteomyelitis; (3) tuberculosis of the shaft and (4) tuberculoid reactions in bone.

Tuberculosis of the spine is almost invariably a combination of tuberculous arthritis and osteomyelitis. Since the paper describing this disease by Sir Percivall Pott in 1779, the condition is widely known as Pott's disease. The organisms reach either the joint tissues or the spongiosa of the vertebral body through the blood stream. They usually spread from an involved area to a healthy site beneath the anterior longitudinal ligaments but they may advance directly by necrosis from one vertebral body to the next. At times a normal body or joint may intervene between two foci of infection.

The infection develops slowly, spreading from the joint synovia to destroy the discs and from the cancellous tissue of a vertebral body to the supportive compacta. Lysis of cartilage and necrosis of bone occur. The trunk is shortened by collapse of the vertebrae and discs and by interference at the growth centers.

With destruction of the discs and bodies severe distortion of the normal spinal curves and alignment occur. The lower thoracic and lumbar regions are the usual sites of involvement. The anterior portion of the vertebral body is commonly most severely involved and necrosis at this site produces a kyphotic angulation, a kyphosis (Fig. 228). The normal anteroposterior curves must increase to compensate for this angulation. Muscle spasm and weakness are early symptoms; later there is distortion, pressure upon spinal nerves and spread of the infection to the soft tissues to produce "cold abscesses."

The latter are slowly developing, necrotizing abscesses which result from tuberculous channels which emerge from the bone or joint. They dissect along fascial planes and come to the surface in the paraspinal region or dissect along the sheath of the psoas muscle to appear in the inguinal region or on the medial aspect of the thigh. They may rupture spontaneously to cause a chronic sinus. They may produce large, fluctuant, subcutaneous masses which persist for a long period. If they remain uncontaminated by pyogenic organisms the whole process may be the site of an extensive precipitation of calcium salts. Sinuses may rupture through the dura and drain into the spinal canal. A tuberculous meningitis usually follows with a high mortality. Angulation and distortion of the vertebral column may cause pressure on the cord but actually this complication occurs less commonly than one might expect. The infection usually stimulates a considerable growth of granulation and this tissue may sufficiently narrow the canal to produce symptoms of a transverse myelitis.

Tuberculous infections in cylindrical bones are usually found in the metaphyses and there is almost always an infection in the corresponding joint. Thus the disease is a combined arthritis and osteomyelitis. The regions of the hip and knee are the most commonly involved. The joints are destroyed by a replacement of the synovial lining with tuberculous granulation. The articular cartilages undergo lysis, particularly about their peripheries. A tuberculous abscess develops within the metaphysis and sinuses develop and open onto the surface. Sequestration is less common than in suppurative osteomyelitis. A well established infection rarely heals without considerable bone and joint destruction. If large amounts of cancellous tissue are involved over a long period, secondary amyloidosis of the liver, kidney and spleen may develop.

Tuberculous infection of the shaft without joint involvement is much less commonly encountered. It heals more readily and extensive bone destruction is unusual. The writer has seen but one instance of multiple tuberculous infection of the metacarpals, a condition which

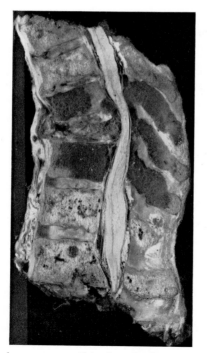

FIG. 228.   Tuberculous osteomyelitis. A sagittal section of a portion of the vertebral column. Two vertebrae are involved and have collapsed, causing kyphotic angulation with compression of the spinal cord.

earlier writers called spina ventosa. Infection of the entire shaft of one or more bones occurs with expansion of the shafts by subperiosteal apposition of bone.

When the joint tissues are involved in a tuberculous infection, the contiguous end of a long bone often reveals evidence of deossification which is out of proportion to the disuse atrophy one might expect. Surgical investigation at this site reveals a disappearance of cancellous bone tissue, thinning of the compacta and replacement with what grossly appears to be tuberculous granulation without actual necrosis or abscess formation. The process is apt to be sterile to culture and the pathologist is unable to find the granulomas which characterize the disease. This occurs often enough to have impressed earlier writers with the difficulty of demonstrating the microscopy of tuberculosis in these cases. In pulmonary tuberculosis the patient may develop what is known as an "id" reaction in the skin. This is a sensitivity response in the skin to a remote infection. Without laboring the matter, it has occurred to the author that some of our bone lesions which are sterile and fail to reveal granulomas on biopsy may be a similar type of reaction within the bone to an infection in a nearby joint. This may account for some of the cases of "tuberculosis sica" of the earlier writers.

ROENTGENOGRAPHIC MANIFESTATIONS

The roentgenographic manifestations of tuberculosis of bone are those of bone destruction usually associated with a minimum of bone reaction and little or no formation of sequestra. Osteoporosis may be a prominent radiographic feature, as well as involvement of the related joint. Where a joint is affected, the destruction of articular cartilage is much slower than is the case with suppurative infections because proteolytic enzymes are not present in the exudate. Joint involvement is manifest by widening of the joint space followed by destruction of the subchondral cortex, particularly where the joint surfaces are not opposed. Later, narrowing of the joint space occurs.

Involvement of the spine is characterized by destruction of one or more intervertebral discs and apposition of the adjacent vertebral bodies, accompanied by destruction of one or more vertebral bodies (Fig. 229). The destruction is especially apt to occur anteriorly with resultant formation of a gibbus. A soft tissue swelling is usually evident around the area and a soft tissue mass of varying size is commonly associated; this mass, which is often pear-shaped and which may calcify, represents a cold abscess. At times, the disease spares the intervertebral disc but produces destructive lesions in the vertebral body,

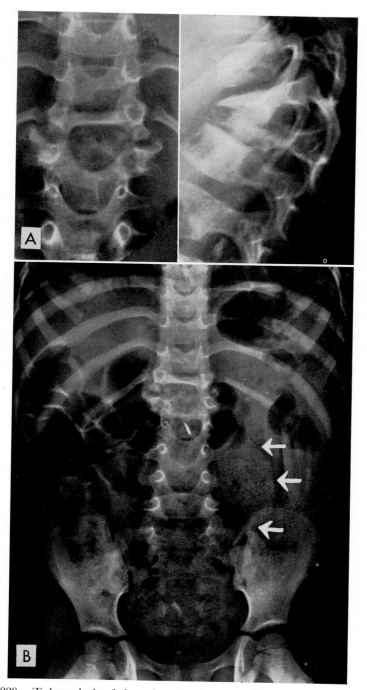

FIG. 229.   Tuberculosis of the spine. Involvement of T12 and L1 is illustrated. The intervertebral disc spaces are narrowed and the affected vertebrae have lost stature, resulting in a gibbus. A cold abscess (arrow, *B*) is evident; speckled calcification is present in the abscess.

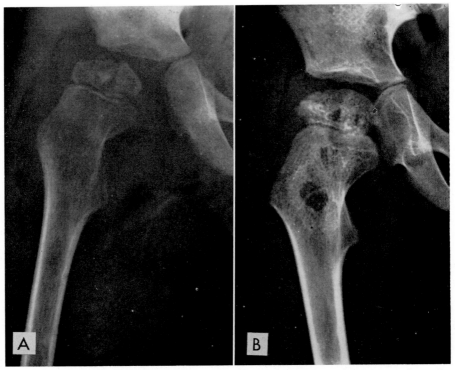

FIG. 230.   Tuberculosis. *A* shows displacement of the proximal femur from the acetabulum as a manifestation of joint involvement. Destructive lesions in the femoral capital epiphyseal center are present and marked osteoporosis is apparent. One year later (*B*) destructive lesions in the femur are present but there is little bone reaction. The joint in this case did not suffer permanent damage.

the pedicles or lamina that do not result in collapse of vertebral bodies and deformity.

In the long bones there is usually severe osteoporosis of the involved area. The response of the surrounding bone is often minimal so that destruction in the spongiosa may not be surrounded by reactive bone and there is little or no periosteal reaction. In some instances, however, the process may resemble pyogenic osteomyelitis and a definitive diagnosis of tuberculosis is usually not possible radiographically.

THE MICROSCOPY OF TUBERCULOSIS

Tuberculous infection, whether it be in lung, bone or anywhere else in the body, characteristically manifests itself as a granulomatous inflammation.

The very earliest evidence of tissue damage by the tubercle bacillus is a focal area of necrosis with an aggregate of polymorphonuclear leukocytes, but within a very short time the epithelioid cell becomes dominant. The term "epithelioid cell" is used here to avoid a term which would more exactly designate the origin of these cells. They resemble macrophages or histiocytes and are phagocytic with nuclei characteristic of the "endothelial" elements of the reticulum. They appear to arise from the young fibroblasts at the periphery of the lesion. It is probable that the latter may become motile and phagocytic if the infection is severe enough to call forth this response. In this instance the margins of the lesion advance, epithelioid cells are formed and in turn form giant cells and perish in the necrotizing reaction at the vortex of the struggle. As the offending organisms are mastered, the peripheral fibroblasts remain fixed and lay down collagen to wall off the quiescent process. Lymphocytes infiltrate the margins. The result is a fairly well delineated lesion which is called a granuloma (Fig. 231).

The term "granuloma" should not be confused with granulation. The former is a specific reticuloendothelial tissue reaction to a specific type of reagent. The latter is a non-specific repair phenomenon found in any tissue and called forth by any injurious agent. Most fungi cause a granulomatous response. Some bacteria, the tubercle bacillus for example, a few viruses, a few parasites and some chemical substances,

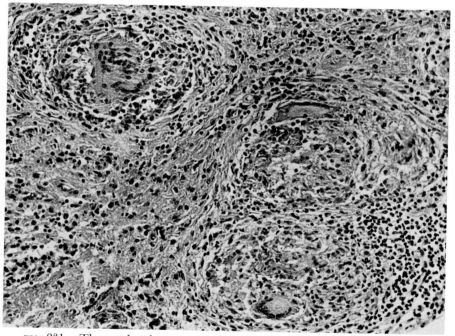

FIG. 231.   Three tubercles are seen. The ones in the upper left and lower right each contain a giant cell in the central area. About this there is an epithelioid cell reaction, lymphocytic infiltration and a peripheral zone of fibrosis. ($\times$ 186.)

especially the lipids and waxes, produce this granulomatous reaction. One cannot, with absolute assurance, name the specific agent on the evidence found in a tissue section. The granuloma (tubercle) of tuberculosis and that of Boeck's sarcoid often cannot be distinguished. If an acid-fast tissue stain is done and characteristic organisms found (less than 50 per cent of granulomatous reactions in bone are positive for organisms), it is probable that these organisms are pathogenic and the cause of the reaction. Even then it may be necessary to do definitive culture work to be sure that the acid-fast organisms found in the tissue are pathogenic tubercle bacilli.

SYPHILIS OF BONE

The Treponema pallidum infects bone just as it does the soft tissues of the body. It may be acquired in utero (congenital syphilis) from an infected mother or in postnatal life by contact (acquired syphilis). The modern treatment of syphilis by antibiotic therapy in its early stages has greatly lessened the incidence of acquired bone syphilis, and effective therapy plus compulsory premarital and prenatal serologic examinations has made congenital syphilis something of a rarity in enlightened communities.

Acquired Bone Syphilis

The spirochete is carried to the site of infection by the blood stream. Bone syphilis occurs late and is usually classified as a tertiary form of the disease. In some instances subperiosteal lesions may be noted along with the skin manifestations of secondary lues. It should be remembered that systemic syphilis is a blood-borne infection and the walls of the arterioles are the primary sites of involvement. A luetic osteomyelitis of cancellous tissue is rarely seen. As a rule the periosteum is involved first, and lacking treatment the infection may spread to the cortex and even through the cortex to the medullary tissues. Both long and flat bones may be involved, predominantly the large bones of the lower leg and the bones of the skull. Alteration of the blood supply secondary to involvement of arterioles induces both necrotizing and proliferative reactions in the tissues involved.

The necrotizing reaction may be circumscribed and surrounded by a zone of collagenized connective tissue. The central portion of the lesion undergoes a characteristic degenerative process which transforms it into a moderately firm, gray, amorphous mass. This lesion is called a gumma. More often the reaction merges imperceptibly into the surrounding tissues producing a type of granulation in which

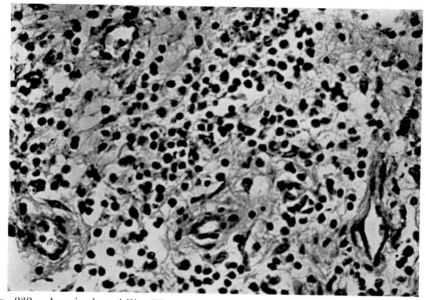

FIG. 232.   Acquired syphilis. The section reveals a perivascular infiltration with lymphocytes and plasma cells.

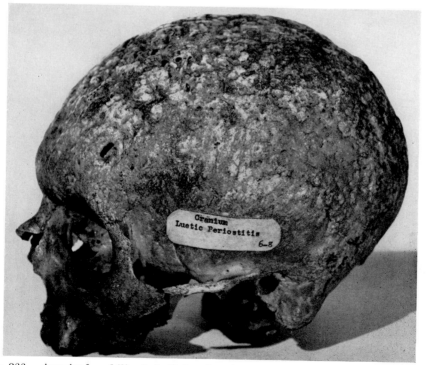

FIG. 233.   Acquired syphilis. A skull showing the roughened outer surface due to the apposition of bone by a periosteum, the site of luetic infection.

there are areas of necrosis, fibrosis and exudative cell reaction. The exudate is composed largely of lymphocytes and plasma cells. The microscopist encountering any chronic inflammatory lesion of bone composed of granulation with large numbers of plasmacytes (Fig. 232), particularly if the latter have a perivascular arrangement, should always think of syphilis, though in most instances the diagnosis will eventually turn out to be something else.

The proliferative reaction is interesting because there are very few infections which provoke the formation of an excessive amount of the tissue involved. New bone may be apposed to both the inner and outer cortical surfaces. Thus a thickening of the bone and sometimes narrowing of the medullary area are achieved. The subperiosteal new bone formation is quite irregular so that the cortical surface becomes roughened by numerous irregular craters and jagged linear depressions (Fig. 233). The interstices are filled with syphilitic granulation.

Congenital Syphilis

The spirochete characteristically attacks the epiphyseal areas in skeletal syphilis of the unborn. Any or all cylindrical bones may be

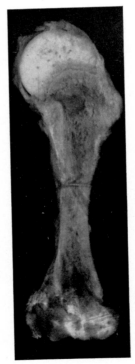

FIG. 234.   The femur of a syphilitic newborn cut in sagittal section. At the upper end the white line represents the juxta-epiphyseal zone of granulation caused by the infection.

involved. The normal metaphyseal tissues are replaced by syphilitic granulation. The infection prevents the emergence of the osteoblasts from the fibroblast pool and consequently osteoid production is inhibited or prevented. Since the epiphyseal cartilage is avascular the organisms are unable to gain access to this region and so the hyalin scaffolding is usually produced. However, since a regular pattern depends upon the invasion of the foot of each column of chondrocytes by a tongue of granulation, and since the latter is replaced by infected granulation, the hyalin masses are irregularly shaped and dispersed. Since the mineralizing mechanism is unaffected, these cartilage masses become densely infiltrated with opaque calcium salts. Thus a broad, dense "epiphyseal line" which is often quite irregular (Fig. 234) in contour appears on the roentgenograms. Since osteoid production is inhibited there is a paucity of cancellous bone in the subchondral area which produces a zone of abnormal translucency. This lack of spongiosa causes the area to be weakened and fractures through this site are common. The epiphysis may be displaced or more often crushed down into the defective ends of the shaft.

Sections through this region disclose a replacement of normal tissues with infected granulation (Fig. 235), an absence of or poor osteoid production and a scrambled pattern of irregular masses of

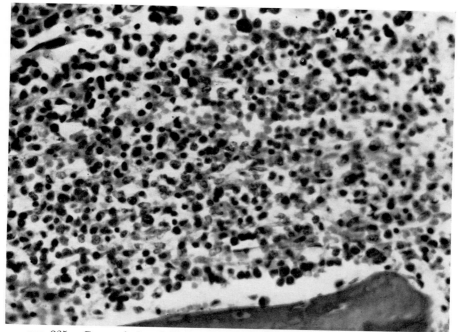

FIG. 235.   Congenital syphilis. A higher magnification of a section from the area shown in Figure 234. The normal tissues are replaced by infected granulation in which the plasmacyte predominates. ($\times$ 450.)

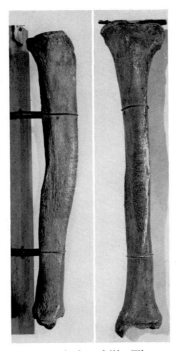

FIG. 236.   The "saber shin" of congenital syphilis. The anterior bowing is illustrated on the left. The prominent, sharp margin is seen on the right.

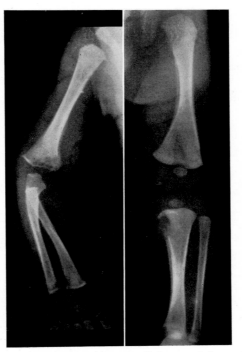

Fig. 237.   Congenital syphilis of bone. Radiolucent defects adjacent to the zones of provisional calcification are present as well as periosteal new bone about the diaphyses. The defect in the proximal tibia was symmetrical (Wimberger's sign). The zones of provisional calcification are prominent.

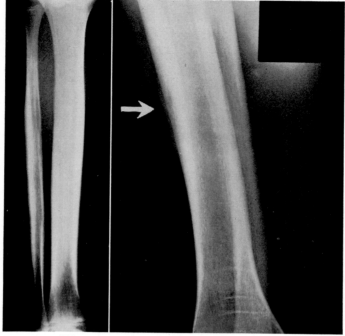

FIG. 238.   FIG. 239.

FIG. 238.   Late congenital syphilis of bone. Periosteal reaction about the tibia and fibula is marked. Endosteal thickening of the cortex of the tibia is evident with encroachment on the medullary canal.

FIG. 239.   Acquired syphilis. A destructive lesion in the tibia associated with periosteal new bone is evident (arrow).

densely mineralized hyalin. The spirochete can often be demonstrated in florid cases if the proper silver staining technique is employed.

The periosteal reaction is not unlike that of acquired syphilis. A proliferative reaction most often predominates. Since this reaction is slowly progressive and most active after birth, it is usually not noted until early childhood. The tibia is most often affected and the subperiosteal apposition of bone to the anterior cortical surface produces a forward bowing and sharpening of the anterior margin, the saber shin of congenital syphilis (Fig. 236).

MISCELLANEOUS INFECTIONS IN BONE

FUNGUS INFECTIONS

A number of fungi may establish growth within bony tissue. These diseases are referred to as mycotic osteomyelitis. Actually they make up a very small percentage of bone infections. The four fungi most often reported in skeletal infections are Actinomyces bovis producing actinomycosis, Coccidioides immitis causing coccidioidomycosis, Blastomyces dermatiditis, blastomycosis, and Sporotrichum schenckii, sporo-trichosis. All of these fungi affect soft tissues more often than bone and the latter is usually invaded by extension of the primary infection. Coccidioidomycosis is an exception in that bone is sometimes involved as part of a generalized infection due to hematogenous dissemination of the organism.

Actinomycosis usually involves the soft tissues of the head and neck and may spread to the mandible, to the lungs involving the ribs or dorsal vertebrae, or to the appendiceal region and extend to the pelvic bones. If the organisms gain access to the bone they form multiple abscesses which are connected by sinuses. The ray fungus has a powerful lytic action on all tissues and the sinuses are formed by liquefaction necrosis with a wall of granulomatous inflammatory tissue. Colonies of the fungi removed in the pus may appear as amorphous, yellow granules which are referred to as sulfur granules. Actinomycosis is a chronic type of infection and when it involves bone it is difficult to eradicate. Surgical measures have been used in the past but recently antibiotic therapy in infections of soft tissues has been so successful that a trial of this type of therapy is warranted.

Coccidioidal infections are usually contracted in the southwest part of the United States, most often in the region of the San Joaquin Valley. When the infection spreads to involve bone there are usually multiple foci and the prognosis is grave. The granulomatous reaction is much like that of tuberculosis and can be differentiated only by finding the fungus forms in the sections.

BOECK'S SARCOID IN BONE

Boeck's sarcoid is a peculiar, granulomatous inflammatory reaction which is usually seen in the lymph nodes, spleen, lungs and liver. A combined involvement of the eyes and parotid glands has been called uveoparotid fever. Involvement of several soft tissue sites is usual and bone lesions, rarely seen independently, are usually a part of a systemic infection.

The cause of Boeck's sarcoid is unknown. For many years it was widely believed to be a manifestation of a benign type of hematogenous tuberculosis. However, the Mycobacterium tuberculosis cannot be isolated from proven sarcoid lesions, the tuberculin skin test is negative in uncomplicated Boeck's sarcoid, tuberculous involvement to the extent of a multiple sarcoid dissemination has a much higher mortality than the latter and a specific skin reaction, the Nickerson-Kveim test, can be obtained in sarcoidosis. Boeck's sarcoid and tuberculosis have frequently been reported in the same patients, but it must be added that sarcoidosis, a relatively benign disease, often is found associated with several other conditions.

Almost no tissue is invulnerable to this disease but the deposits of reticuloendothelial tissue appear to be the favorite media for the etiologic agent. Even with massive involvement of large amounts of tissue the ultimate prognosis is relatively good, though occasionally infection of the lungs, liver, spleen and kidneys may cause death. The marrow tissue of bones is involved in perhaps 10 per cent of cases.

The skeletal parts most commonly affected are the small bones of the hands and feet, particularly the metacarpals, metatarsals and phalanges. The large bones are much less frequently involved.

Sometimes the disease is symptomless but often the patient will complain of malaise and will run a fever. The diagnosis may be exceedingly difficult to make and can be substantiated only by biopsy. If an enlarged superficial node can be found it should be sampled. Roentgenograms of the mediastinum may disclose bilateral lymph node enlargement which is highly suggestive. The lung fields are sometimes characteristic, having the appearance of hematogenous miliary tuberculosis except that the multiple opacities are often coarser. Needle aspiration of the liver should be done[2] and the sarcoid lesions may be obtained in a surprisingly high number of cases. The author had the opportunity of studying the liver aspiration biopsies of 21 cases of sarcoidosis which were initially thought to be tuberculous. Positive material was obtained in 16 of these. Biopsy of the skin lesions may be diagnostic.

Analysis of the serum proteins, calcium, phosphorus and alkaline phosphatase levels should always be done. The globulin level is frequently elevated, usually with a reversal of the albumin-globulin ratio. The serum phosphorus level is usually not disturbed but it may be a little high. Most characteristic is the elevation in the levels of calcium and phosphatase. The former has been investigated[3] and it is thought that, though there is bone involvement, the calcium levels are out of proportion to the amount of deossification. It is postulated that the patient with sarcoidosis metabolizes a substance which is, or has an action like, vitamin D. These patients are sometimes sensitive to vitamin D therapy, and moreover if the fecal calcium is bound by a phytate so that it cannot be absorbed, the serum calcium level falls. The elevated serum alkaline phosphatase level may be due as much to the involvement of the liver as of bone.

Actually the high serum calcium level may be one of the most troublesome features of the disease since it leads to metastatic calcification of soft tissues, particularly of the kidneys. Nephrocalcinosis and urinary tract stones may cause the symptoms that bring the pa-

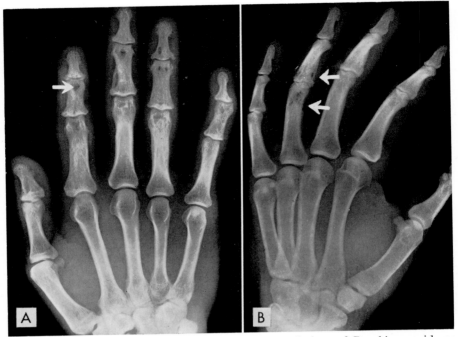

FIG. 240.   Boeck's sarcoid in bone. The osseous lesions of Boeck's sarcoid are illustrated. Round, "cyst-like" radiolucencies are evident in the phalanges of *A*. A reticular pattern of destruction is evident in the phalanges of *B* (arrows).

tient to see his physician. Snapper[4] emphasizes the frequency of lesions in the skin over the involved bone site.

Roentgenographic Manifestations

The osseous lesions of Boeck's sarcoid most frequently involve the phalanges. The granulomatous process in the marrow cavity destroys bone but causes no bone reaction. Radiographically, the lesions may present as small focal areas of radiolucency or the process may be diffuse within the involved bone to cause destruction of smaller trabeculae and irregular erosion of the cortex, resulting in a coarse reticular trabecular pattern.

Microscopy

The lesions of Boeck's sarcoid are found in the interspicular marrow tissue. The microscopic appearance of the lesion depends upon its age. It begins as a minute area of necrosis measuring less than a millimeter in diameter. At first there is little cellular reaction but soon there is an infiltration of macrophages, epithelioid cells. Often the center of the lesion is occupied by a small mass of acellular, pink-staining material which has the appearance of amyloid but which does not take the amyloid stain. It is probably what Teilum calls para-amyloid. Giant cells are frequently seen among the epithelioid cells. They may contain cytoplasmic condensations which if stellate and pink-staining are called asteroid bodies and if blue and laminated are called Schaumann bodies. It was once thought that these structures were pathognomonic of the disease but they have since been demonstrated in giant cells of a variety of granuloma types. There is a tendency for the granulomas to merge (Fig. 241) but their peripheral outlines usually remain discernible because of the reserve cells which develop into collagenoblasts and lay down collagen. As the lesions age the latter cells become more prominent until they eventually replace the epithelioid cells. Necrosis does occur but it is usually not as prominent as that in the tuberculous granuloma and it is rarely if ever caseous. There is usually a sprinkling of lymphocytes about the

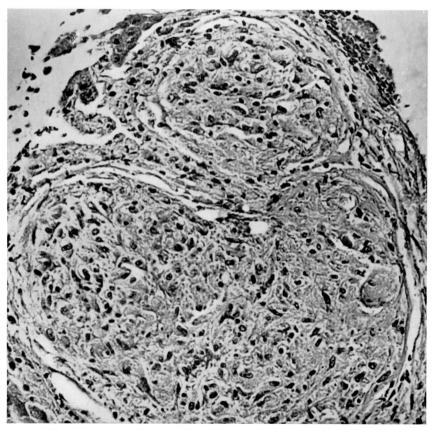

FIG. 241.   Three granulomas of Boeck's sarcoid. The top lesion is quite discrete. All are composed of an epitheloid cell reaction surrounded by a fibrous collar. (× 267.)

periphery of the lesion. The granuloma of Boeck's sarcoid cannot be differentiated from those of a host of other diseases, but if granulomas are found with typical clinical and laboratory findings and roentgenograms the diagnosis can usually be established with a fair degree of certainty.

INFANTILE CORTICAL HYPEROSTOSIS (CAFFEY)

The cause of this curious disease is entirely unknown. It is placed among the inflammatory diseases of bone because it has all of the clinical attributes of such, though careful search on numerous occasions for an etiologic agent has been fruitless and the disease does not respond to the usually effective anti-infection type of therapy.

Cortical hyperostosis is a disease of infants, usually making its appearance before the sixth month of life, but cases have been reported as late as a year and a half. It runs an irregular course, often with remissions, and is usually completely healed within one year.

Caffey and Silverman described a small series of cases[5] in 1945, and provided a name for the condition. Since then it has commonly been referred to as "Caffey's disease." There are less than a hundred reported cases but these have been collected in little more than a decade so it is apparent that the condition is not rare.

The onset is usually suggestive of a systemic infection. There is fever, leukocytosis and an increase in the erythrocyte sedimentation rate. The child is irritable and obviously unwell. In a matter of days or weeks soft tissue swellings are noted over flat bones, particularly the mandible and clavicle, and the shafts of long bones. These masses are often firm, even brawny and obviously tender. They are not red or hot. Bone changes may be present at this time or they may be lacking but appear when the apparent acute phase of the disease is subsiding. When the swellings have disappeared the child may seem to have recovered but the same process may then recur at another site. Lesions have been described in almost every bone of the skeleton except the vertebrae and pelvis. They are apparently rare in the small bones of the hands and feet. The serum alkaline phosphatase is said to be elevated in most instances.

ROENTGENOGRAPHIC MANIFESTATIONS

Infantile cortical hyperostosis is manifest radiographically by marked proliferation of bone by the periosteum. The metaphyses and epiphyses of the tubular bones are spared. The periosteally produced new bone surrounds the shaft and, as the process progresses, this new

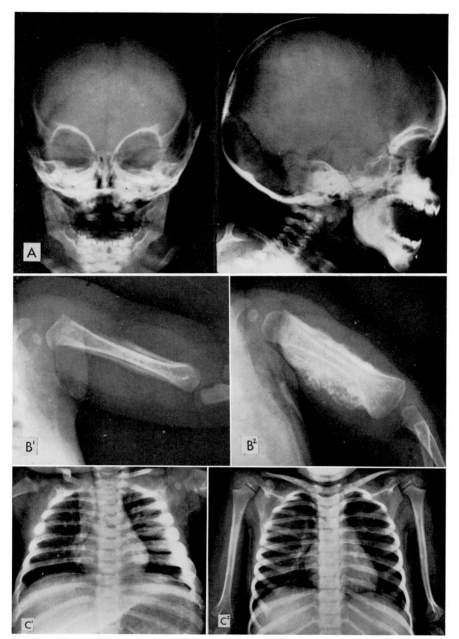

FIG. 242.   Infantile cortical hyperostosis. *A*, Abundant new bone is evident about the entire mandible as well as prominence of the soft tissues (13 weeks of age). *B*[1], The humerus (11 weeks of age) shows periosteal new bone about the diaphysis. This progressed markedly over the following 2 weeks (*B*[2]). *C*[1], The left ribs (3 through 8) are involved. *C*[3], A radiograph exposed at the age of 3 years reveals no residual enlargement of the humerus or of the ribs.

bone is produced in larger amounts so that its external surface may be quite coarse and irregular in outline. Early in the course of the process the underlying cortex is usually visible but later it blends with the surrounding newly formed bone. The diameter of the involved bones may become quite large. When healing commences, the new bone becomes lamellated and over a period of months the bone resumes a normal contour.

In longstanding cases after remissions and exacerbations, the involved bones may show a large medullary canal and thin cortices as healing progresses. In time, however, the bone returns to a normal contour and the cortex becomes normally thick.

PATHOLOGY

Since infantile cortical hyperostosis is a self-limiting disease and since the diagnosis is usually made on the clinical findings and the roentgenograms, there is inadequate material for conclusive descriptions of the organic changes. There is always subperiosteal bone formation. Fine spicules of new bone are laid down by the cambium on the outer cortical surfaces. In the author's limited material the arrangement is orderly, the axes of the spicules at right angles to the axis of the bone (Fig. 243). Several microscopists have failed to find

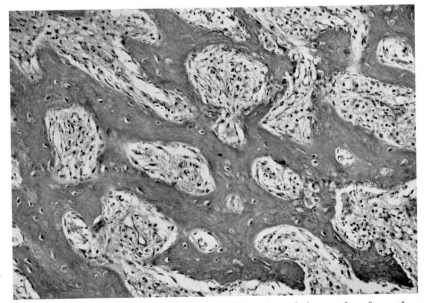

FIG. 243.   Infantile cortical hyperostosis. A section of tissue taken from the subperiosteal area of the mid-shaft region. This bone has been laid down by the cambium and apposed to the normal cortical surface. Between the bone spicules there is a fibroblastic reaction. Note the lymphocytes scattered through the latter. ($\times$ 124.)

the expected inflammatory reaction in these tissues. In at least one case of the author's there were very definite aggregates of lymphocytes which gave the impression of a low-grade chronic productive periostitis. The roentgenograms in this case were classic and the clinical course was in every way compatible with the diagnosis of cortical hyperostosis. At least one report describes degeneration and fibrosis of the overlying muscle tissue.

The greatest difficulty in this disease is the exclusion of other entities such as hypervitaminosis A, syphilitic periostitis, trauma and scurvy. Careful analysis of the roentgenograms and of the history is usually adequate for differentiation. The rare entities, multiple hereditary diaphyseal sclerosis of Ribbing and progressive diaphyseal dysplasia of Engelmann, may be more difficult to exclude. Indeed, there is in the author's files a case which has been debated for months by numerous orthopedists, roentgenologists and pathologists without sufficient agreement to include it under any of the three categories.

SCLEROSING OSTEITIS (GARRÉ)

In 1893, Garré described a type of osteomyelitis as a low-grade, chronic, diffuse inflammatory reaction which caused thickening and increased density in cortical and cancellous bone. Several reports stress the lack of suppurative exudate, the increase in bone mass, sometimes with fibrous replacement of the interspicular tissues, and the usual inability to culture organisms from the lesion. The process is said to involve the shafts of long bones particularly, causing a fusiform thickening. Mild to moderate bone pain, especially at night, is said to be the chief and sometimes only symptom.

Other writers, unable to identify a causative agent for the condition, have suggested that the lesion may be caused by an interference with the blood supply. They point out that if the normal oxygen tension in bone is reduced but still adequate for bone cell viability, organic osteoid will be laid down and soon becomes mineralized. They suggest that the increase in bone mass produces tension which could cause pain. They fortify their argument by stating that surgical incision or drilling frequently relieves the pain. This presumably is brought about by the formation of granulation and thereby an increase in the blood supply to the area.

There are many orthopedists today who feel that if the lesion which appears on clinical and roentgenographic evidence to be sclerosing osteitis is carefully studied it will be found to be one of a variety of other conditions. They suggest that there is no such entity as Garré described. Since the roentgenographic findings might be produced by a number of sclerosing conditions and since the microscopic structure is certainly far from pathognomonic, there is no way of proving whether or not the entity exists. It is certain that the diagnosis is much less frequently made today than it was in the past in many large clinics.

VILLONODULAR PIGMENTED SYNOVITIS

The descriptive term for this condition was supplied by Jaffe, Lichtenstein and Sutro in 1941.[6] They described a proliferative reaction of the synovial lining of tendon sheath, joint or bursa which is characterized in the early phase by inflammatory reaction, giant cell formation and the presence of xanthoid cells and hemosiderin. The lesion may be nodular or villous in character. As it ages the inflammatory reaction becomes less and less conspicuous, synovial cells proliferate and form sinusoid spaces which often contain giant cells. The lesion which eventually evolves has been described as an inflammatory reaction, as a xanthoma, as a sclerosing hemangioma and as a true neoplasm, benign synovioma. This lesion is most commonly encountered as a small mass, usually not larger than a centimeter in diameter in the proximity of the joints of the metacarpal bones and phalanges of the hands. Much less often it occurs in the joint synovia,[7] almost always of the knee, where it produces a bulky brown or red mass which may be mistaken for a malignant tumor. Occasionally it occurs within a bursa.

An association with alterations in bone was unknown to the author until recently when two cases of this condition, one in the hip joint and the other in a bursa near a humeral fracture with delayed union, were presented at a combined meeting of orthopedists, radiologists and pathologists.[8] In these an associated inflammatory reaction in the metaphysis beneath the articular cartilage of the involved joint was demonstrated. This reaction had caused roentgenographic deossification. Carr and Davis reported a case[9] of villonodular pigmented synovitis of the hip in which the process had penetrated the articular cartilages of the femoral head and acetabulum and produced tumor-like masses within bone. They cite another report of a similar case.

Recently, still another case of synovitis of the hip with involvement in the subarticular femoral metaphysis has come to the author's attention. In this case, sections purported to be made from metaphyseal tissue reveal changes which are quite characteristic of the so-called benign synovioma (Fig. 244).

It appears that this process is a type of inflammatory reaction which may spread through the capsular lymphatics to involve the subarticular metaphysis or it may penetrate the articular plate and grow

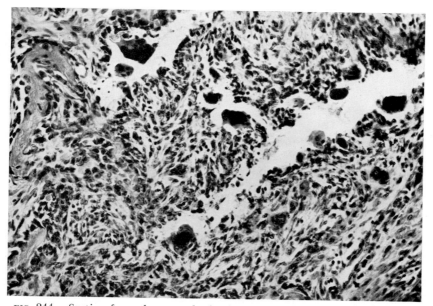

FIG. 244.   Section from the metaphysis of a patient with villonodular pigmented synovitis in the hip joint. Compare this section with one of typical synovitis within a joint seen in Figure 246. (× 170.)

into the adjacent supportive cancellous tissue. The cause of the condition is unknown though several hypotheses have been offered. It is said to be the result of bleeding into the joint cavity. Similar lesions in experimental animals have been produced by the infection of blood by one group and failed to appear in a similar experiment by others.

MICROSCOPY

In the early stages of villonodular pigmented synovitis one finds a non-specific inflammatory reaction (Fig. 245). The synovia is thickened by edema and an infiltrate with lymphocytes. In some cases large amounts of hemosiderin darken the tissue to a red-brown color. There may be considerable fibroblastic reaction which if it enlarges the villous processes gives the lesion a shaggy or bearded appearance. As the proliferative reaction becomes more dominant, nodules of solid tissue are produced. Eventually the composition is one of fibroblastic and synovial cell hyperplasia (Fig. 246). Spaces and clefts are formed many of which are lined with synovial cells. Within the spaces are found giant cells which appear to have arisen from the contiguous lining cells. Small groups of lipid-bearing macrophages, xanthoid cells, are usually found scattered through the fibrous stroma. The stromal cells may be so immature that they suggest undifferentiated mesenchymal tumor cells. When the stroma is young and active this lesion

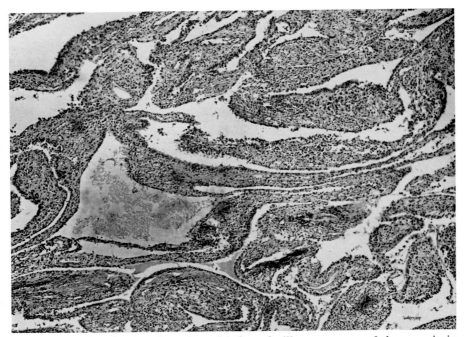

FIG. 245.   Section showing the enlarged inflamed villous processes of the synovia in early villonodular pigmented synovitis. (× 40.)

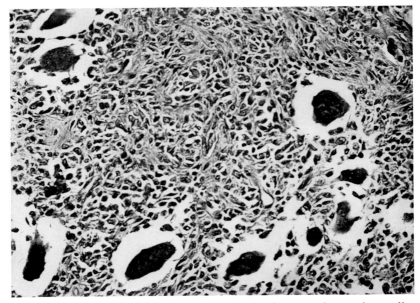

FIG. 246.   Villonodular pigmented synovitis (benign synovioma, giant cell synovioma). In the terminal stage the proliferation of synovial cells predominates in the section, producing a tumor-like mass. Irregular sinuses are formed in which lie giant cells. (× 170.)

may quite easily be mistaken for a giant cell tumor and it is probable that at least a few of the "benign giant cell tumors" of the past were, in reality, examples of this condition. When the lesion is composed of sheets of rather undifferentiated synovial cells in which giant cells have failed to appear, there is a temptation to consider this a malignant tumor.

The term "benign synovioma" is an unfortunate one because it infers that the lesion is a true tumor and moreover related to a neoplasm with a high mortality. In all probability this condition is a type of chronic proliferative inflammatory reaction. The tendon lesions are apt to erode bone from without and they may recur after surgical removal. One such lesion in the ankle region involved most of the soft tissues about the tarsal bones but eventually these proliferating cells matured and the lesion became static, still allowing function. To the writer's knowledge no such lesion has ever metastasized.

REFERENCES

1. Hughes, J. G., and Carroll, D. S.: Pediatrics, *19*:184, 1957.
2. Shay, H., Berk, J. E., Sones, M., Aegerter, E., Weston, J. K., and Adams, A. B.: Gastroenterology, *19*:441, 1951.
3. Henneman, P. H., Dempsey, E. F., and Albright, F.: J. Clin. Invest., *35*:1229, 1956.
4. Snapper, I.: Bone Diseases in Medical Practice. Grune and Stratton, New York, 1957.
5. Caffey, J., and Silverman, W. A.: Am. J. Roentgenol., *54*:1, 1945.
6. Jaffe, H. L., Lichtenstein, L., and Sutro, C. J.: Arch. Path., *31*:731, 1941.
7. Atmore, W. G., Dahlin, D. C., and Ghormley, R. K.: Minnesota Medicine, *39*:196, 1956.
8. Deakens, J. S., Wohl, G. T., and Pietrolugongo, A. L.: Personal communication.
9. Carr, C. R., and Davis, W. C.: J. Bone & Joint Surg., *36A*:1007, 1954.

Tumors and Tumor-like Processes

16

General Consideration of Tumors

The most important section in orthopedic pathology is that dealing with tumors. The incidence of primary bone tumors does not compare with that of the carcinomas of the breast, cervix, lung and stomach, yet, excluding the leukemias and lymphomas, the primary bone tumors constitute the most important single group of tumors in patients under the age of 20 years.

Also, a thorough knowledge of the primary bone tumors is absolutely essential because the differential diagnosis arises in practically all lesions which cause focal bone destruction. Because the malignant bone tumors must be treated radically, often necessitating amputation, it is paramount that the diagnosis be made early and correctly in order that the patient may have the maximum chance for survival in the case of tumor and in order that a needless sacrifice of a part be avoided in non-neoplastic lesions.

The number of entities usually classified under the heading of bone tumors is uncommonly large. The most valuable asset in consistent diagnostic accuracy is a thorough knowledge of the possibilities. Thus, every clinician, radiologist and pathologist must be familiar with this rather formidable array of lesions and their features which apply particularly to his specialty. The following discussion is a general survey of the entire field including a classification. Following this survey each of the cytogenic groups will be considered in greater detail.

The term "primary bone tumor" cannot be satisfactorily defined at present because as yet we cannot define either a tumor or the various

401

so-called types, benign and malignant. At best we can only say that a primary bone tumor is one which arises in one of the various tissues which compose the skeleton. But the definition is not strictly accurate since we include the myelomas as bone tumors and do not include the leukemias which may form tumor masses within the marrow tissue. The definition of tumor is even less informative. In the name of accuracy the word "neoplasm" has been suggested to separate the true tumors from inflammatory and traumatic masses. The substitution does not materially ease the dilemma since no one has been able to define neoplasm.

To shorten a discourse in semantics one may say there are four types of new growth. We may have an excessive reparative proliferation of cells which ultimately mature, as exemplified by the keloid. Or we may have a "spontaneous" proliferation of cells in which maturation is incomplete or lacking. Such is the nature of the lesion which we call fibroma. Or we may encounter a hyperplasia of cells which fail to mature completely and which have the added ability to invade. An example of this on the epithelial side is the basal cell epithelioma and on the mesenchymal side, the desmoid. Finally, there is the non-maturing hyperplasia of cells which not only invade but have the ability to set up independent growth, metastases. The inability of a group of cells to achieve maturity probably implies progression. A progressive hyperplasia is one which proceeds, though not necessarily at a constant rate, until intervention by some agent whether it be surgery, irradiation, chemotherapy or, in rare instances, interference with the blood supply.

The progressive, invading, metastasizing hyperplasia is obviously a true tumor, or neoplasm. How far one may extend this category to the non-invading or even non-progressive groups depends upon the inclination of the writer. This author chooses to include in the category of neoplasms only those lesions which are at least progressive, believing that our knowledge of the etiology of malignant tumors implies that the hereditary pattern of a cancer cell has been changed unalterably, causing it to reproduce before it reaches maturity, thus setting up an endless chain of reproduction, progressiveness. Those spontaneous growths which produce an excessive number of cells beyond the normal, which cells reach maturity and cease to reproduce except for the normal replacement caused by necrobiosis, are called hamartomas. Hamartomas exceed the normal limits of growth but eventually cease growing because their cells mature. A true tumor has the potential of infinite growth as long as its host can supply it nourishment. In short, it is progressive.

The criteria for judging a group of cells malignant are still more nebulous. All microscopists agree that increased nuclear-cytoplasmic ratio, irregularity of nuclear border, excess chromatin particularly if it is found in rough aggregates, the prominence of the nucleolus and an increase in mitotic figures are features which accompany malignant behavior. Yet every experienced microscopist has found some or all of these features in normal, young, rapidly growing cells whose growth has been altered by inflammation, environment or change in blood supply. This constitutes the greatest hazard for the orthopedic pathologist who must judge a lesion on the basis of the microscopic sections alone, for injury and repair in skeletal tissues may mimic every feature of malignant tumor.

The line which separates malignant from benign tumors, if it exists, is especially vague. The microscopy of a tumor is immensely helpful in this respect but it must be admitted that all the morphologic features of malignancy may be found in tumors which do not metastasize and in a few which are non-invasive. There is a modern school which is of the opinion that all true tumors are malignant, though demonstrating variable degrees of malignancy, and that there is no such thing as a benign tumor. The latter they would classify as hamartomas, choristomas or simply hyperplasias of known or unknown etiology such as the viral papillomas. There is much to be said for this contention but our knowledge is as yet too incomplete to make more than presumptive statements in this field.

In the search for the cause of cancer we have learned much concerning its physiology. A basic understanding of these mechanisms is fundamental to a working concept of bone tumors. A digression into the theories of the cause of general cancer may be warranted at this point.

Though there is still disagreement on the subject, most oncologists believe that the characteristics of cancer are transmitted from one cell to its offspring through the genetic equipment in the nucleus. It is probable that the heredity pattern is dictated by the arrangement of the molecular constituents of the genes and the spacial relationship of these molecules. It has been shown that desoxyribose nucleic acid is the principal fabric of the gene. Its constituents, the most important of which are adenine, thymine, guanine and cytosine, are probably arranged in a double helix allowing a variability in pairing patterns. These patterns apparently establish the template for the copying process which dictates the genetic equipment of the new cell.

The desoxyribose nucleic acid of the nucleus is synthesized through ribose nucleic acid in the cytoplasm. Here, enzymic activity manufactures the nuclear requirements and passes them on to the nucleus in preparation for cell division. It is probable that the genetic equipment of a nucleus, once mature, is stable and constant until it is being prepared for division. Thus the offspring of a normal cell must be normal cells but as the genes are constructed in the latter, abnormal enzymatic activity in the cytoplasm may result in abnormal molecular patterns in the gene. This cell is still a normal cell for practical purposes as long as it does not divide but, in dividing, its offspring are different cells and one of the probably many different types which may result is a cell which undergoes replication before it matures, a cancer cell.

It is apparent then that cancer can arise from any cell or groups of cells whose genetic equipment bears a certain type of abnormal structure. The cancer stigma may lie latent until the cell divides, either in the course of normal tissue replacement or secondary to an outside influence. The abnormal gene may have come from the parent, primary hereditary factor, or it may have been constructed by abnormal enzymatic activity of the cell which it replaced, somatic factor. The activity of the enzymes may be influenced by viruses, which are themselves very similar to enzymes, by metals which may inhibit enzymes, by any substance which competes for enzymic activity or by cancerogenic agents. Beryllium has been used to produce osteosarcomas in the experimental animal. A knowledge of these mechanisms is helpful in building a classification of bone tumors.

It was stated earlier in this chapter that the greatest help in making a diagnosis is a knowledge of the possibilities. The very essence of such knowledge is a classification, one that is simple enough to remember yet complete enough to embrace all possible entities. The only perfect classification is that one constructed by its author but certainly some are more useful than others. Until approximately twenty years ago all malignant bone tumors arising from the fibroblastic stem cell, i.e., those of the osteogenic, chondrogenic and collagenic series, were usually classified as osteosarcomas. This has made it most difficult to use the older literature since in many instances the reader cannot be sure which entity is being discussed. In 1939, Ewing constructed a classification for the Bone Sarcoma Registry but, though it was an improvement on the older system, it was soon realized by nearly all who tried to use it that it was hopelessly inadequate. Several better classifications have been prepared by individual writers. The one offered here is a modification of these and, though seemingly complex is, we believe, the easiest to use and retain. Actually two classifications are given here (pp. 405 and 410). Because several of the entities included in the standard classifications are reactive lesions or hamartomas, they are so entered in the second classification.

Bone tumors are best divided into four groups, each group arising

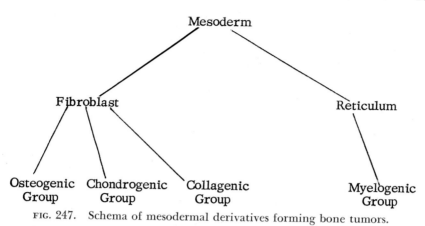

FIG. 247.   Schema of mesodermal derivatives forming bone tumors.

from one of the four stem cell types which are derived from the mesoderm. Figure 247 is a schema indicating these lines of derivation. The primitive fibroblastic cells (see Chapter 1) come from the mesenchyme which also gives rise to fat and muscle. The fibroblasts are so named because they are the progenitors of three types of cells each of which is related to a specific type of intercellular ground substance, the osteoblasts to osteoid, the chondroblasts to hyalin and the collagenoblasts (fibrous connective tissue cells) to collagen. Each tumor group is made up of a number of entities each of which is characterized by the type of ground substance of the group. The members of the fourth group, the myelogenic tumors, probably come from the various derivatives of the marrow reticulum.

CLASSIFICATION OF PRIMARY BONE TUMORS

A. Osteogenic series
 1. Osteoma
 2. Osteochondroma
 3. Osteoid osteoma
 4. Osteoblastoma
 5. Osteosarcoma
 6. Parosteal sarcoma
B. Chondrogenic series
 1. Benign chondroblastoma
 2. Chondromyxoid fibroma
 3. Enchondroma
 4. Chondroma
 5. Chondrosarcoma

C. Collagenic series
 1. Non-osteogenic fibroma
 2. Subperiosteal cortical defect
 3. Ossifying fibroma
 4. Angioma
 5. Aneurysmal bone cyst
 6. Giant cell tumor
 7. Fibrosarcoma
D. Myelogenic series
 1. Plasma cell myeloma
 2. Ewing's tumor
 3. Reticulum cell sarcoma

THE OSTEOGENIC SERIES

The lesions usually classified in this series are six in number. All but the last two, osteosarcoma and parosteal sarcoma, always produce an intercellular substance which, though it may be abnormal, is recognizable as osteoid. Osteosarcoma usually produces at least some osteoid but it is our contention that it need not, thereby allowing the inclusion in this class of a group of tumors whose cells have the appearance of osteoblasts and whose behavior is like that of osteosarcomas. To place these tumors among the fibrosarcomas because they produce no osteoid is to resort to a completely morphologic classification without consideration of the effect the tumor has upon the patient. Fibrosarcomas are slowly growing tumors, invasive and frequently recurrent, but they metastasize late and the metastases, like the primary neoplasm, grow slowly. Osteosarcoma usually grows rapidly and in most instances has sown seeds of metastasis before diagnosis is made. Metastatic deposits grow rapidly and therefore the fatal outcome is earlier and the mortality higher than that of fibrosarcoma. It is the behavioristic rather than the morphologic characteristics which should dictate the classification of these tumors, accounting for inclusion of the rapidly growing, non-osteoid-producing tumors in the osteogenic series.

The parosteal sarcoma occurs much less commonly than the osteosarcoma. It appears to arise from cells within or near the periosteum. These cells apparently have the capacity to form collagen, osteoid or cartilage and in most instances produce all three in the same lesion. When such is the case they might be called mesenchymomas of bone, following the precedent set by Stout for the name he applies to tumors in soft tissues which are made up of a variety of mesenchymal derivatives. But to do so would introduce a new name into the already crowded terminology of the field and the importance of this tumor probably does not warrant it. Admittedly, the lesion might be placed in the collagenic or chondrogenic series with as much logic as it is placed in the osteogenic group. Since it is frequently mistaken for an osteosarcoma, perhaps its contiguity in classification with that tumor may serve to emphasize their differences.

The osteoblastomas are a nebulous group. Lichtenstein[1] places here all of the benign, bone-forming lesions considered by him to be neoplasms which do not conform to the characteristics of the other bone-forming lesions. Such benign, bone-forming neoplasms are occasionally encountered, but if those ossifying fibromas which occur in the jaw and less frequently elsewhere in the skeleton are excluded as non-neoplastic lesions, the term benign osteoblastoma will rarely be needed. Since the author knows too little about the benign osteoblastoma to exclude it on the basis that it does not exist, the term is retained in the above classification, serving presently only as a monument to our ignorance.

Assuming the benign osteoblastoma to be a true neoplasm, these three entities, the osteoblastoma, the osteosarcoma and the parosteal sarcoma, are the only ones which can be included in the classification of tumors. The osteoma is a hamartomatous production of bone by periosteum. The bone is always formed by intramembranous ossification and represents a simple exaggeration of a normal, physiologic process. The formation of this lesion is quite different from the progressive, invasive proliferation of cells which characterizes true tumor; therefore this lesion cannot logically be accepted in a tumor classification.

Like the osteoma, the osteochondroma is a hamartomatous overgrowth. But in this instance the excess bone is formed by enchondral ossification. The bony pedicle is laid down in much the same manner as the primary cortex of a normal cylindrical bone in the metaphyseal region, the cartilaginous cap serving as the enchondral plate. Most osteochondromas mature and cease growing at the time the nearest ossification center closes. Their growth is orderly and limited and so they must be considered hamartomas rather than tumors. A small percentage serve as the sites of true neoplastic growth arising in one or another of their cellular components. These tumors are not a part of the original process and represent a neoplastic accident superimposed on an aberrant growth process. The fact that the incidence of tumor development is higher in osteochondroma than in normal bone can be explained by comparing this incidence with that of tumor formation in other ectopic tissues.

The nature of the osteoid osteoma has been much debated. To some it appears to be an inflammatory reaction caused by an unknown etiologic agent. Others have described it as a disturbance in bone caused by an alteration in blood supply. Whatever its exact nature it does not have the qualifications of a tumor. Its productive pattern is regular and its growth period is limited. Since we cannot yet define the morbid physiology which results in this lesion it is best to include it in a third class of lesions which must be designated simply as reaction in bone.

Thus, in the standard classification of tumors of bone which form osteoid we have two hamartomas, osteoma and osteochondroma; one idiopathic type of bone reaction, osteoid osteoma; and three true bone tumors, the benign osteoblastoma, the osteosarcoma and parosteal sarcoma.

THE CHONDROGENIC SERIES

The only entity in the standard classification of the cartilage-forming tumors which is unequivocally a true neoplasm is the chondrosarcoma. There is some evidence to suggest that the benign cartilage-forming lesions which are called chondromas are in reality a mixed group, some being cartilage-forming hamartomas like the enchondroma and the others, chondrosarcomas which lack the cellular characteristics of malignancy. The clinician has learned to distrust the microscopist's diagnosis of benign chondroma because so many of these tumors have eventually shown the aggressive behavior of malignancy. It is easy to explain this behavior by assuming that the malignant tumor represents a superimposed change on the benign one. If the pathologist admits that not all malignant tumors have the cytologic characteristics of malignancy, then some malignant tumors may be posing as hamartomas. A more careful analysis of the clinical features of these lesions, the age incidence and the skeletal region involved may help us to clarify this matter.

The enchondroma is a true hamartoma, i.e., an excessive proliferation of cells which eventually reach maturity and cease to reproduce. The enchondroma obeys the laws of body growth and becomes static at about the time the bone involved reaches its maximum size. It remains static for the duration of life unless some stimulus for neoplastic growth changes its character. Only then can it be included in a classification of true tumors.

The benign chondroblastoma and the chondromyxoid fibroma are lesions about which more knowledge is needed before they are designated a permanent place in the classification of bone tumors. Some of these lesions have given the author the impression that they too are hamartomatous cell proliferations, but in each group there has been one which showed the aggressive characteristics of true tumor. For that reason they are being placed here in the category of benign cartilaginous neoplasms. Certain similarities (both clinical and microscopic) suggest that they may be closely related or perhaps even the same entity conditioned by the area in which it arises. The benign chondroblastoma always arises in the epiphysis or in relation to it while the chondromyxoid fibroma arises in the metaphysis or shaft.

The term fibroma for the latter tumor is probably inappropriate since the cartilage which it produces is one of its most distinctive features.

In the standard classification of cartilage-producing tumors there are five entities one of which is unquestionably a tumor, chondrosarcoma; one of which is possibly a mixture of hamartomas and low grade chondrosarcomas, chondroma; two of which are probably tumors, benign chondroblastoma and chondromyxoid fibroma; and one hamartoma, the enchondroma.

THE COLLAGENIC SERIES

This group includes seven entities three of which are probably reactive lesions in bone, two of which are hamartomas and the remaining two true tumors.

The non-osteogenic fibroma is no longer considered a neoplasm by most clinicians and roentgenologists. By some it is considered a type of ischemic necrosis and in this book it is discussed in the chapter dealing with circulatory disturbances. Whatever it is, it is quite certainly not a true tumor and until its exact nature is known should be classified as a type of bone tissue reaction. The subperiosteal cortical defect is probably the same lesion as non-osteogenic fibroma except that it occurs along the outer surface of the cortex rather than the inner.

The ossifying fibroma is the term used for a group which has been a scrap basket for a variety of lesions. If there be such an entity as the benign, bone-forming tumor called benign osteoblastoma, it has been included until recently under this head. The bone-producing fibrous lesions of the jaw are probably reparative reaction to injury in most instances.

The angioma and the aneurysmal bone cyst are placed in the collagenic series because they originate from the fibroblastic cell which may produce connective tissue of blood vessels depending upon its environment and stimulus. The angioma of bone, like the angioma of soft tissues, is a hamartomatous multiplication of vessel units. Angiomas are often multiple throughout a variety of tissues including bone, are congenital, and obey the laws of growth of the part which they affect. Angiosarcoma rarely develops from a preceding hemangioma.

The aneurysmal bone cyst is an entity produced by an unknown mechanism. The osteolysis and reparative shell of newly formed bone may be caused by an excessive supply of blood to the area. The extra blood may be the result of alterations of pressure gradients or of congenital arteriovenous fistulae. Whatever the mechanism the process is not a tumor and is rarely classified as such. It is placed in the following classification among the hamartomas because it consists of an abnormal mass of vascular channels.

The term "giant cell tumor" has been used to cover a multitude of entities. Besides the true giant cell tumor, benign synovioma, the giant cell reparative granuloma of Jaffe,[2] giant cell reaction to metaphyseal hemorrhage and aneurysmal bone cyst, among other lesions, have been wrongly included in this group. It is probable that some of these non-neoplastic lesions are still being included and possibly account for all the so-called giant cell tumors which have a completely benign behavior. Whatever the status of the Grade I group, the Grade III lesions are unequivocally neoplastic.

The fibrosarcomas arising from the medullary connective tissue or the outer periosteum act like other extraskeletal fibrosarcomas.

THE MYELOGENIC SERIES

The three entities of this group are all malignant tumors. The exact cell of origin is known in none of them though various cytogenic theories have been offered. From rather sketchy data it appears to this writer that the Ewing's tumor may arise from one of the early forms of the myelogenous granulocytes and the reticulum cell sarcoma from an analogous cell in the lymphogenous series. The exact cytogenesis of the plasma cell myeloma is completely unknown but it is tempting to hypothesize that it may come from a forerunner of the erythrocyte. It is probable that all three types are derived eventually from the marrow reticulum. If such is the case they might all be called myelomas of the plasma cell, Ewing's and reticulum cell types.

REVISED CLASSIFICATION OF BONE TUMORS AND TUMOR-LIKE LESIONS

I. Reactive Bone Lesions
   A. Osteogenic
      1. Osteoid osteoma
      2. Ossifying fibroma
   B. Collagenic
      1. Non-osteogenic fibroma
      2. Subperiosteal cortical defect
II. Hamartomas Affecting Bone
   A. Osteogenic
      1. Osteoma
      2. Osteochondroma
   B. Chondrogenic
      1. Enchondroma
   C. Collagenic
      1. Angioma
      2. Aneurysmal bone cyst

III. True Tumors of Bone
    A. Osteogenic
        1. Benign osteoblastoma
        2. Osteosarcoma
        3. Parosteal sarcoma
    B. Chondrogenic
        1. Benign chondroblastoma
        2. Chondromyxoid fibroma
        3. Chondroma
        4. Chondrosarcoma
    C. Collagenic
        1. Giant cell tumor
        2. Fibrosarcoma
    D. Myelogenic
        1. Plasma cell myeloma
        2. Ewing's tumor
        3. Reticulum cell sarcoma

If one insists that a true tumor must, by definition, be progressive, i.e., that the replication of its cells is due to a fundamental alteration in its genetic character, then only the entities entered in category III can be accepted as actual neoplasms. Thus the standard classification of bone tumors becomes immensely simplified. By excluding the hamartomas, the reparative reactions to bone injury and other idiopathic lesions of unknown mechanism, the number of primary bone tumors becomes relatively few and easy to remember. Such simplification, we believe, makes for a clearer concept of the subject and a more workable classification for diagnoses.

A most interesting concept of bone tumors has recently been proposed by Johnson.[3] It is based on the premise that the morphology and behavior of this group of neoplasms is dictated not only by the cell of origin but by the area within the bone affected, the region of the skeleton, and the age of the host at the time of growth. It concedes that the primary bone tumors arise from a variety of cells, the osteoblasts, chondroblasts, collagenoblasts (fibroblasts), marrow cells and osteoclasts (a transitional stage of osteoblasts), but suggests that all these cells have a common denominator, the stem cell from which they arose, the mesenchymal cell. These cells may be divided broadly into three groups. Those which normally produce an extracellular substance which is composed predominantly of a "collagenic" material include the reticulum cell, collagenoblast (fibroblast) and osteoblast. Those which normally produce a predominantly glycoprotein substance, the marrow cells (apparently excluding the reticulum cell), make up the second group, and finally those cells which are predominantly osteolytic in function, the osteoclasts, are placed in a third group. The metabolism of the tumors which arise from these cells, i.e., the chemical constituents of their cellular products, will be determined by the cell of origin, but since the cells are all related by a common ancestor, the functions, perverted by neoplastic alteration, may become mixed with wide overlapping. Since morphology is closely related to metabolic activity the appearance of any one tumor may show variations which characterize other types. This kinship is enhanced by the normal predominant activity of the area involved, since matrix synthesis dominates the subepiphyseal metaphysis and osteoclasis preparatory to bone reconstruction occurs towards the shaft. As a tumor enlarges and spreads from one area to another, its morphology is correspondingly changed. Tumor incidence and rate of growth are influenced by what Johnson calls the metabolic gradient within the bone and the position of the bone in the skeleton. Metabolic activity is lowest in the epiphysis, next in the mid-diaphysis and becomes greater as the subepiphyseal metaphysis is approached. Moreover, this activity is greater in a cylindrical bone at the end of maximum growth—lower end of the femur, upper end of the tibia, upper end of the humerus and lower end of the radius. Also, the activity rate declines in direct proportion to the distance from the vertebral axis. The metabolic activity is also influenced by the age, being high in the last "reconstruction spurt" of adolescence and decreasing thereafter.

Johnson's concept is boldly comprehensive and refreshingly new. Whatever may be said about it, his approach disregards a burdensome mass of preconceived ideas and starts afresh with behavior rather than morphology as the correlating feature. Such a concept will be hard for morphologists to accept or even to contemplate but this does not necessarily make it erroneous. In the author's material, the frequency and the age and site incidence are compatible with Johnson's thesis. Also the association of growth rate and the relation of non-neoplastic lesions and superimposed tumors are consistent. The hypothesis fails when one attempts to find the variety of forms within a single neoplastic lesion. It is true that a rare tumor from a very early stem cell may diverge into numerous morphologic types but this is the exception, and most evidence of diversity within a single lesion can usually be accounted for on the basis of reparative response of injured tissue. It is true that the chondroblast in certain instances may resemble a plasmacyte to some extent but similarity in appearance does not justify the conclusion that there is similarity in metabolic activity. Moreover, though the relationship of tumors deserves more emphasis than it has enjoyed in the past, "over-lumping" may blur the sharp focus of identity which is so important for diagnostic acuity. The behavior of bone tumors varies according to type. In most instances this behavior, if the tumor is correctly diagnosed, is predictable. To deemphasize this predictability would be unwise. However, whatever its merit, everyone interested in bone tumors should read Dr. Johnson's paper carefully.

TUMORS METASTATIC TO BONE

The great preponderance of the metastatic tumors in bone are of epithelial origin. A few sarcomas manifest this behavior. Ewing's tumor metastasizes to one or more bones in something less than half the cases. Osteosarcoma may rarely metastasize to another bone. Bone involvement may be found in less than one quarter of the cases of leukemia, malignant lymphoma and Hodgkin's disease.

Practically any tumor, with the exception of the primary tumors of the central nervous system, may occasionally metastasize to bone, but this phenomenon is unusual in some instances, as in squamous cell carcinoma of the skin, and highly characteristic in others, as in cancers of the breast and prostate. From a half to two thirds of the latter two carcinomas will, some time in their course, metastasize to bone. Other cancers which frequently develop secondary deposits in bone are those of the thyroid, kidney and lung. Bone metastasis is also very common in neuroblastoma.

Emboli of viable tumor cells are carried by both the blood vascular and lymphatic systems. Since the latter method is exceedingly common in breast and prostate cancers the pattern in these lesions is often highly suggestive. The thoracic vertebrae, the ribs, sternum and clavicle are most commonly involved in breast cancer whereas the lumbar and sacral vertebrae and the pelvic bones are the ones usually affected in carcinoma of the prostate. When transport is by the blood stream the metastases may occur anywhere in any bone, but as a rule the flat bones are more often involved than cylindrical bones and metastases in bones distal to the elbows and knees are somewhat unusual.

The principal symptom and sign of metastatic bone tumor are pain and pathologic fracture. The pain may be insidious at the onset with periods of remission but eventually it usually becomes extreme. The layman's concept of cancer as a disease of agonizing pain is largely derived from the cases with multiple bone metastases. Most metastatic carcinoma causes bone lysis so that it is not surprising that pathologic fracture is common. The fracture may be the first evidence of neoplastic involvement, either metastatic or primary. This is especially true of carcinoma of the prostate. Fracture may stimulate the remaining normal skeletal tissues to produce callus and eventually achieve healing even in the presence of the tumor which caused the fracture. Secondary deposits of breast cancer may lie quiescent within the bone for years.

It is not highly unusual to find bone metastases suddenly manifesting themselves twenty symptomless years after a radical mastectomy for breast cancer.

Some metastatic tumors produce characteristic changes in the serum chemistry. The most important of these is the elevation in acid phosphatase that occurs in bone metastasis of prostate cancer. Acid phosphatase is produced by the cancer cells but for some as yet unsatisfactorily explained reason the serum levels are not appreciable until metastasis has occurred, or at least until the cancer has invaded the prostate capsule. It would seem logical that the amount of acid phosphatase in the blood is directly proportional to the number of cancer cells which produce it. A cancer confined to the prostate gland apparently is not large enough to cause a significant elevation in total serum acid phosphatase. However, with L. tartrate inhibition of non-prostatic acid phosphatase, the increase in prostate acid phosphatase may be appreciated. Invasion of the capsule probably means that the tumor has actually spread elsewhere, and though the early bone deposits cannot be demonstrated the cells are sufficient in number to produce a measurable increase in the total enzyme.

Any cancer which destroys a considerable amount of bone may initiate sufficient osteoblastic reparative activity to produce a rise in the serum alkaline phosphatase. This is particularly true of prostatic cancer which is often of the osteoblastic or sclerosing type. Excessive amounts of mineralizing osteoid are characteristically produced in response to the presence of carcinoma of the prostate and rarely in other cancer types, especially those from the breast. The serum alkaline phosphatase level may sometimes be used as a guide in treating these metastases. Since alkaline phosphatase is excreted by the liver, abnormal serum levels may mean liver disease rather than osteoblastic activity. Considerable difficulty is encountered in this respect when the liver is the site of metastatic growth as it so frequently is in adenocarcinomas.

Blood calcium levels may be altered in extensive skeletal metastases. This may be due to actual bone destruction and the freeing of bone salts into the blood stream and it may be enhanced by disuse atrophy secondary to pain. High serum calcium levels may lead to metastatic calcification of soft tissues. Nephrocalcinosis is especially prone to occur in these situations. The excess calcium may spill into the urine and urine calcium levels may be indicative of the progress of the disease. In osteoblastic metastases sufficient calcium may be taken up by the excess osteoid to keep the serum level normal or even lower than normal. In rare instances dangerously low calcium levels may be induced by this mechanism. Excessive osteoid production is usually induced by the tumor but irradiation and hormone therapy may also stimulate new bone formation.

THE RADIOLOGY OF TUMORS METASTATIC TO BONE

The radiographic manifestation of tumor metastatic to bone is related to destruction of bone. Sometimes, as with metastatic carcinoma of the prostate, the destruction is obscured by the osteoblastic response provoked by the tumor. In contrast, carcinoma of the breast usually causes frank destructive, radiolucent defects but may at times cause an associated osteoblastic response with resultant areas of opacification. Metastatic neuroblastoma results in small destructive foci, usually in the long bones, which grow rapidly and which may be associated with periosteal new bone overlying the involved cortex. In any event, radiographic appearance of the osseous lesions of metastatic malignancy will not permit positive differentiation of metastatic neoplasm from primary neoplasia of bone, nor will it be specific for any given primary site of origin of the metastatic disease.

The surrounding trabeculae are destroyed by the emboli of neoplastic tissue which grow in the marrow. Metastatic neoplasms which are confined to the marrow are thus associated with round or ovoid areas of radiolucency without associated reactive bone. In metastatic carcinoma of the prostate, the osteoblastic response results in round or ovoid areas of opacification which are homogeneous but fuzzy in outline. In the pubic bones, the slowly growing metastases of carcinoma of the prostate may result in actual widening of the bone as the periosteum is stimulated to lay down new bone. This appearance is readily confused with that of Paget's disease.

Bones may be eroded and invaded by direct extension of carci-

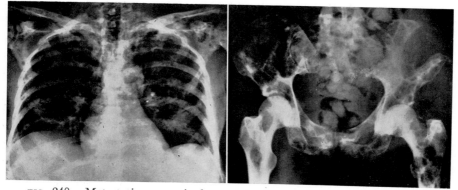

FIG. 248. Metastatic tumor in bone. There are diffuse areas of radiolucency secondary to carcinoma of the breast. The lesions vary in size but tend to be round or ovoid with no surrounding bone reaction

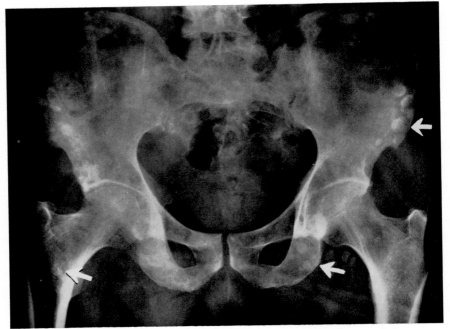

FIG. 249. Metastatic tumor in bone. Metastases from carcinoma of the prostate have evoked an osteoblastic reaction in bone. There are multiple rounded opacities evident (arrows) as well as thickening and diffuse opacity of the right ischium.

noma involving the adjacent tissues. The cortex is then irregularly destroyed from without, with little or no periosteal reaction. When extensive invasion has occurred, the appearance may be identical with that of a growth originating in the medullary cavity and extending outward through the cortex.

PATHOLOGY OF BONE METASTASES

Tumor emboli may be deposited anywhere within bone but the hematopoietic marrow appears to be the most fertile soil for survival and growth. In the cancellous tissue the metastatic tumor must reach sufficient size to destroy considerable spicular or cortical bone before it can be appreciated. Thus, we must presume that most metastatic deposits in bone are present for some time before they are apprehended. Most metastases are focal, destroying bone by pressure and by interfering with its blood supply. At times viable tumor cells may be seeded diffusely throughout an entire bone or the major portion of the skeleton. The general deossification that occurs then may be hard to distinguish from osteoporosis or diffuse myelomatosis.

Diagnosis of metastatic tumor should always be made by microscopic section even though there is a history of primary cancer and the roentgenograms are typical. Many instances of expected metastases have been found to be innocuous, coincidental lesions, thus altering the prognosis and allowing a more intelligent attack on the primary neoplasm. Biopsy by open surgical approach may seem unjustified in the face of the clinical evidence for metastasis. Here the needle aspiration method is invaluable. One of a variety of needles with a cutting edge may be used and numerous samples removed by multiple punctures if necessary. If the procedure is properly done and the material correctly handled the efficiency of the method is high and may sometimes yield results after an open biopsy has failed. The slides are relatively easy to interpret even though minute quantities of tissue are withdrawn. Most osseous metastases are carcinomas made up of cells which are entirely foreign to the normal tissue area. Even a few of these cells can give the microscopist assurance of the presence of metastatic tumor.

Since adenocarcinoma is the commonest tumor type metastasizing to bone and since the primary lesion may arise in any epithelial or glandular tissue in the body, it is quite often impossible for the pathologist to name the site of origin from examination of material removed from bone. One exception is the tubule lining cell carcinoma primary in the kidney. The metastatic deposits usually faithfully reproduce the original and because of the distinctive cellular morphology and pattern can be readily identified. Carcinomas from the prostate frequently present cells which show none of the nuclear characteristics of malignant tumor. Carcinomas from the intestinal tract usually show some evidence of mucin production within the cells. The metastatic neuroblastoma may be impossible to distinguish from the Ewing's tumor on microscopic sections alone. Metastatic tumor from the thyroid may be identified if its cells are sufficiently differentiated to take up radioactive iodine.

REFERENCES

1. Lichtenstein, L.: Cancer, 9:1044, 1956.
2. Jaffe, H. L.: Oral Surg., Oral Med. & Oral Path., 6:159, 1953.
3. Johnson, L. C.: Bull. N. Y. Acad. Med., 29:164, 1953.

17

Tumor-like Processes

Reactive Lesions in Bone

OSTEOID OSTEOMA

The osteoid osteoma is a small (usually not greater than 2 cm. in diameter), circumscribed lesion occurring in bone. It is characterized clinically by pain out of proportion to its size, radiologically by a translucent sphere surrounded by an exaggerated zone of sclerosis, and pathologically by a nidus of osteoid surrounded by a network of fine, new-bone trabeculae in a vascular fibrous matrix.

Henry Jaffe recognized the lesion as a distinct entity, suggested the name "osteoid osteoma" and gave a thorough and lucid description of five cases in 1935.[1] Several more recent papers have cited instances of earlier descriptions, but, with the exception of Bergstrand's cases reported in 1930, they were thought to belong to other bone disease categories. Bergstrand considered the lesion non-inflammatory and non-neoplastic and by exclusion arrived at the conclusion that they were congenital rests. Five years later Jaffe defined the lesion as a benign neoplasm and his beautiful descriptions and illustrations established the criteria for its diagnosis. More recently several workers have expressed dissent from the theory of neoplastic genesis but there can be no doubt that osteoid osteoma is a clinical, radiologic and pathologic entity.

Osteoid osteoma is a rather common bone lesion. There are well over three hundred cases reported and most active orthopedic clinics can cull fifteen or more cases from their files. It has probably been reported in every bone of the skeleton though about half the lesions are found in the bones of the lower extremity and most of these in the femur. In at least one series[2] the vertebrae were involved in 25 per cent of the cases. Unlike most bone lesions, osteoid osteoma may occur anywhere in the bone rather than just in the metaphysis. It is true that the diaphysis is usually involved but at least one case has been reported in the epiphysis. It may be surrounded by cancellous bone, it may lie against the inner cortical surface, it may be located entirely within the compacta or, as in a few recently reported cases,[3] it may be found on the outer cortical surface directly beneath the periosteum. The author has seen two cases of the last.

The most important clinical characteristic of osteoid osteoma is pain. The patient first becomes aware of a minor, nagging discomfort and frequently attributes it to muscle stiffness, joint disease (if the lesion is at the end of a cylindrical bone) or previous trauma (about 25 per cent). At first the discomfort is usually intermittent but in time it becomes more persistent and sharply defined. After weeks or sometimes months the pain often becomes intense and point tenderness develops. As in many other bone lesions the pain is usually worse at night. Many patients volunteer the information that aspirin is effective in relieving the symptoms. Usually the pain is at the site of the lesion but if the osteoid osteoma is in the upper end of the femur, particularly the neck, it may be referred into the leg and mask as a herniated intervertebral disc.

Diagnosis is rarely made before several months of symptoms have elapsed, and since diagnosis depends upon roentgenographic evidence, this suggests that symptoms antedate demonstrable morphologic change. Pain in a few instances has become severe enough to cause threats of suicide and it has been known to persist for as long as six years. Often there is disability and disuse atrophy of muscle. Eventually, a swelling or mass due to bone thickening may become obvious but the lesion does not achieve the redness and heat of an infectious inflammation.

Osteoid osteoma is somewhat more than twice as common in males than in females. The age group of predilection is 10 to 25. In a series of 30 cases reported by Jaffe and Lichtenstein,[4] all but 5 fall in this age group, and in a series of 22 cases studied by the author there were 17 cases of this age. But in the same series there is a case of 4 years and one of 54 years, so neither youth nor age precludes the diagnosis though they may make it unlikely.

ROENTGENOGRAPHIC MANIFESTATIONS

Since the osteoid osteoma is relatively constant in its pathologic features, one would expect the radiographic manifestations to be uniform. The nidus of osteoid tissue in a vascular fibrous matrix produces a radiolucent zone which contrasts sharply with the surrounding sclerotic, opaque bone; if the osteoid tissue calcifies, an opaque shadow may be visualized within the radiolucent nidus. The sclerotic bone about the lesion is lamellated and when the lesion involves the cortex, multiple layers of new bone may be apparent. More frequently, however, the lamellations are not apparent and the dense sclerotic bone

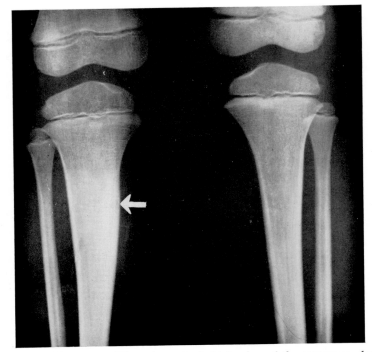

FIG. 250.   Osteoid osteoma. There is marked thickening of the cortex on the medial aspect of the right tibia. A central radiolucent nidus (arrow) is evident.

casts a homogeneous shadow which may be responsible for eccentric thickening of the shaft. The nidus may not be seen unless special projections of the involved area are made. When the lesion arises in spongy bone, peripheral sclerosis tends to be less marked than when compact bone is involved.

MORBID ANATOMY

The osteoid osteoma is a sharply circumscribed (Fig. 251), spheroid or ovoid lesion which rarely reaches a diameter greater than 2 cm. The term "giant osteoid osteoma" has been used to designate an osteoid-forming lesion which is often larger than osteoid osteoma and lacks the characteristic microscopic pattern of the latter. In the words of these authors,[5] "It is distinctly different from ordinary osteoid osteoma and should not be classed with it." We agree with Lichtenstein[6] that it belongs with the other bone-forming lesions which he designates as "benign osteoblastoma."

Many osteoid osteomas have been removed en bloc and studied both grossly and miscroscopically in their entirety. The principal mass consists of an aggregate of deep red, brown, purple or gray tissue with a decidedly gritty consistency, encased in a wall of massive spicules or nearly solid bone. The surrounding area of sclerosis may be many times that of the lesion proper, particularly if it lies within or contiguous to the compacta. If isolated in cancellous bone the zone of sclerosis is less impressive. When the lesion is curetted the wall of he remaining cavity is fairly smooth.

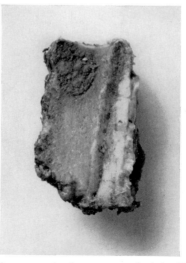

FIG. 251.   An osteoid osteoma in the upper end of the fibula. The lesion is round, about 1 cm. in diameter, sharply demarcated and gray-brown in color. Its sharp, regular delineation is almost pathognomonic.

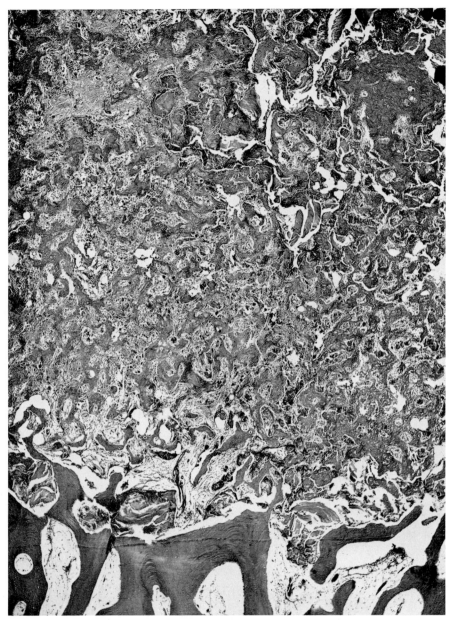

FIG. 252.   A quarter segment of a section through the center of an osteoid osteoma. The central nidus of mineralized osteoid is in the right upper corner, the
peripheral zone of sclerotic cancellous bone is at the bottom. An orderly arrangement
of microspicules forms a wide zone around the nidus. ($\times$ 20.)

If full sections are made through the mid-center a highly characteristic microscopic morphology is apparent. The central area is made up of one or more nidi of irregular masses of osteoid (Fig. 252). It may or may not be calcified. The osteoid dominates the field but in the interstices between its ramifications there is a moderately loose, rather vascular matrix of elongated and spindled cells which appear to be fibroblasts undergoing transition into the more cuboidal cells which form a layer of osteoblasts over the solid osteoid nucleus (Fig. 253). As one progresses toward the periphery the crude osteoid merges into a network of very fine spicules of more mature bone. Osteoblastic activity is often quite apparent about these structures. These miniature spicules are arranged radially around their respective nidi. At the extreme edge they appear to press against but do not merge with the massive spicules of lamellated bone that run in the opposite direction to surround the lesion (Fig. 254). In the peripheral zone, measuring approximately one third of the radius, one may find fairly normal appearing osteoclasts and the spicules are even more delicate than those toward the center. There is little or no evidence of fat and no hematopoietic marrow. The density of the matrix tissue varies but it is never highly collagenized. There may be a few scattered lymphocytes, suggesting a mild inflammatory reaction, but never enough exudate to imply infection. Cartilage appears to play no role in the genesis of this lesion. Here and there one may find granules of hemosiderin but there is not enough to suggest hemorrhage as a factor. The pattern is

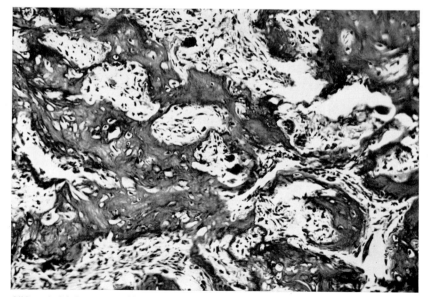

FIG 253. A higher magnification of the central osteoid nidus seen in Figure 252. (× 130.)

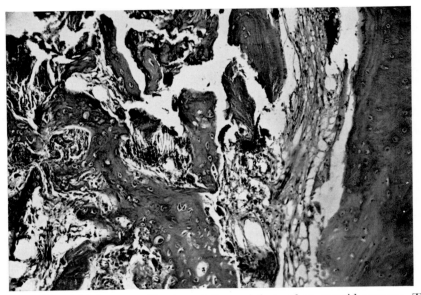

FIG. 254.   A higher magnification of the periphery of an osteoid osteoma. The surrounding zone of sclerotic cortex is seen on the right. The microspicules approach the encasing shell but in most places are separated from it by a zone of granulation. (× 115.)

rigidly dictated and, except for the apparent confusion where the alignment around one nidus intrudes upon that of another, in cases where multiple nidi are present, the microscopy is marvelously consistent. When the lesion is removed intact and so sectioned the diag- nosis is clearly apparent to anyone but the uninitiated. More often, however, the pathologist must depend upon sections made of curetted fragments of the lesion mixed with pieces of the surrounding bone and even marrow tissue. Under these unfortunate circumstances, un- less the diagnosis has been strongly suggested by the clinician and roentgenologist, the nature of the lesion as demonstrated in the sec- tions can only be surmised since a firm diagnosis depends so strongly on pattern.

PATHOGENESIS

The pathogenesis of osteoid osteoma is unknown. Before the definitive paper by Jaffe in 1935, it was categorized as traumatic, as infectious, as ischemic and as a congenital rest. Jaffe marshaled the facts against these theories and concluded that the lesion was none of these and, therefore, it must be neoplastic. Whether one accepts this hypothesis depends upon one's concept of true neoplastic growth. Most oncologists today believe that a cell becomes neoplastic only after its nuclear hereditary mechanism becomes unalterably changed so that ultimate maturation can no longer occur. Thus, these cells must divide and their daughters divide until some mechanical or metabolic influence causes their death. Therefore, a true neoplasm cannot, by definition, reach a static growth plateau and all lesions which do are not true tumors.

If one accepts this definition, then osteoid osteoma is not a neoplasm. There is serious question in the mind of the writer whether it grows at all. It is a most difficult point on which to gather dependable data but it appears that once a diagnosis is made radiologically, the lesion proper does not enlarge. On the contrary, it sometimes appears to diminish in size. This suggests that it appears, full blown, like an infarct or a fracture and then, though reaction about it may develop and seemingly enlarge the area, the lesion does not increase in volume or mass. There is no evidence at present to suggest that osteoid osteoma is the result of either fracture or infarction but failure of growth is strong evidence against a neoplastic genesis.

Another bit of evidence supports this thesis. Several writers have followed a growing number of cases which have undergone spontaneous healing. The first of these[7] reported two cases which regressed to a healed state in seven years and there are others[8] which described a similar behavior. Admittedly, more data is needed since an ultimate diagnosis can only be made on section, and section eradicates the lesion. But the remarkably consistent clinical and radiologic features coupled with a familiar behavior pattern are rather convincing.

Finally, there is one more characteristic about osteoid osteoma which makes its classification as a neoplasm hard to accept. The microscopy of the lesion describes a set and predictable pattern which is decidedly unlike that of the random growth of a tumor. This pattern suggests that something happens to a circumscribed area of bone. In an attempt at repair a mass of osteoid, microspicules and granulation are substituted for the affected normal tissue. The central area appears younger and more active, suggesting that the lesion heals centripetally. If this is the case it would explain why the primary lesion does not grow in size. The cause of the surrounding zone of sclerosis is equally debatable. Perhaps, as Golding suggests, it may be due to pressure causing a relative ischemia, this in turn causing a laying down and mineralization of an abnormal amount of organic matrix.

PROGNOSIS

Osteoid osteoma may be a self-limiting disease. There is some evidence, quoted above, that such is the case. But spontaneous healing is a long-protracted and painful process and no surgeon would knowingly impose this type of management upon his patient. The almost instantaneous relief of pain following excision of the lesion is ample testimony of the virtue of early surgery.

Osteoid osteomas have been known to recur and it is said that this may be expected if the nidus is not removed. If the surgeon wishes to comfort himself with the assurance that the entire lesion has been removed in toto, he may x-ray the removed block and find on the film the nicely delineated nidus. When the primary focus is removed, the patient may expect complete and absolute recovery.

OSSIFYING FIBROMA

Within the entire framework of the classification of bone tumors there is no entity which is so nebulous, so ill-defined and so elusive as the one which has been called ossifying fibroma, osteogenic fibroma, osteoid fibroma, fibrous osteoma or benign osteoblastoma. It is purported to be a benign tumor of osteoblastic origin producing a fibrous matrix in which are embedded masses and spicules of osteoid and bone. At least one of the reasons for this dilemma is that there are a variety of bone lesions, neoplastic, reactive, vascular and metabolic, which are characterized by this microscopic picture. Since the clinical and radiologic features of these conditions may differ widely, the poor pathologist who rarely has the opportunity of examining all aspects of the case has had a tendency to lump together a variety of entities because their microscopic picture appears to be the same. As a result, it is almost completely futile to obtain a lucid concept by analysis of the literature.

At the outset it should be stated that the reparative action of bone tissues which have been damaged by a number of processes including mechanical trauma, hemorrhage, ischemia and neoplasm can, under the right conditions, produce fields of fibroblastic proliferation with osteoid and bone production. If the primary cause remains hidden, a diagnosis of benign bone-forming tumor may be made and any one of the above terms applied. The writer has had the experience on two occasions of receiving material with every feature of benign giant cell tumor only to find later that the tissue came from the vicinity of two quite dissimilar lesions which had nothing to do with true giant cell tumor and which, when proper samples were obtained, were readily diagnosable on the sections.

It is impossible to avoid this unhappy experience altogether but certain precautions should be taken by the pathologist when he is presented with a microscopic picture of this type. First, he should insist that he have all the facts of the case as obtained by the clinician and the radiologist before he gives his ultimate diagnosis. Second, if the roentgenogram clearly indicates a malignant neoplastic process, the microscopist should be chary about pronouncing the lesion a benign ossifying fibroma. Third, if the diagnosis is not reasonably clear, a second and more ample biopsy, preferably consisting of samples taken from various parts of the lesion, will not hurt the patient as much as the protracted hospitalization or delay in therapy of a malignant tumor which may result from a mistaken initial impression.

If reaction to bone injury can be firmly ruled out, then there are several other conditions which must be considered:

Fibrous dysplasia is one of the most frequent problems. It is a relatively common condition, it can occur anywhere in any bone and at any age though the great preponderance occurs in late childhood and adolescence. Fibro-osseous metaplasia is said to be the hallmark of fibrous metaplasia but fibro-osseous metaplasia is not always easy to be certain of, it may be absent in mature fibrous dysplasia and it may occur in lesions which have been diagnosed as ossifying fibroma. Indeed, some writers[9] have expressed the opinion that most of the so-called ossifying fibromas of the jaw are, in fact, monostotic fibrous dysplasia. The difficulty cannot always be resolved on microscopic sections alone.

Osteosarcoma may have to be considered when examining a lesion of this sort. The differences in the cellular morphology of a malignant tumor and a benign tumor are known to every pathologist, and yet in certain instances those differences may shrink to the vanishing point if one is comparing a young and vigorous osteoblastic reaction with a sedentary and mature type of osteosarcoma.

Giant cell tumor of bone has already been mentioned. Though it may seem radical to suggest it, the writer believes that many lesions which have been diagnosed as benign giant cell tumors have been nothing more than bone reaction to an occult or hidden primary lesion.

Osteoid osteoma may simulate the microscopy under discussion. If the osteoid osteoma is received in fragments, the over-all pattern which is so helpful to the pathologist is almost sure to be lacking. The clinical and roentgenographic aspects are apt to be most helpful.

The giant osteoid osteoma recently described by Dahlin and Johnson[10] is thought by Lichtenstein[11] to be a type of what he calls "benign osteoblastoma," and since this seems to be a reasonable conclusion it will be discussed under that heading.

The lining of a solitary bone cyst may exactly simulate the microscopy of a benign bone-forming tumor. The description of a cystic lesion by the surgeon will clinch the differential since ossifying fibromas are not truly cystic.

A fractured aneurysmal bone cyst may produce all the features of a benign ossifying fibroma both grossly and under the microscope. It is probable that some of the lesions of the vertebrae bearing the diagnosis of ossifying fibroma are, in reality, aneurysmal bone cysts.

When all these conditions have been excluded one may entertain the diagnosis of ossifying fibroma, if indeed there be such an entity. The writer feels that there probably is and it will be discussed under the heading of benign osteoblastoma (see page 446).

NON-OSTEOGENIC FIBROMA

The non-osteogenic fibroma is a focal area of deossification replaced by collagenous fibrous tissue. It is difficult to estimate its incidence since more than half of the known cases have been symptomless and discovered only on skeletal surveys done for other reasons. It, with subperiosteal cortical defect, constitutes the most common type of delineated translucency found in the skeleton. The name "non-osteogenic fibroma" was applied by Jaffe and Lichtenstein in 1942[12] in their paper in which they established the identity of this lesion. They believed it was a neoplasm and classified it with the fibromas of bone. Because it is self-healing, often multiple and occasionally bilaterally symmetrical and usually asymptomatic, it is difficult for this author to accept it as a true tumor and so it is considered more fully along with similar lesions in another section (see page 277). A brief summary is included here only because it is still classified in some texts as a tumor.

So-called "non-osteogenic fibroma" occurs most commonly in the age group 10 to 15 years, though characteristic lesions are not uncommonly found in younger children and less often in young adults. It occurs with greatest frequency in the large bones of the lower extremity, the femur being most often affected. Other parts of the skeleton may be involved, however, and it has been seen, though rarely, in flat bones.

It makes its appearance in the metaphysis a few centimeters proximal to the epiphyseal line. It usually begins at the inner surface of the metaphyseal compacta and causes lysis of the contiguous cortical and cancellous tissues. It expands slowly over a period of months to reach a diameter of 3, 5 or even more centimeters. Because its growth is slow, the normal tissue along its advancing frontier manifests a reaction sclerosis which sharply delineates it on the x-ray film from the adjacent cancellous bone. It erodes the overlying cortex from within and the periosteum responds by laying down a lamina of bone on the outer cortical surface, thus producing the picture of eccentric expansion. In slender bones it may occupy the entire diameter and cause a fusiform enlargement.

Because the process is so insidious there is no pain unless the cortex becomes so thinned that infractions occur or minor trauma results in a pathologic fracture. Practically all of the symptomatic lesions are diagnosed on this basis.

MORBID ANATOMY

When the surgeon removes the thin shell which often covers the non-osteogenic fibroma, he finds a mass of yellow, gray or brown soft tissue without spicules of bone. This tissue often has a rather tough, stringy character.

When sectioned, it is found to consist of fields of spindled cells resembling moderately immature fibroblasts. There is a tendency for them to weave irregularly in a broad ribbon pattern, often producing whorls of poorly palisaded forms. Intermixed, one can usually find, either singly or in aggregates, large macrophages whose cytoplasm contains lipid granules and vacuoles. It is this lipid which apparently lends the yellow color to the lesion as it is seen grossly. Hemosiderin granules are usually quite prominent and if they are present the lesion may be brown. The fourth feature of note is the appearance of giant cells. Intercellular collagen is usually present but rarely dominates the picture. Osteoid is never found and if present, by definition, the lesion cannot be designated "non-osteogenic fibroma."

The microscopy is not pathognomonic since there are many types of reaction to bone injury which will produce an identical picture. The pathologist should have the advantage of viewing the roentgenograms or knowing the clinical diagnosis before he commits his diagnosis of non-osteogenic fibroma. If the lesion is young and the fibroblastic reaction florid, one may be mislead into a diagnosis of fibrosarcoma, but the xanthoid reaction, the pigment, the collagen and the giant cells will usually save the pathologist from this pitfall. The differential diagnosis of solitary cyst, giant cell tumor, fibrous dysplasia, lipid reticuloendotheliosis, chronic osteomyelitis and bone infarct is dealt with in another section (see page 283).

SUBPERIOSTEAL CORTICAL DEFECT

The lesion which we choose to call "subperiosteal cortical defect" appears to be an erosion of the outer cortical surface of the ends of long, cylindrical bones in children and adolescents. It is seen with such frequency in roentgenographic surveys of otherwise normal skeletons that one suspects that it is a variation in normal bone growth. The importance in correctly recognizing the lesion stems from the danger of mistaking it for a process with a more serious prognosis and consequently overtreating a quite innocuous alteration. Should it be diagnosed as sarcoma, and at least one such lesion has been so diagnosed, the mistake may lead to the tragedy of a needlessly amputated extremity.

Subperiosteal cortical defect is not a tumor. It is considered in this section only because it is most important that it be differentiated from a tumor. A more complete discussion may be found in another section (see page 284).

The condition affects males about twice as often as females. It occurs most commonly in the first six years of life and less frequently up to the age of 15. To date, it has been reported only in cylindrical bones, usually in the lower extremity. The most common sites of involvement are the posterior and medial surfaces of the distal end of the femur. The next most common sites are the posterior and anterior surfaces of the proximal end of the tibia.

The lesion probably always starts at or near the epiphyseal line. As the involved bone grows the affected area appears to pull away from the epiphysis and drift deeper into the metaphysis. There may be more than one area in a single bone but more commonly a second lesion will be found on the opposite side involving an analogous situation.

On roentgenograms the affected area appears as a dish-like erosion beneath the periosteum. The deep and advancing edge of the lesion may reveal a limiting zone of sclerosis and the overlying periosteum may produce a thin layer of bone which roofs the cortical defect.

MORPHOLOGY

When the periosteum is reflected or the eggshell-like roof is removed, a disc of yellow, gray or reddish brown tissue is found filling a concave defect in the compacta. This tissue is apt to be tough and fibrous. When sectioned it is found to consist of a fibrous stroma often with a suggestion of trabeculation. Scattered through this matrix one can usually find xanthoid cells, giant cells and hemosiderin pigment. In the limited material at hand (these lesions are infrequently biopsied) we have found small masses of osteoid and primitive cartilage. It is difficult to ascertain whether these components are the products of the lesion itself or the result of periosteal reaction.

The microscopy appears to be, within the limits of variation, identical with that of non-osteogenic fibroma. This leads to the interesting speculation that together they constitute a single lesion type, one occurring within the metaphysis and the other outside. The radiology of the two lesions supports this thesis since unless the roentgenograms are taken at various projections by rotating the part, it may be impossible to differentiate them.

The etiology and pathogenesis of subperiosteal cortical defect are unknown. It may be an ischemic lysis of bone which is then replaced by the cheaper fibrous stroma or it may be a reaction in the periosteal cambium which brings an abnormal supply of blood to the part and thereby deossifies the area. It is probable that the lesion from the outside may perforate the cortex and enter the cancellous metaphysis and that the non-osteogenic fibroma may progress in the reverse manner, making it impossible to state where the lesion started.

PROGNOSIS

Subperiosteal cortical defect is a self-limiting condition. A number of cases have been followed throughout the course of the process[13] and have eventually healed in from two to five years. At least one lesion is reported to have been excised and later recurred deeper in the metaphysis at the site where it would have been had it been allowed to remain. Since the lesion is symptomless its only importance is in recognizing it for what it is rather than as a condition which would necessitate therapy.

Hamartomas

OSTEOGENIC HAMARTOMAS

OSTEOMA

The osteoma is usually classified as a bone-forming tumor. Actually, it is no more than a localized exaggeration of intramembranous bone formation. It is a mass of bone tissue which is laid down on the surface of its host bone, matures and becomes static and can be considered an idiopathic hyperplasia or osteogenic hamartoma. Since it is strictly intramembranous in origin it is never complicated by the formation of cartilage and is found only where bone is normally produced directly by fibrous tissue. Thus we may expect to find osteomas involving those bones which are formed predominantly by intramembranous ossification, and such is the case. Most osteomas are found on the inner or outer surfaces of the head bones, though occasionally they arise from the bones of the extracranial skeleton.

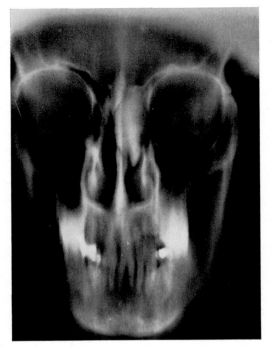

FIG. 255. A planigraphic roentgenogram of an osteoma in the outlet duct of the frontal sinus.

The term osteoma has been applied to any excrescence or protuberance of fibrous or cartilaginous tissue which becomes ossified and predominantly bony. Such usage should be discouraged. Osteophytes are formed by the calcification and later ossification of tendinous tissue at the site of its insertion. This process is known as dystrophic calcification and is caused by a chemical or physical change in collagen which increases its affinity for calcium salts. Pointed "stalagmites" or ridges are formed thusly but the mechanism of formation is quite different from that of osteoma or osteochondroma. Proliferating, reactive fibroblasts may acquire the ability to form bone but here again these are not osteomas but osteoid osteomas or ossifying fibromas.

True osteomas usually occur on the inner or outer tables of the bones of the calvarium or bones of the face or mandible. In certain conditions such as hyperostosis frontalis interna and senile hyperostosis they may be multiple. More often they occur singly and when they arise on the outer surface of the skull they may constitute a torus.

Osteomas are usually symptomless unless they protrude into a paranasal sinus or its drainage channel (Fig. 255), on the hard palate where the lesion may interfere with a dental prosthesis, on the internal surface of the mandible where it may handicap the movement of the tongue, or into the orbit.

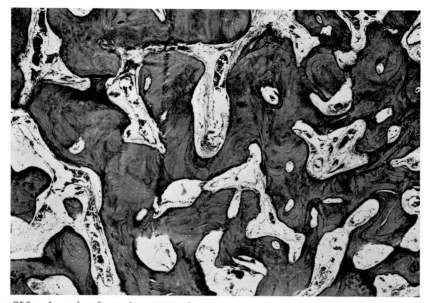

FIG. 256. A section from the center of an osteoma. It consists of cancellous tissue composed of massive spicules. This is covered with normal appearing compacta. (× 20.)

Osteomas are formed by the apposition of osseous tissue upon the surface of the host bone. As the compacta is thickened there may be resolution of the normal cortex with the formation of massive spicules of lamellated bone which forms the cancellous tissue of the protruding mass (Fig. 256). The ratio of bone mass to interspicular space is greatly increased over normal. Hematopoietic marrow may form in the spaces or they may fill with fibrous tissue. The outer surface may be bosselated. It is always covered by a layer of periosteum.

Osteomas may form at any age but they are usually discovered some time during adult life. Once formed they remain without evidence of activity. They have never been known to exhibit truly neoplastic growth. They should be removed only if they intrude upon and disturb the function of nearby normal parts.

OSTEOCHONDROMA

The solitary osteochondroma is identical in every respect to the lesion which continutes hereditary multiple exostoses. For a more general discussion see page 139. The abnormality is essentially a perversion in growth direction. It always arises at or near an epiphyseal line and protrudes at a right angle to the long axis of the host bone. Osteochondromas are always formed by enchondral growth, and since the bone substance produced is normal in every respect it may be considered not a tumor but rather an enchondral hamartomatous hyperplasia.

The cartilaginous portion of the osteochondroma acts as the enchondral plate for this abnormal growth. It persists only as long as there is growth activity and then becomes dissipated by the utilization of its chondrocytes to form a thin layer of hyaline cartilage over the top, or disappear entirely. The mature portion of the lesion consists of bone and therefore it should not be called a chondroma, or even an osteochondroma. A better name would be enchondral osteoma to associate it with the intramembranous osteoma which is its counterpart.

The osteochondroma may be a solitary manifestation of hereditary multiple exostoses or more likely, since there appear to be no hereditary features involved, it may be an accidental occurrence of the same forces which are inherited in the general disease.

It may occur on any bone which is predominantly formed by enchondral ossification. A bit of the periphery of the enchondral plate of a normal bone apparently becomes separated from the main epiphyseal mass and retains its growth potential. It forms an epiphysis of the parasite lesion and is similar in all respects to the normal epiphysis except that it has no osseous nucleus. An irregular epiphyseal line is established and bone laid down over a hyalin lattice. The cartilaginous cap is pushed outward over a cylinder of normal cortical bone which surrounds a "metaphysis" of cancellous tissue coextensive with that in the normal metaphysis. Interspicular hematopoietic marrow is formed with the same regulation as normal marrow. The same laws of growth that govern the normal skeleton also apply in the osteochondroma. Hamartomatous ossification slows and stops at the same time as normal ossification at the nearest epiphyseal line. At this point most of the lesions remain static. If they impinge on tendon movement, bursae form over them. A bursitis may develop or they may press upon vessels or nerves and thus give cause for removal.

Because of a failure of modeling of the host bone the metaphysis may remain wider than normal, giving a characteristic roentgenographic picture. If viewed perpendicularly a ring of translucency representing the defect in the cortex at the base of the lesion may appear on the film surrounded by a zone of opacity caused by the pedicle. Unless taken at another projection this may lead to confusion in diagnosis. For a more complete description of the x-ray findings, see page 142.

Morbid Anatomy

The osteochondroma is a cylindrical bony projection from the outer cortical surface of a normal bone. Its metaphysis is continuous with the cancellous tissue of the host. It is usually fin-shaped, flattened from side to side and leans toward the diaphysis and away from its epiphyseal center of origin. During its growth period its cartilaginous cap often extends down over the epiphyseal margin of the pedicle, a finding to be taken into consideration if surgical removal is contemplated since a certain percentage recur, perhaps because the germinal cartilage has not been completely removed.

When sections are made one finds the structure to consist of normal cortical and cancellous bone covered with an enchondral plate and a simulated epiphyseal line. One can judge whether the lesion is progressing or quiescent by the degree of activity in this area.

Prognosis

The osteochondroma should cease growing at the time of maturation of the nearest epiphyseal center. The great preponderance then remains inactive throughout adult life. Occasionally reactivation occurs and the reason is usually not apparent. There may be a history of trauma with fracture of the pedicle. When renewed growth occurs the lesion must be considered a sarcoma until proven otherwise. It should be remembered that the cartilage and bone of osteochondroma are ectopic and like misplaced tissue anywhere in the body—embryonal rests, undescended testis—are prone to take on a neoplastic character. It is assumed that a foreign environmental influence is responsible for this new growth potential. Since the three types of fibrous tissue are involved, the tumor may be a chondrosarcoma, osteosarcoma or fibrosarcoma. Or it may be made up of all three fibroblastic derivatives and as such produce a parosteal sarcoma.

CHONDROGENIC HAMARTOMAS
ENCHONDROMA

The solitary enchondroma is a circumscribed mass of cartilage cells occurring in the metaphysis of cylindrical bones, including the ribs. Both radiologically and cytologically the lesion is the same as that of enchondromatosis (see page 133). Solitary enchondroma is rarely seen in children and in our own material of 16 patients there were only two under the age of 28 years, with an average age incidence of 35. Of 8 patients with enchondromatosis, there were none over the age of 22 with an average of 14. These data suggest that the solitary enchondroma is not a congenital lesion. Since it is morphologically and behavioristically identical with the lesion of enchondromatosis, one must assume that it is an accident of bone development which in enchondromatosis occurs in a congenital pattern, probably beginning in utero.

Solitary enchondroma probably begins in childhood or adolescence. A group of cartilage cells from the epiphysis apparently is not utilized in the process of hyalin lattice formation and is by-passed by the advancing epiphyseal line until it becomes isolated in the metaphysis. One might hypothesize that these are epiphyseal cells which fail to mature and, lacking the glycogen and enzymatic complements which are necessary for utilization in the line of provisional calcification, are ignored by the normal process of enchondral ossification and end up, viable and proliferating, in the metaphysis. They multiply slowly and it takes a long time for them to produce a mass sufficient to displace enough metaphysis to be identifiable on the roentgenogram. Eventually, they may occupy enough space to erode the cortex from within and cause the overlying periosteum to compensate with an apposition of bone on the outer surface, giving the appearance of expansion.

The great preponderance of solitary enchondromas are found in the short, cylindrical bones of the hands and feet. Here they may cause lysis and replacement of the entire medullary tissue of the host bone. Less often they occur in the large, long bones of the extremities, the humerus and femur being most commonly involved. It is possible that solitary enchondromas may occur in the flat bones such as the ilium, but they are exceedingly rare and any abnormal aggregate of cartilage cells within a flat bone should be regarded as a true neoplasm until disproven by adequate biopsy. Enchondromas probably always begin near a cartilaginous epiphysis. A cartilage mass in the mid-diaphysis should always arouse the suspicion of the diagnostician. It may be a benign neoplasm or a chondrosarcoma but it is almost certainly not an enchondroma and cannot be expected to behave like one.

MORPHOLOGY

The solitary enchondroma is a spheroid mass of cartilage which replaces cancellous tissue and may erode the cortex. Because it grows so slowly it almost never produces symptoms until the overlying compacta becomes so thin that infractions or pathologic fracture occurs. Grossly it appears as a pale, bluish, glistening, elastic substance often with a lobulated or scalloped periphery. It never invades bone but pushes it aside or by pressure causes its lysis. Almost always one can find areas of sticky, semi-liquid or gelatinous material within its substance and sometimes the major portion of the lesion may have this consistency. This suggests that the normal cartilage cell function of hyalin production is deranged and the so-called "myxomatous material" is the best that it can produce.

Through the microscope one finds fields of hyalin in which are caught the chondroblasts. Their nuclei are small, uniform, darkly staining and young in appearance. Some fields may consist almost entirely of cells, other fields may be entirely hyalin and always the arrangement of the cells is much less regular than that of normal cartilage. Mitotic figures are usually lacking and if nucleoli are found they are small.

PROGNOSIS

To foretell the behavior of an enchondroma from its microscopy alone is difficult or impossible, the reason being that the appearance of the cartilage cell, at least by present-day staining methods, gives us only an imperfect idea of what the cell is doing. The cytology of an ecchondroma or a central chondroma may be identical. Yet these are progressive and aggressive tumors, growing until outside intervention is applied, whereas the enchondroma grows to a certain size and then ceases to enlarge. The fact that all three lesions have an identical microscopy is no reason to insist that they are all the same lesion. In final analysis, the behavior of a tumor is far more important in its classification than its morphology, the latter being only a means, and often a poor one, of prognosing the former. The central chondroma and the peripheral chondroma or ecchondroma are true tumors, the enchondroma is a hamartoma. That we as yet have no means of absolutely differentiating the two types does not dispute this fact. It is possible that a central chondroma begins in the metaphysis as often as elsewhere in bone, and when it does it is diagnosed as an enchondroma and its behavior denigrates the reputation of the latter. Or perhaps the enchondroma alone begins in the metaphysis and, being ectopic to the area, has a penchant for changing into a true neoplasm.

To the knowledge of the writer there is no means by which the clinician, the radiologist or the pathologist may be absolutely sure whether he is dealing with a neoplasm or a hamartoma, though there are certain features which are helpful. If the lesion is in a small bone of the hands or feet, it is almost surely an enchondroma. If it is in the metaphysis of a large, cylindrical bone, in the middle third of any bone or in a flat bone, it is more apt to be a central chondroma. If the microscopist can demonstrate invasion, or evidence of rapid growth (numerous mitoses) or cellular pleomorphism, a diagnosis of neoplasm is warranted. In most instances the problem remains a problem until subsequent behavior of the lesion defines its character. Consequently it is justifiable to treat a problematic case more radically than one would recommend for a known enchondroma.

COLLAGENIC HAMARTOMAS
ANGIOMA OF BONE

The capillaries and the small afferent and efferent channels in relation to them are made up of a variety of cell constituents. Lining the vessel is a single layer of endothelial cells supporting which there is a thin layer of fibrocytes. Spiraling about the latter are the hemangiopericytes of Zimmerman, curious cells which like muscle have the capacity of contracting. These three cell types apparently have a common stem cell genesis, mesenchymal fibrous tissue. In newly formed granulation one can see evidence of transition of fibroblasts into endothelial cells and the reverse, and it is assumed that the hemangiopericytes have a like origin. The morphology and activity of the three types of cells appear to depend upon environment and functional demand. It should not surprise us, therefore, that developmental and neoplastic alterations in the components of vessels produce a variety of lesions. These lesions fall into two large classes, the neoplasms and the hamartomas. Since both arise from fibrous tissue they are placed in the collagenic group for the sake of convenience.

The appearance of the vasculature neoplasms depends upon the type of cell which is predominantly involved. If the proliferation is largely endothelial these lesions are best called hemangioendotheliomas (Stout), if the fibrous element predominates they may be called hemangiosarcomas (Kaposi) and if the hemangiopericytoma is principally concerned they are best called hemangiopericytomas (Stout).

The developmental lesions of vessels are less simply classified. Usually all structural elements are represented so that recognizable vascular channels form the unit of the lesion. If the channels are large and thin-walled they are called cavernous hemangiomas, if small and thick-walled, capillary hemangiomas. If the channels become obliterated by fibrous tissue they are called sclerosing hemangiomas. In the skin they may be called vascular nevi or birthmarks. These are simple overgrowths of tissues native to the part and as such are true hamartomas. The lesions enlarge at the rate of growth of the surrounding tissue and cease to grow at maturity. Since they are not progressive they should not be considered neoplasms.

A cumbersome nomenclature of eponyms has grown up to designate various complexes of vascular lesions of developmental nature. Various combinations of skin, visceral and brain involvement have been designated as Sturge-Weber disease, Rendu-Osler-Weber disease and von Hippel-Lindau disease. A combination of multiple hemangiomas and enchondromatosis is sometime called Maffucci's syndrome.

Vascular hamartomas called angiomas have been found in practically every tissue of the body. They are often multiple. In the cavernous type the arteriovenous communications (referred to in some areas, particularly the lungs, as arteriovenous fistulae) may be sufficient to cause hypertrophic arthropathy, cyanosis and polycythemia. One of the hazards of these lesions if they involve an internal surface is hemorrhage.

Angiomas occur in muscle and bone. No one knows the incidence of the latter because apparently the majority are symptomless and can be found only on sectioning the bone. Others produce areas of bone lysis large enough to show up on x-ray films which have been taken for other reasons. Still others produce bone destruction and give rise to symptoms. These last are quite unusual.

The mechanism by which bone angioma produces lysis is unknown but one can presume that since there may be arteriovenous communications, an excess of arterial blood flows through the part.

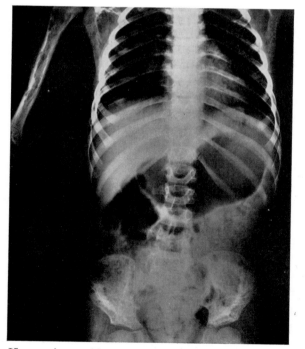

FIG. 257. Hemangioma of bone. Extensive skeletal involvement is evident. The bones are somewhat osteoporotic with many areas of circumscribed radiolucency. Both compact and spongy bone are involved.

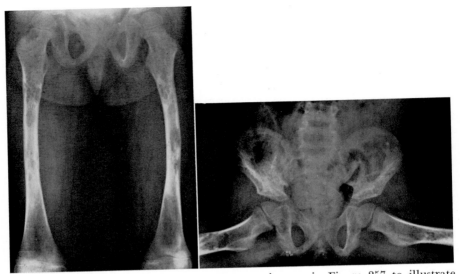

FIG. 258.   Hemangioma of bone. Same patient as in Figure 257 to illustrate better the individual lesions and the general abnormality of architecture and density.

This alteration in other lesions produces a leaching of the bone involved and the same mechanism may apply in angioma.

Angiomas may occur in any bone but the vertebra is the site most frequently reported. They are usually found in children and adolescents. Massive involvement of a vertebral body may eventuate in collapse with pressure upon the cord or the nerve roots. The pattern of bone destruction and reaction is often sufficiently characteristic to allow a diagnosis from the roentgenogram.

There is a condition which has been called massive osteolysis, disappearing bones, acute absorption of bone or phantom clavicle in which, usually following trauma in adolescents and young adults, there is a progressive resorption of one or more bones in a skeletal area. The clavicle is most often involved but the scapula, jaw, pelvis, femur and bones of the hands and feet have been reported. All or a major portion of an entire bone may gradually disappear from the roentgenograms over a period of months and years. Only a few cases have been adequately studied but in some of these[14] the bone has been found to be involved in what is called angiomatosis, that is, a permeation by an excessive number of small, thin-walled capillary type vessels. Since these do not progress to neoplastic growth it is assumed that they are a type of hamartomatous angioma. The bone or several related bones may be converted to a residual fibrous band showing no evidence of the former normal structure.

Morbid Anatomy

The highly vascular nature of the angioma of bone and its capacity for hemorrhage on incision may give the surgeon considerable difficulty. There are reports of patients who exsanguinated on the operating table.

The diagnosis on the sectioned tissue is usually simple. Most of these lesions are cavernous hamartomas (Fig. 259) consisting of large,

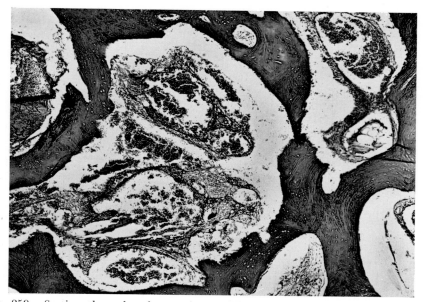

FIG. 259. Section through a hemangioma of bone. Between the spicules of bone there are numerous large, thin-walled, vascular sinuses filled with blood. (× 27.)

irregular spaces filled with red blood cells and surrounded by thin walls lined with endothelium. There are a number of situations in which the microscopy may be imitated by telangiectasis or varicosities of otherwise normal vessels. Inflammatory granulation or highly vascular tumor may occasionally mimic angioma. If the lesion is not quite apparent the cautious pathologist should use restraint in making the diagnosis.

Prognosis

The angiomas are highly vulnerable to irradiation therapy. If thrombosis can be produced, sclerosis may be initiated. The angiomas of bone are more difficult to reach than those of soft issue and the therapist must weigh the possibility of damage to the enchondral centers in growing bone.

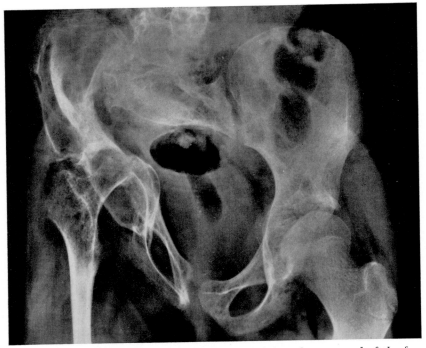

FIG. 260.   Angiomatosis involving the right pelvis and upper end of the femur. There is a congenital, hamartomatous proliferation of vessels which inhibited normal growth. The left pelvis and femur have grown normally.

True vasculature tumors of bone are exceedingly rare though hemangioendotheliomas have frequently been reported. These usually run a rapid malignant course with fatal termination due to wide spread metastasis.

Angiomas are often congenital and not infrequently multiple. If several bones are involved the condition is known as angiomatosis of bone (Fig. 260). The lesions may be monomelic, unilateral or widely scattered and general. Any portion of the bone may be involved. The great majority of patients with angiomatosis of bone will reveal angio-hamartomas in the soft tissues, especially the skin. Angiomas of the viscera, the eye, mucous membranes of the pharynx and the coverings of the brain are apt to rupture and bleed. Other than large lesions of the vertebrae, most bone angiomas remain symptomless.

ANEURYSMAL BONE CYST

The aneurysmal bone cyst is a shell-like protrusion from the corti-cal surface of a bone, surrounding a soft tissue mass of convoluted vascular channels bearing a blood flow in communication with the normal circulation. Since it causes bone destruction and a tumor-like mass it is frequently classified as a neoplasm. Neither its behavior nor its microscopy is that of neoplastic growth so it is considered here under the heading of tumor-like processes. Actually, it is a circulatory disturbance and is discussed more fully in that section (see page 259).

Aneurysmal bone cyst, as an entity, has been reported only since 1950, though several accounts of the lesion may be found in the earlier literature under the title of aneurysmal cyst, bone hemangioma, aneurysmal giant cell tumor and telangiectatic osteogenic sarcoma. The lesion is a type of angiomatous hamartoma. It differs from ordinary angioma of bone in that the sinuses are not true vascular walls and the angioma does not produce the saccular outpouching of cortical bone.

Aneurysmal bone cyst has been reported over a wide age range from childhood to old age, but it occurs prevalently in the second and third decades. Both flat and cylindrical bones may be involved with perhaps one quarter of the cases occurring in the vertebrae, often involving the laminae or the pedicles.

The process starts within cancellous or medullary tissue and erodes the cortex from within. The progress is slow enough to allow the periosteum to deposit bone over the affected area. Continuous erosion from within and apposition on the outside cause an expanding lesion whose silhouette is not unlike that of a saccular aneurysm of the aorta—hence the name. Eventually stress or trauma is likely to cause fracture of the protective shell of bone and blood may be extravasated into the surrounding soft tissues. A hematoma with consequent organization, fibrosis, calcification and ossification may mask the primary lesion and produce a picture very similar to that in secondary myositis ossificans. Diagnosis of aneurysmal bone cyst before cortical outpouching takes place or after fracture and hemorrhage have occurred may be difficult or impossible. Misdiagnosis has all too frequently in the past resulted in overtreatment.

The only consistent symptom of aneurysmal bone cyst is pain, probably due to lifting of the periosteum, pressure upon contiguous normal structures or fracture. A firm mass may be palpated if the involved bone is superficial. Roentgenograms are frequently diagnostic though massive bone destruction and secondary hemorrhage may mask the saccular profile.

The morbid physiology of aneurysmal bone cyst is unknown. Because the structure is an alteration in vascular anatomy and because it is known that an excessive blood flow to a given region of bone will cause lysis, one is tempted to use this mechanism as an explanation. The lesion has been so incompletely studied from the anatomic standpoint that confirming data are lacking. Perfusion x-ray studies would be most helpful but as yet they have not been reported. It is unknown whether the lesion represents a congenital arteriovenous fistula, an organized hematoma with arterial and venous communications, or simply an alteration in pressure dynamics.

GROSS AND MICROSCOPIC APPEARANCE

When the covering shell of bone is incised, a profusely and steadily bleeding mass of soft tissue is encountered. Much of the lesion consists of blood lakes traversed by a meshwork of fibrous walls in which are embedded larger, irregular fields of solid tissue. Sections of the latter show them to be basically fibrous, usually with large numbers of giant cells, xanthoid cells and degenerating blood pigment. This is the same microscopy that one finds wherever there has been extravasation of blood within bone. The walls are composed of fibrous septa. It is impossible to say whether the lining cells are endothelial or merely swollen components of connective tissue. Wherever a fluid-filled space is created within solid tissue one can find the surrounding fibrous tissue adapting itself, with the production of a lining of cells indistinguishable from those of normal vascular channels. In the walls one may find the same giant and xanthoid cells and hemosiderin granules that characterize the larger masses of solid tissue. In addition, there are often long, fragile spicules of osteoid which may be partially mineralized. One must assume that the fibrous tissue is stimulated to produce bone in an environment which is supercharged with calcium salts being freed from the surrounding bone which is being destroyed. The vascular channels are large and tortuous and the walls much thicker than those of normal vessels. If proper tissue is obtained by the surgeon the diagnosis is obvious at a glance. If small bits of the solid tissue are obtained the appearance may be that of "giant cell tumor" or brown tumor of parathyroid adenoma.

PROGNOSIS

The lytic activity of the lesion is apparently controlled if flow of blood through the sinusoids is prevented. This may be done by thrombosing and sclerosing the channels with irradiation or mechanically interrupting the flow by curettage. Either method appears to be effective without completely destroying the lesion.

REFERENCES

OSTEOID OSTEOMA

1. Jaffe, H. L.: Arch. Surg., *31*:709, 1935.
2. Sherman, M. S.: J. Bone & Joint Surg., *29*:918, 1947.
3. Johnson, G. F.: Am. J. Roentgenol., *74*:65, 1955.
4. Jaffe, H. L., and Lichtenstein, L.: J. Bone & Joint Surg., 22:645, 1940.
5. Dahlin, D. C., and Johnson, E. W.: J. Bone & Joint Surg., *36A*:559, 1954.
6. Lichtenstein, L.: Cancer, *9*:1044, 1956.
7. Moberg, E.: J. Bone & Joint Surg., *33A*:166, 1951.
8. Golding, J. S. R.: J. Bone & Joint Surg., *36B*:218, 1954.

OSSIFYING FIBROMA

9. Schlumberger, H. G.: Military Surgeon, *99*:504, 1946.
10. Dahlin, D. C., and Johnson, E. W.: J. Bone & Joint Surg., *36A*:559, 1954.
11. Lichtenstein, L.: Cancer, *9*:1044, 1956.

NON-OSTEOGENIC FIBROMA

12. Jaffe, H. L., and Lichtenstein, L.: Am. J. Path., *18*:205, 1942.

SUBPERIOSTEAL CORTICAL DEFECT

13. Sontag, L. W., and Pyle, S. I.: Am. J. Roentgenol., *46*:185, 1941.

ANGIOMA

14. Gorham, L. W., Wright, A. W., Schultz, H. H., and Maxon, F. C.: Am. J. Med., *17*:674, 1954.

18

Osteogenic Tumors

BENIGN OSTEOBLASTOMA

The term "benign osteoblastoma" was recently supplied by Lichtenstein[1] to denote a group of neoplasms with a fibrous matrix which
produces osteoid and bone. It is a worthy term since it specifies osteoblastic activity and as a new term it clears the mind of such encum-
brances as ossifying fibroma, osteogenic fibroma and fibrous osteoma
(many lesions so diagnosed are not true tumors) and giant osteoid osteoma, which is a bad term because the lesion is not an osteoid osteoma.

There is very little that one can learn by an analysis of the
literature on the subject of ossifying fibroma. One finds that the name
has been used for a variety of lesions and that the clinical and radiologic aspects of the cases are so incompletely given that it is impossible
to tell exactly what disease the author is describing. In our own material we find but 10 cases under this heading. Seven of those are lesions
with a remarkably similar cytology, all having a rather mature fibrous
matrix in which one finds considerable quantities of osteoid, usually
calcified, and some recognizable bone spicules (Fig. 261). It is interesting that of these 10, five are in the mandible and two in the maxilla.
All of these but one (age 67) are in the age group 15 to 30. Four
patients are males and three females.

In the remaining three patients, all females, ages 6, 17 and 35,
two lesions are located in the sacrum and one in the greater trochanter
of the femur. These last show a less mature fibrous stroma, very
little osteoid and more bone spicules.

It appears that there is an entity which occurs in the jaw of
adolescents and young adults, often in relation to the socket of an
infected or recently extracted tooth. It is debatable whether the lesion

in the tooth is the cause or the result of the entity. It produces a circumscribed mass of rather loose, highly vascular fibrous tissue in which are embedded irregular spheroids and fragments of osteoid, some of which mature into recognizable bone. Fibro-osseous metaplasia is not apparent. A few giant cells may be scattered through the field. Almost certainly some cases of monostotic fibrous dysplasia have been diagnosed as ossifying fibroma but in others the diagnosis of fibrous dysplasia is not tenable. Whether these lesions represent true tumor is another matter. We are inclined to think of them as a type of reactive fibrosis.

There is a true fibrosarcoma of the jaw which must not be confused with the above lesion. We have 9 such cases in our material. All are in the age group of 21 to 38. These tumors run an aggressive, rapidly invasive course with a very high mortality. They may be confused with ossifying fibroma of the jaw because of their deceptively mature-appearing cellular components (Fig. 262).

The remaining three cases in our material, two in the sacrum and one in the proximal femur, healed with a minimal amount of therapy. One of these, a large, poorly defined lesion in the sacrum of a six year old girl, was presented at a pathologists' symposium on bone tumors and was diagnosed as almost everything from fibrous dysplasia to osteosarcoma. Dr. Henry Jaffe considered it an ossifying fibroma

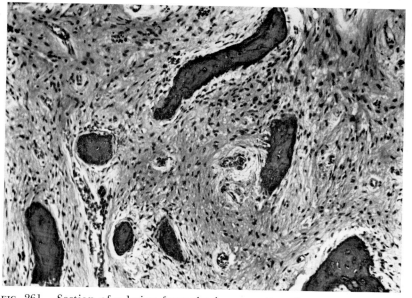

FIG. 261. Section of a lesion from the jaw revealing fibrous proliferation and osteoid production. It may be an ossifying fibroma or a benign osteoblastoma. It was related to a tooth socket, was circumscribed and in places shows osteoblastic activity, features which seem to set it apart from fibrous dysplasia. (× 130.)

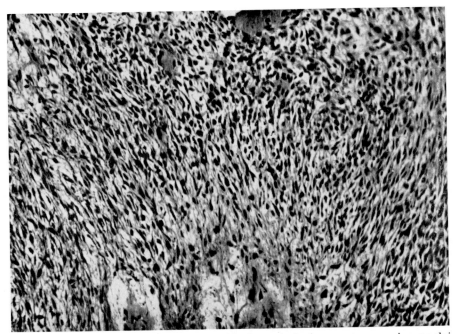

FIG. 262. Fibrosarcoma of the jaw with deceptively innocent appearing nuclei. These tumors have an unusually high mortality because of the difficulty in accomplishing adequate resection. (× 200.)

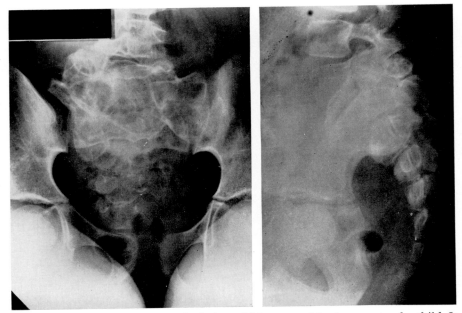

FIG. 263.   Roentgenogram of a lesion which occurred in the sacrum of a child. It was thought to be an osteosarcoma but it healed spontaneously, thus suggesting the diagnosis of benign osteoblastoma.

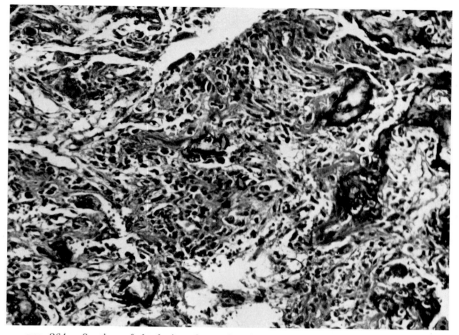

FIG. 264.   Section of the lesion shown in Figure 263. There is a brisk osteoblastic activity suggesting the diagnosis of osteosarcoma. It may fall in the group called benign osteoblastoma. (× 200.)

(Figs. 263 and 264). After a regimen of rest it healed completely and a ten-year follow-up reveals the patient to be entirely well. Instances of this kind make the experienced pathologist extremely cautious about pronouncing a fibrous, bone-forming lesion a true neoplasm.

At the time of this writing there are four reports deserving of the consideration of one who is interested in the diagnosis of ossifying fibroma or benign osteoblastoma. The case reported by Jaffe and Mayer[2] certainly has all the attributes of a neoplasm. The two cases of Golding and Sissons[3] appear to be tumors but the possibility of certain other lesions such as aneurysmal bone cyst cannot be completely excluded. The cases of Dahlin and Johnson[4] and of Lichtenstein[1] may be true tumors. Our material represents over a thousand lesions usually classified as bone tumors. In none of this material do we find a case which with complete certainty we can give as an example of a true neoplasm called benign osteoblastoma.

OSTEOSARCOMA

The osteosarcoma is a malignant neoplasm arising from the undifferentiated fibrous tissue of bone. It is more generally called osteogenic sarcoma. Ewing used the term "osteogenic" to indicate that the tumor is of osseous genesis but other writers use it to mean that it forms bone tissue. Since the cells of osteosarcoma may be less mature than the bone-forming osteoblast and since they may or may not form osteoid, many recent writers prefer to use the non-committal term "osteosarcoma."

Until relatively recently the term "osteogenic sarcoma" was used to include all primary malignant tumors of bone with the exception of malignant giant cell tumors and those arising from marrow elements. Thus, osteosarcomas, chondrosarcomas and fibrosarcomas of bone were all grouped together. Since these three tumors have quite different age and site incidence, radiologic and cytologic features and mortality statistics, this unfortunate situation has led to confusion and quite inaccurate reporting. Recently a more definitive classification has led to clearer concepts and more trustworthy prognostication.

Once the importance of establishing the primary malignant bone tumors as entities is established, further classification becomes largely a matter of taste. Osteosarcoma has been subdivided into many categories, the most generally used being sclerosing, osteolytic, subperiosteal, medullary and telangiectatic. The author holds that any classification of a disease which is not concerned with the manner and extent to which the patient is affected is tedious pedantry. The above classification may be of some use to the radiologist but since it in no way indicates the behavior of the tumor type, its general usage should be abandoned.

With the exception of plasma cell myeloma, osteosarcoma is the most commonly occurring primary malignant tumor of bone. It is encountered nearly twice as often as chondrosarcoma and, excluding the special type in the jaw, about three times as often as fibrosarcoma. In almost all reported series its incidence in males is greater than in females and in some, twice as great. The age incidence of osteosarcoma is most interesting. If one analyzes the various available series one finds that there is a preponderance in the age group under 30 years, but a rather bountiful scattering throughout the ages over 30. However, if one considers the type of bone involved, one sees a more distinct separation of two types of osteosarcoma. In our first 50 cases with data sufficient to allow analysis, 35 of the tumors occurred in cylindrical bones and 15 in flat bones. Of the 35 in cylindrical bones, 29 were in patients 30 or under and only 8 in the older age groups. Of the 15 occurring in flat bones, 14 were in patients over 50. Thus, it appears that osteosarcoma is more frequent in those under 30 and usually occurs in cylindrical bones. A second and smaller rise occurs in the age incidence curve after 50 and these tumors are almost always found in flat bones.

The most common bone to be involved in all series is the femur; in fact, nearly 50 per cent of all osteosarcomas occur in this bone. The humerus and tibia are next most commonly involved, and since the usual area is distal femur and proximal tibia about 75 per cent of all osteosarcomas occur in the region of the knee. The upper end of the humerus is much more commonly involved than the lower end. It will be noted that these are the sites of principal growth in these bones. Of the flat bones the ilium is most often involved but the sacrum, sternum, ribs and skull are not invulnerable. Osteosarcoma rarely affects the small bones of the hands and feet. There are none in our material and not more than a half dozen in the entire literature. The tumor has been reported recently in the phalanges following irradiation; these are presumably secondary tumors. A number of lesions commonly occurring in these short cylindrical bones may mimic osteosarcoma and it is well to remember that this diagnosis in these bones is almost certain to be wrong.

When osteosarcoma affects the cylindrical bones, it usually is the metaphysis that is involved. The tumor arises very near the epiphyseal line, practically always within 5 cm. of it. Only two long bone osteosarcomas in our material have occurred outside the metaphysis (Fig. 265). Most osteosarcomas arising in the medullary shaft are those

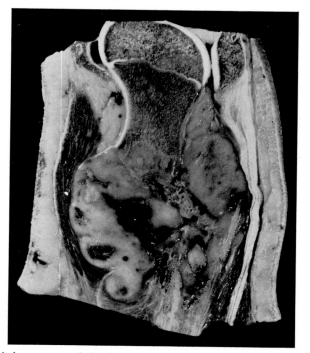

FIG. 265.   This is an unusual site for an osteosarcoma. The tumor apparently started several centimeters shaftward from the metaphysis.

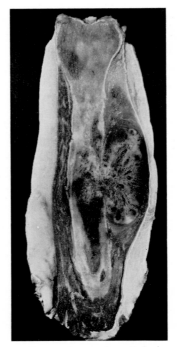

FIG. 266.   Osteosarcoma superimposed on a Paget's lesion. In this instance the tumor may be found in any part of the bone rather than in the usual site, the metaphysis.

following osteochondroma, Paget's disease or irradiation or they are metastatic. Two extrametaphyseal osteosarcomas in our material appeared to arise in the periosteum. The literature contains numerous instances of primary osteosarcoma of the diaphyseal shaft and the validity of these reports will not be denied, but it is worthy of mention that any lesion in a long bone involving other than the metaphyses should be very carefully considered before a diagnosis of osteosarcoma is made.

There is a peculiar and rare type of multiple osteosarcoma which involves many sites simultaneously. Both cylindrical and flat bones are involved and the reported cases[5] have all been in young patients under 15 years of age. It is unknown, of course, whether the tumor is multicentric or whether the many lesions represent bone metastases. Bone metastasis is unusual in osteosarcoma, lending credence to the former idea.

Extraosseous osteosarcoma is a rare tumor. Fine and Stout[6] collected 12 cases and reviewed those in the literature. Seven out of 46 cases apparently began in myositis ossificans. The preponderance of the tumors occurred in the muscles of the extremities, most frequently in the legs. They behaved very much in the same manner as do osteosarcomas of bone. Most of them ran a rather rapid course and metastasized to the lungs. There was only an 8.8 per cent five-year cure rate among the cases on which there was sufficient data for analysis. These authors urge caution in diagnosis of a group which they term "pseudo-malignant," stating that this lesion is a type of myositis ossificans.

Osteosarcoma, chondrosarcoma, fibrosarcoma and, much less frequently, malignant giant cell tumor may be superimposed on Paget's disease (Fig. 266). In the series of Thomson and Turner-Warwick,[7] of 32 cases of osteosarcoma, 5 were associated with Paget's disease. In our material there were 9 cases. All of these patients were over the age of 50. Putting it another way, of the combined series there were 26 patients with osteosarcoma over the age of 50. Fourteen or slightly over half of these had Paget's disease. Paget's disease is common, and if one estimates the percentage of associated osteosarcoma the figure must be very low. Indeed, an authority on Paget's disease has stated that no case of Paget's which he has followed has ever developed osteosarcoma. However, osteosarcoma in patients over the age of 50 is quite uncommon and the figure of 50 per cent is probably not far wrong in expressing an association, especially if occult monostotic Paget's disease is considered.

Osteochondroma predisposes to osteosarcoma. It is impossible to give an accurate estimation of the number of osteochondromas which eventually develop into malignant tumors, almost always either chondrosarcoma or osteosarcoma, but the figure has been variously stated as 5 to 15 per cent. In our series of 50 osteosarcomas, there was evidence that three had developed at the site of a preceding osteochondroma.

Recently, it has been shown that osteosarcoma may evolve at a site affected with fibrous dysplasia. A recent paper[8] reviews the literature on four cases and reports a fifth. The osteosarcoma, which may be multicentric, runs the usual rapid course with death in about eighteen months.

Massive irradiation of bone tissue appears to increase the incidence of bone sarcomas. Osteosarcomas, chondrosarcomas and fibrosarcomas have been reported following x-ray therapy for other lesions in bone or contiguous soft tissue. Hatcher reviewed the literature[9] and found 24 cases, 15 of which were osteosarcoma. One osteosarcoma of the ilium in our material followed irradiation therapy for a genital carcinoma. In most cases, though not in all, excessive doses have been administered. The sarcoma has usually appeared in the area of bone most heavily irradiated rather than in the customarily involved sites. Its course is not unlike that of primary osteosarcoma. There is some evidence that not only is the dosage important but that divided doses administered over an extended period, such as a year, are more apt to be cancerogenic. The interval between therapy and the advent of symptoms of sarcoma has averaged about eleven years. It has been stated that in cases in which sarcoma appears within three years of irradiation, the latter probably has no etiologic relation. Martland studied the cases of 800 girls[10] who had worked in a luminous dial factory and who had ingested significant amounts of zinc sulfide combined with radium and mesothorium. Several of these girls developed osteosarcomas. He found the lethal dose to be in the neighborhood of 10 to 180 micrograms. These cases are reminiscent of the lung cancers which were reported in the Schneeberg cobalt and Joachimsthal pitchblende miners.

X-ray, radium and mesothorium have been used to induce osteosarcoma in experimental animals. Typical osteosarcomas can also be induced in rabbits[11] with intravenous injections of zinc beryllium silicate. Beryllium causes a rather extravagant cellular proliferation of any body tissue in which it becomes lodged. Apparently the bones have a greater affinity for beryllium than other tissues and when a certain concentration is reached, a neoplastic proliferation of osteogenic tissue results. It is not suggested here that either radiant energy or beryllium is an important causative agent of osteosarcoma in humans but the possibility of causing a bone sarcoma by giving irradiation for soft tissue tumors must be kept in mind.

Pain is the only consistent symptom of osteosarcoma. It is often insidious in onset and at first there are usually remissions. Later, the pain becomes severe, deep, boring and constant. Osteosarcoma is a destructive tumor. It infiltrates and causes lysis of the overlying cortex and then lifts the periosteum. It is probably the latter which causes much of the pain. Soon a palpable tumor mass develops (Fig. 267). Since osteosarcomas of long bones are near a joint the pain may be referred into this area. Soon there is limitation of motion and disability. A pathologic fracture is apt to occur because of the cortical destruction. The tumor mass often becomes erythematous, hot and exquisitely tender, suggesting acute inflammation. The superficial veins in relation to it may become dilated and prominent. Eventually there is apt to be fever, malaise, weight loss, anemia and progressive debilitation. The systemic signs and symptoms of osteosarcoma probably arise because of the destruction of normal tissue and the degeneration within the tumor itself. Though it is a highly vascular tumor it is rapidly growing and it is probable that large fields become necrotic because of loss of adequate blood supply.

The serum alkaline phosphatase level depends, among other things, upon osteoblastic activity. It has been shown that tumor osteoblasts contain and probably secrete phosphatase. Serum phosphatase levels are usually elevated in osteosarcoma[12] and a level of 20 Bodansky units is not infrequently noted. It should be remembered, however, that the amount of phosphatase depends upon the number of osteoblasts which produce it. The number in an early and small tumor may be inadequate to elevate the level above normal or an osteosarcoma of immature cells may produce no osteoid and no phosphatase. An elevated level in suspected osteosarcoma is highly significant; a normal level is without meaning. The level often falls following the ablation of a large, osteoid-forming tumor. Periodic serum analysis has been used to guide the prognosis when pulmonary metastases are to be expected. The level may or may not rise with metastasis depending upon the degree of maturity and function of the tumor cells.

The diagnosis of osteosarcoma may be considered all but certain because of clinical and radiologic findings but it must be certified by biopsy before therapy may be undertaken. This rule is absolutely infallible since there are numerous benign and innocuous lesions which precisely mimic the clinical and roentgenographic characteristics of osteosarcoma. The treatment of osteosarcoma, whatever it is, must always be radical, and overdiagnosis and overtreatment without a biopsy is inexcusable and indefensible. It has been stated by a prominent authority that biopsy delays the advent of therapy, increases the growth rate, predisposes to pulmonary metastasis and hastens the death of the patient; therefore, treatment should be administered without

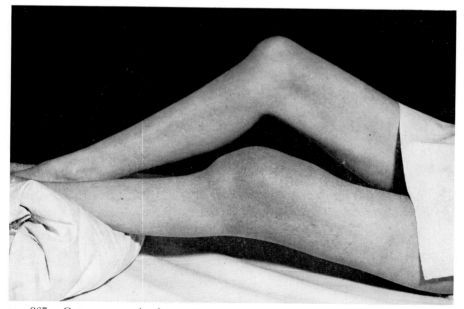

FIG. 267.   Osteosarcoma in the most common site, the lower end of the femur. After penetrating the cortex it produced a bulky soft tissue tumor.

it. It would be difficult to argue the veracity of most of the premises of the first part of this statement. Biopsy often delays the advent of therapy, though if properly done the delay need not be more than twenty-four hours. It is questionable whether it increases the rate of growth though such might be argued. Almost certainly, the cutting through viable tumor tissue, lymphatic and blood channels increases the probability of metastasis and hastens the death of the patient. But the most important point has been ignored. The mortality of osteosarcoma, no matter how it is treated, is probably somewhere around 95 per cent. The patient with osteosarcoma has only one chance in twenty, at best one in ten, of surviving his disease. To amputate the extremity of a patient with an innocuous lesion which was thought to be a sarcoma is certainly less defensible than failing to amputate an osteosarcoma which would almost certainly have caused death no matter what the treatment.

The biopsy of choice is a frozen section taken with tourniquet applied. Unfortunately this is not always possible. The presence of bone may make it impossible to section biopsy tissue without demineralization. And just as often, the nuclear detail upon which the pathologist depends so greatly in making the diagnosis of osteosarcoma may be impossible to retain with the frozen technique. Frozen section should be attempted but in the majority of cases it will be necessary to withhold the diagnosis until paraffin-embedded tissue may be examined.

The taking of the biopsy is exceedingly important. If cut from the superficial portion of what grossly appears to be tumor, nothing more than bone reaction may be obtained. If such material consisting of actively proliferating young osteogenic tissue is obtained from an innocent lesion suspected of being sarcomatous, the pathologist may be misled into the diagnosis of malignant neoplasm. If a deep biopsy is obtained the material may be so necrotic that cellular clarity has been destroyed. It is best to take at least two samples of tissue and better four from different levels of the tumor. And the pathologist should remember that if a definite opinion cannot be given on frozen section, the patient is probably better off waiting for paraffin technique than taking the gamble which is necessary without cytologic guidance.

ROENTGENOGRAPHIC MANIFESTATIONS

The roentgenographic manifestations of osteosarcoma are those of bone destruction alone or in combination with the formation of new bone. The tumor usually begins in the metaphyseal end of a bone and results in irregular, ill-defined radiolucent defects as a result of de-

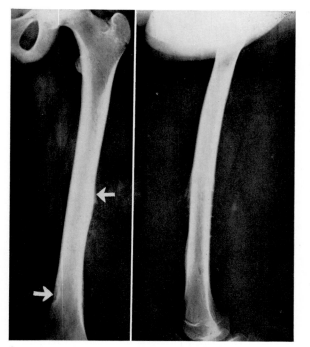

FIG. 268.   Osteosarcoma. Irregular destruction is evident in the medullary canal. Periosteal new bone is evident perpendicular to the cortex and at the junction of the elevated periosteum and the cortex (arrow). A subperiosteal cortical defect is present in the distal shaft (lower arrow).

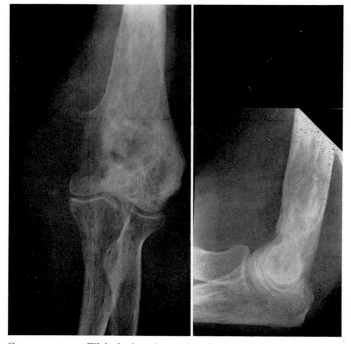

FIG. 269.   Osteosarcoma. This lesion is arising from an area of Paget's disease in the distal humerus. Bone destruction and a soft tissue mass are evident.

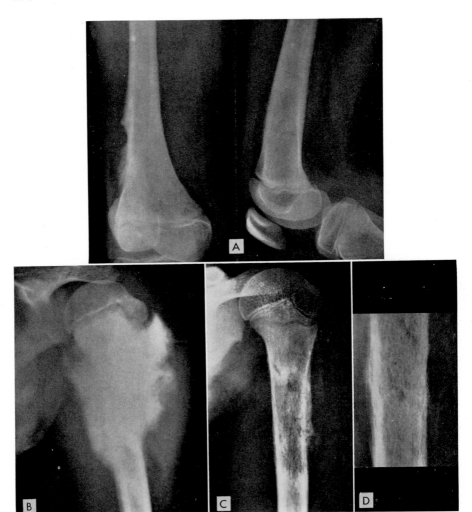

FIG. 270.   Osteosarcoma. *A, B* and *C* illustrate this tumor in three patients. *A* shows very minimal evidence of medullary involvement. Bone production is marked in *B*. There is marked destruction of spongy and compact bone in *C* with areas of sclerosis (new bone). *D* represents a portion of the involved shaft of *C,* magnified to show the tiny areas of destruction and the periosteal new bone.

struction of trabeculae of bone. Periosteal new bone formation may be the first manifestation of cortical involvement and may be apparent before there is recognizable destruction of the cortex and in some instances before macroscopic evidence of destruction of trabeculae. Codman's triangle and the "sunburst" appearance are manifestations of periosteal elevation and as such are not specific for this neoplasm. The former refers to the triangular-shaped area where the elevated periosteum rejoins the cortex; the "sunburst" appearance results from the formation of reactive and/or neoplastic new bone which is laid down perpendicular to the shaft along vessels passing from the periosteum to the cortex. In time, the periosteum is ruptured and a soft tissue mass becomes apparent. Osteoporosis often accompanies the lesion, possibly as a result of increased vascularity secondary to the presence of this vascular tumor.

If the neoplastic cells do not produce osteoid or bone in any appreciable amount, the radiographic appearance will be primarily the result of bone destruction (radiolucency), and sclerosis within the neoplasm will not be a feature. Even in these neoplasms, however, reactive periosteal new bone may be formed. The most common type of osteosarcoma (Class I) both forms and destroys bone, so that bone destruction and periosteal and neoplastic new bone formation are apparent. The density of the mass of neoplastic tissue extending into the soft tissues is again dependent upon the ability of the neoplastic cells to form bone. Accordingly, this mass may be of the density of soft tissue or it may be irregularly opaque as the result of the presence of multiple masses of neoplastic bone.

GROSS PATHOLOGY

In the great majority of cases, osteosarcoma has destroyed a portion of the cortex and involves both intracortical and extracortical tissues by the time an anatomic examination can be made. A few bone-forming tumors will be encountered which appear to be arising from the periosteum and growing outward into the soft tissues with little or no cortical destruction. In the experience of the writer the microscopy of these latter tumors is usually different from that of true osteosarcoma and, moreover, from the available data it appears that they behave somewhat differently. Some writers, including the author, place these in a separate category variously called juxtacortical sarcoma, periosteal osteosarcoma or parosteal sarcoma. Some writers have concluded that all true osteosarcomas arise in intracortical tissues. This conclusion is not justifiable and until it is, we must admit of the possibility that an osteosarcoma rarely may spring from the bone-forming elements of the periosteum.

Since osteosarcoma grows rapidly it has almost always reached a considerable size by the time it is examined. In long bones, primary osteosarcoma almost always begins in the metaphysis. It usually replaces the metaphyseal cancellous tissue before it destroys the cortex. Since, in long bones, it usually occurs in adolescents, the enchondral plate is often still unossified. Apparently cartilage is less readily invaded by osteosarcoma than cortical bone for it often remains intact until quite late (Fig. 271). If the enchondral plate is violated, the

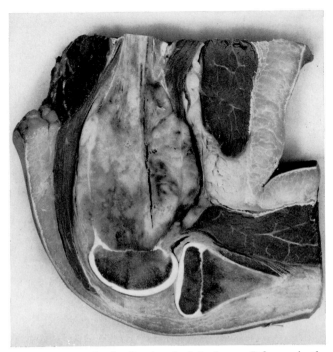

FIG. 271.   Osteosarcoma in the distal end of the femur. It began in the metaphysis and destroyed the compacta on both sides. It elevated the periosteum which remains intact. Note that it has not violated the enchondral plate.

tumor grows through the ossified nucleus of the epiphysis to the articular plate which usually restrains the neoplastic process. Osteosarcoma permeates the haversian canals of the cortex and interferes with the blood supply. Soon the cortex gives way and great portions of it simply disappear. As the tumor reaches the outer surface the periosteum is stretched over it but for some time it remains intact (Fig. 272). In pulling away from the cortical surface the periosteum drags along the small vessels which pass from it into the cortex and these take a vertical direction to the cortical surface. About these vascular channels columns of new bone are laid down, perhaps because of the abundant blood supply. These trabeculae of bone account for the sunburst effect which is so often seen in the roentgenogram. Most of the bone so formed is reactive and non-neoplastic, or so it appears through the microscope. Moreover, other non-bone-forming tumors such as carcinoma and even non-neoplastic processes may produce this identical picture. At a point near where the periosteum rejoins the cortex, the bone that it lays down is annealed to the cortical surface, causing a localized area of thickening. This produces the Codman triangle which, though it characterizes tumor elevation of the periosteum, particularly by osteosarcoma, is itself not a neoplastic prolifera-

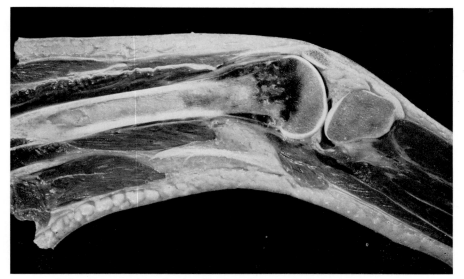

FIG. 272.   Osteosarcoma in the distal end of the femur. Though a rather small tumor it has caused marked destruction of the overlying bone. The elevated periosteum is still intact.

tion. Though the periosteum may be greatly distended over the tumor before it gives way, eventually it is penetrated and the tumor infiltrates wildly through the soft tissue structures.

Most osteosarcomas are highly vascular. Thus, the gross appearance is that of a frankly hemorrhagic tumor. About half of them produce considerable amounts of osteoid which soon becomes mineralized. In the more sclerotic lesions it may be necessary to chisel out a block for section. Others produce only enough bone to give a gritty consistency and in still others there is no palpable evidence of bone. Necrosis is usual and often extensive. This involves not only the tumor but the tissue which it destroys.

The classification of osteosarcoma into medullary and subperiosteal types has already been commented upon. Separating this tumor into sclerosing and osteolytic varieties is also quite futile on an anatomic basis. One usually finds sclerotic and lytic areas in the same tumor, the former being inside and outside the cortex and the latter in the area where the process has broken through the compacta.

MICROSCOPIC PATHOLOGY

Though the diagnosis of osteosarcoma on the basis of microscopy is usually a fairly simple matter because of the malignant characteristics of the cells, in some instances it can be exceedingly difficult. In bone reaction where there is very active osteogenesis it may be necessary to carefully evaluate the possibility of malignant growth. This is because an occasional osteosarcoma is composed of relatively mature bone-forming cells, and also because all too frequently the biopsy material actually submitted for osteosarcoma may consist not of tumor tissue but of bone reaction about it. Thus, the microscopist has a difficult time in establishing his criteria for osteosarcoma.

In analyzing a group of primary bone tumors the author was struck by the variation in cellular pattern. A cytologic classification was made with the hope that the recognition of at least some varieties might help in the planning of therapy and in prognosis. A series of 20 cases was selected in which there was a reasonably good clinical record and a five-year follow-up in the survivors, adequate roentgenograms and ample histologic material. The clinical and radiologic data were analyzed by a participating worker and the coded slides were examined by the author. By microscopy the cases fell quite naturally into four fairly distinct groups. There was a certain amount of overlapping between classes in some cases and a few showed transition from one class to another in which biopsy and autopsy samples were both available, but in general there were four dominant cytologic pictures.

When the clinical data was considered in relation to the histologic types it became apparent that no correlation could be made. Regardless of whether the tumor was bone-forming, cartilage-forming or was too immature to form either, there was no relation to the rate of growth, the advent of metastasis or the length of the survival period. It was deemed impossible to predict the behavior of osteosarcoma on the basis of histology alone.

The grouping of the tumors into the four cytologic classes became a mere academic exercise, useful only to the pathologist in recognizing the lesion and in recording its characteristics. To serve the latter purpose it will be used in the following discussion.

Class I osteosarcoma: In this group the tumor matrix cells are spindled or less frequently pleomorphic. They align themselves along irregular masses of crude bone and are obviously active in the production of osteoid. Tumor giant cells are not unusual. Sometimes the tumor cells orient themselves in relation to spicules of normal bone and form tumor osteoid around it. Where this happens it is not always possible to be sure which is neoplastic and which is normal bone tissue. This is particularly true in the region of the subperiosteal, perpendicular rays where both reactive and neoplastic bone formation occur simultaneously. There is a considerable degree of variation in maturation of the tumor cells and in the architecture of the osteoid they produce. Usually the nuclei are obviously of malignant character

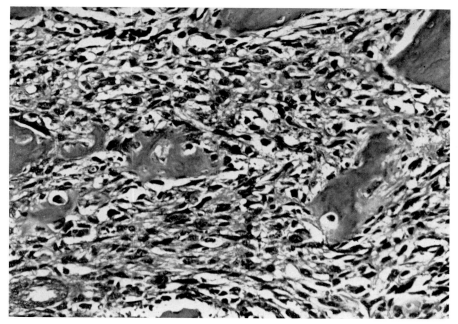

FIG. 273.   Class I osteosarcoma. The matrix is composed of spindled cells with nuclei having all the characteristics of malignant neoplasm—irregularity in size, shape and chromatin content. These cells are producing crude osteoid. (× 200.)

though in some, one has to consider the possibility of fibrous dysplasia and ossifying fibroma.

Tumors of the Class I group (Fig. 273) have all the characteristics of the classic concept of osteosarcoma. Osteoid tissue is formed by tumor osteoblasts directly and without the intermediary of cartilage or collagen. This is the type that Thomson et al.[7] would call osteoblastic sarcoma. Some writers would exclude all other types from the category of osteosarcoma. Class I osteosarcoma is the most commonly occurring type. Practically all of the long bone lesions in adolescents fall in this group.

Class II osteosarcoma produces areas which are identical with the cytology of Class I. In addition, there is cartilage production (Fig. 274). In some lesions the cartilage is minimal and actually hard to find while in others there may be large fields which are totally cartilage. The hyalin is probably an intermediary product in the formation of bone but if the biopsy is limited to this material, a diagnosis of chondrosarcoma is inevitable. These conditions may account for the occasional "chondrosarcoma" which runs a rapid and fatal course, the course which one expects in osteosarcoma.

The criticism has been made that if a tumor contains any considerable amount of cartilage it should not be called an osteosarcoma,

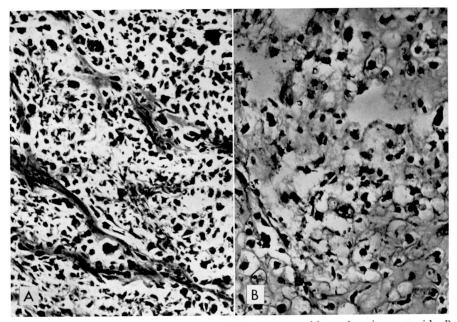

FIG. 274.   Class II osteosarcoma. *A,* Tumor osteoblasts forming osteoid. *B,* Tumor chondroblasts forming hyalin. These two photographs were made from the same section. (× 130.)

but should be classified with the chondrosarcomas or called ostoechondrosarcoma. The writer agrees wholeheartedly with Jaffe and Lichtenstein that if a tumor contains any considerable portion of osteosarcoma it will behave like an osteosarcoma and should be called such. To make another tumor class is making things more complicated than they need be, and to classify a tumor as a chondrosarcoma is to erase the identity of the latter as a clinical entity.

Class III osteosarcoma fails to form either bone or cartilage, but woven among the tumor cell aggregates are strands and bands of what appears to be collagen. The tumor cells tend to line up along the edges of these collagen bands just as osteoblasts line up along osteoid seams. The cells are more uniform and less pleomorphic than those in other osteosarcoma types (Fig. 275). Thus, the pattern may simulate to a certain degree that of the so-called "benign synovioma." The distinction should not be difficult, however, since the cells are usually in greater aggregates, the nuclei have more characteristics of malignancy, the collagen bands have less tendency to form sinusoid-like spaces and the spaces do not contain giant cells.

Most writers contend that if a tumor forms neither osteoid nor cartilage it cannot be classified as an osteosarcoma. They would call such a tumor an intracortical fibrosarcoma. It should be pointed out, however, that the histologic pattern of this lesion is distinct and different from that of fibrosarcoma and, more important, its behavior is that of osteosarcoma and much more malignant than fibrosarcoma of bone.

Class IV osteosarcoma is the least common of the four types. It appears to be incapable of forming any intercellular substance and, therefore, there is no bone or cartilage and very little, if any, collagen. The cells are usually quite pleomorphic and obviously malignant in character. The pattern is scrambled but a characteristic feature about the lesion is slit-like spaces very similar to those seen in malignant synovioma. Sections of one such tumor were submitted to several "name" pathologists about the country. More than one classified it as a synovioma. Later a hindquarter amputation was done, affording an opportunity to examine the tumor in detail. It arose in the cancellous tissue of the ilium and at no point did it extend through the cortex. No tumor was ever found outside of bone until pulmonary metastasis and later widespread visceral metastasis occurred. The course was that of osteosarcoma. Another case almost identical in sex, age group, site and cytology metastasized to the lung. The lung metastases produced considerable amounts of well formed bone (Fig. 276).

In brief, there are four recognizable cell patterns in osteosarcoma:

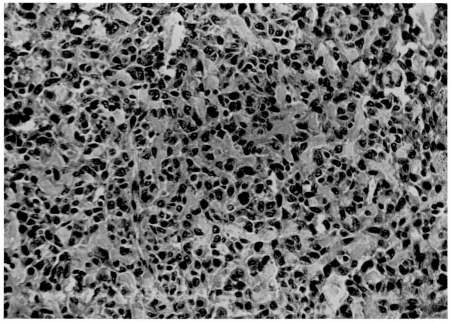

FIG. 275.   Class III osteosarcoma. Irregular cords and islands of tumor cells are surrounded by strands of collagen. There is no osteoid nor hyalin formation. (× 200.)

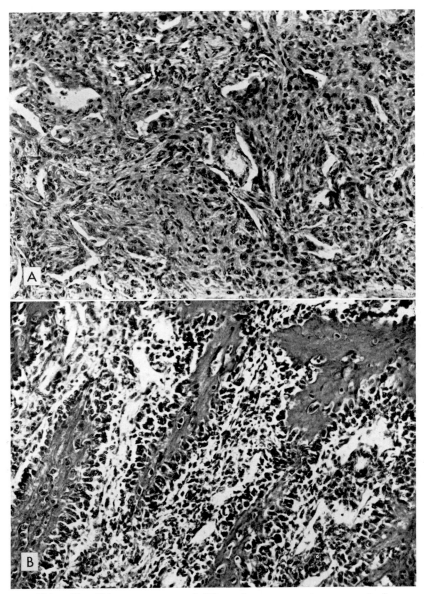

FIG. 276.   Class IV osteosarcoma. *A,* The primary tumor is composed of masses of pleomorphic tumor cells with little or no hyalin, osteoid or collagen. The presence of slit spaces suggests synovioma. *B,* Section of a pulmonary metastatic deposit from the tumor illustrated in *A.* Osteoid production establishes the unequivocal diagnosis of osteosarcoma. ($\times$ 130.)

in one the outstanding feature is osteoid production, another forms both osteoid and cartilage, a third produces neither osteoid nor cartilage but forms collagen, and in the fourth one finds little or no evidence of any of these intercellular substances. Although these cytologic patterns may predominate in many blocks, the classes are not distinct.

A single tumor may contain more than one pattern and the pattern of the metastasis may be different from that of the primary. Whatever the pattern no inference may be made in regard to the degree of malignancy.

Price[13] attempted to classify osteosarcoma in relation to its behavior on the basis of an index of the mitotic figures seen in the sections. Most microscopists with a wide experience in the diagnosis of osteosarcoma would probably not agree that the number of mitotic figures will assist in making a prognosis. At best, the number of mitotic figures is but an index of the rate of growth. There are too many other factors which influence the effect of osteosarcoma upon the patient to make it of considerable prognostic significance.

The cytologic diagnosis of osteosarcoma is exceedingly important and not always easy. There are no special stains which are helpful. Engfeldt[14] has suggested that microradiology has reached a stage of practicability in this field. It is true that certain, apparently characteristic patterns have been defined for osteopetrosis, osteogenesis imperfecta and Paget's disease, but the mineralization pattern in osteosarcoma is so kaleidoscopic that as yet one should hesitate to apply these patterns in cases in which an extremity may be the pawn.

PROGNOSIS

Excluding the myelogenic tumors, osteosarcoma is the most malignant tumor of bone. The expected course is from a few weeks to three months of symptoms before diagnosis is made and a post-diagnosis survival period of approximately eighteen months. Death is almost always the result of pulmonary metastasis. Once pulmonary metastases are demonstrable, life expectancy is not greater than six months. The reason for the grim mortality of osteosarcoma, that is, the reason it metastasizes so consistently and so early, is not known. It is often highly vascular but as yet there are no data to indicate that the so-called telangiectatic type metastasizes earlier than those of the less vascular group. The relation of tumor cells and vascular channels seems to be no more intimate than in some other tumors such as synovioma, which characteristically metastasizes late. The trauma of manipulation before and during diagnosis has been blamed, but although everyone agrees that the suspected osteosarcoma should be handled with all possible gentleness, this precaution has not seemed to prevent or delay the onset of metastasis. It is probable that most or all malignant tumors send showers of viable cells into the lymphatic and blood channels long before the cells are capable of setting up independent growth. Green has shown by the technique of explanting tumor samples that a primary growth must exist for some time before its explant will grow, and that if the explant survives the primary has established the capacity for metastasis. It is unknown whether primary growth eventually imparts independence to its component cells or whether the primary affects the host organism, breaking down an early established immunity. Whatever the factor which prevents or delays independent growth, it is of less importance in osteosarcoma than in most other tumors.

Prognosis in osteosarcoma concerning the behavior of the various types is difficult or impossible. There seems to be some evidence that the nearer the trunk the site of the primary, the higher the mortality and the shorter the course. Most writers agree that a 10 per cent five-year salvage is as much as can be expected today. If allowance is made for those tumors which are mistakenly placed in this category the figure is probably nearer 5 per cent.

It is unusual for osteosarcoma to spread to the regional lymph nodes. If adequately removed, osteosarcoma rarely recurs at the primary site. Almost all osteosarcomas metastasize to the lungs first, usually within nine to twelve months. Terminal widespread metastasis is not uncommon. Metastasis to other bones is unusual but it may occur either early or late. If multiple bone lesions should occur in a case in which one site has been diagnosed as osteosarcoma, the validity of the diagnosis should be challenged.

The osteosarcoma has shown little vulnerability to irradiation therapy. It is better not to use it if surgery can be done. There has been a tendency over the past decade to increase the extent of surgery. In some clinics a hindquarter amputation is considered the proper treatment for an osteosarcoma of the distal femur. Sufficient data is not available as yet to judge whether the salvage has been improved by this method, but since osteosarcoma infrequently recurs and rarely spreads to regional lymph nodes it would seem that not more surgery but earlier surgery is what is needed. It is probable that most osteosarcomas have already metastasized to the lungs, though the deposits are not yet demonstrable, by the time the diagnosis is made. A few cases have undergone resection of a pulmonary metastasis with reported cure.[15] Close scrutiny of these cases reveals that the tumors in question, whether they were osteosarcomas or not, were not behaving like osteosarcomas at the time the lung deposit was removed, because the interval between resection of the primary and the appearance of the metastasis was greatly prolonged. Under these circumstances pulmonary resection is certainly justified, but with the gamble for a good result so great, thoracotomy for a metastasis which appeared within one year hardly seems reasonable.

The public must be educated to seek counsel earlier, the clinician must maintain a higher index of osteosarcoma suspicion and insist on x-ray examination at the outset, the pathologist must be thoroughly acquainted with the differential diagnostic possibilities, and once the diagnosis is made procrastination must be abhorred by all parties concerned. Then perhaps the mortality figures for osteosarcoma can be bettered.

PAROSTEAL SARCOMA

When one studies the radiology and histology of the osteogenic neoplasms and carefully analyzes their clinical behavior and mortality statistics, there emerges a type which over the past few years has come to be recognized as an entity separate from central osteosarcoma. It has been called parosteal osteoma, parosteal osteogenic sarcoma, periosteal chondrosarcoma, juxtacortical sarcoma and desmoid of bone. Geschickter and Copeland[16] used the term parosteal osteoma in a paper in which they reported what they considered to be 16 cases of this lesion in 1951. In 1954, Dwinell, Dahlin and Ghormley[17] reported a series of 15 cases, 14 of which they felt fulfilled all the criteria for the lesion. The following year Lichtenstein,[18] in criticizing the validity of such an entity as described in the previous two reports, described under the heading of periosteal chondrosarcoma one case which, judging from the illustrations of the roentgenograms and the microscopy, is classic parosteal sarcoma. In reviewing our own material we find four cases which are unequivocally parosteal sarcoma, five others which probably fall in this group and two cases which, except that they involve the mandible where it has not yet been reported, cannot be excluded.

We prefer the term parosteal sarcoma to the other names which have been used. By using the word parosteal instead of periosteal we avoid confusion of this lesion with periosteal fibrosarcoma and, if there be such an entity, true periosteal osteosarcoma. The word sarcoma is preferred to osteogenic sarcoma and chondrosarcoma since often one can find in sections of this tumor components of all three mesenchymal tissue types—fibrous tissue, cartilage and bone. In a sense it is a periosteal mesenchymoma but since the same thing can be said of some osteosarcomas, the parosteal sarcoma is considered in this section.

Parosteal sarcoma is considerably less common than osteosarcoma, chondrosarcoma and even fibrosarcoma of bone. It apparently affects females about as frequently as males. There appears to be an age predilection for those between 15 and 35 years. In the very limited material available this tumor has been reported involving only the large cylindrical bones of the extremities. In the author's material there are two lesions arising from the outer surface of the mandible which show a remarkable similarity in both the roentgenograms and sections. The lower end of the femur appears to be the commonest site of involvement, this being the affected area in 25 of 41 cases. The tibia and the humerus claim most of the remainder.

The usual clinical sign of parosteal sarcoma is a firm, smooth mass protruding from the outer cortical surface near the end of a long, cylindrical bone. The patient has often been cognizant of the mass for several months. Pain may or may not be present and usually is late in onset. Since there is little or no destruction of the host bone, fracture does not occur.

ROENTGENOGRAPHIC MANIFESTATIONS

The parosteal sarcoma has a radiographic appearance suggestive of a benign neoplasm. The tumor grows into the soft tissues adjacent to the periosteum and usually does not involve the underlying cortex;

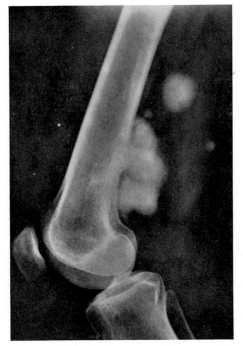

FIG. 277.   Parosteal sarcoma. The neoplasm has resulted in very little change in the femur. Homogeneous opacity is evident within the soft tissue mass of neoplasm. Local recurrence in approximately one year followed removal and necessitated amputation.

in some instances, however, the cortex may be eroded on its external surface. Since there is no differentiation of the neoplastic bone within the tumor into recognizable trabeculae, it tends to be uniformly dense and opaque. The non-ossifying portion of the neoplasm, which may be extensive in amount, is responsible for a mass which has the density of soft tissue.

MORPHOLOGY

Parosteal sarcoma appears to arise in periosteal tissue (Fig 278). Almost all cases to date have involved the metaphyseal region. The posterior cortical surface of the lower end of the femur, the floor of the popliteal space, is the usual site of involvement. The tumor may grow from a broad base or a relatively narrow pedicle. When the base is small the tumor may produce a mushroom head which expands laterally beyond the pedicle, sometimes resting lightly upon the surrounding cortex. The surface is fairly smooth and tends to be lobulated. About half the tumors appear grossly to have a dense fibrous capsule. The parosteal sarcoma is attached to the underlying compacta of the host bone by means of the periosteum. It has been possible to dissect the tumor away without greatly disturbing the cortex in

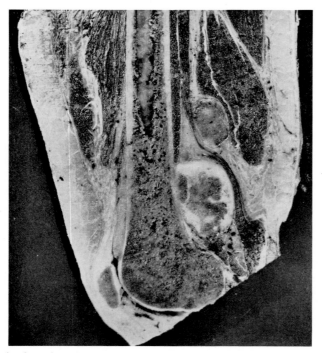

FIG. 278. Sagittal section through a femur with a parosteal sarcoma arising from the periosteum of the distal posterior surface.

some cases. In others there has been erosion of the cortex from without and in a few cases there appears to have been some infiltration.

The parosteal sarcoma is usually firm and may be quite hard, depending upon the amount of mineralized osteoid present. The base and central portions of the tumor often have a bony appearance and consistency whereas a zone beneath the convex surface is usually softer and sometimes frankly cartilaginous. Eventually, there is usually invasion of the contiguous soft tissues; thus muscle bands may disappear into the substance of the tumor. Though the superficial portions or the growing frontier may be soft, to cut blocks from the more mature portions it may be necessary to use a chisel.

From the above description one might conclude that parosteal sarcoma is a type of osteochondroma. Actually they are quite distinct lesions. The parosteal sarcoma does not develop a cylinder of mature bone coextensive with the cortex; it has no intracortical cancellous tissue. Though there may be a zone of cartilage overlying its convex surface, this is neoplastic cartilage and there is no attempt at the formation of an epiphyseal line such as is seen at the junction of the pedicle and cartilaginous cap of the osteochondroma. If the two lesions have any relationship, the parosteal sarcoma is the malignant, neoplastic analogue of the hamartomatous osteochondroma.

The microscopic sections of parosteal sarcoma are more apt to lead to confusion than to clarification of the diagnosis unless the pathologist has samples of various levels of the tumor. It is usual to find fields of fibrosarcoma, others of chondrosarcoma and still others of osteosarcoma all in the same lesion. Or, in some cases, the characteristics of aggressiveness are so minimal that the pathologist concludes that he is dealing with a benign or even a non-neoplastic process. Lichtenstein has stated[18] that many of the lesions described as parosteal sarcoma are in fact no more than examples of heterotopic ossification such as that seen in myositis ossificans. He decries the acceptance of lesions without the microscopic criteria of malignant neoplasia in the category of aggressive tumors. His position is understandable since the adoption and casual application of such a policy would inevitably lead to unnecessary amputation. However, every experienced microscopist must eventually admit that there are tumors of malignant nature which lack the microscopic criteria for their behavior. The cellular criteria of malignancy were laid down long ago and the pathologist is apt to put his faith and stake his reputation on them. He expresses dismay and disenchantment when a tumor, whose cells appear quite mature and innocent, shows aggressive behavior. Just as one cannot always identify the criminal by his physiognomy, so one cannot always predict the activity of a cell by the appearance of its nucleus. The cells of some parosteal sarcomas may have an appearance as innocent as those of a desmoid or keloid, yet the tumor is invasive and may eventually metastasize.

In the fields of fibrous proliferation there may be sufficient collagenization to suggest scar or callus formation (Fig. 279). In other fields neoplastic proliferation may be obvious. In material obtained from recurrent lesions, the sections may resemble those of the most pleomorphic fibrosarcomas. Some sections are apt to show fibrocartilaginous metaplasia and it may be assumed that the cartilage constituents of parosteal sarcoma are of fibroblastic genesis. Here again, the cartilage may appear quite innocent or one may encounter the typical microscopy of chondrosarcoma (Fig. 280). Irregular trabeculae of cartilage are usually seen at the periphery of the fields of osteoid and it is apparent that much of the latter is formed by chondro-osseous metaplasia. Other fields show fibro-osseous metaplasia and in still others there may be osteoblastic osteogenesis (Fig. 281). The appearance of the bone may be quite respectable and innocent and one may be misled into the opinion that one is dealing with material from a callus or myositis ossificans.

The first two cases studied by the author were thought to be benign processes. Both recurred and in both the microscopic appear-

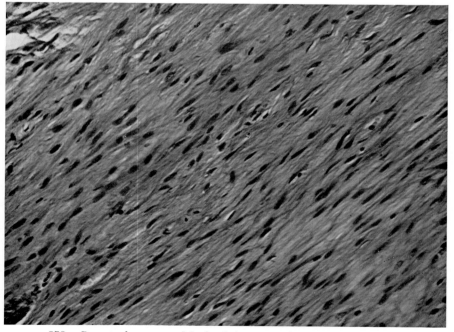

FIG. 279.   Parosteal sarcoma. Much of the tumor is made up of adult bone in a fibrous matrix. The cells of the latter are quite orderly in arangement, and their nuclei are fairly mature. ($\times$ 200.)

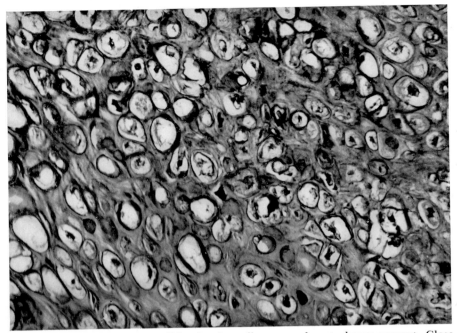

FIG. 280.   Parosteal sarcoma. Islands of cartilage are almost always present. Close examination reveals the cellular evidence of malignancy. (× 200.)

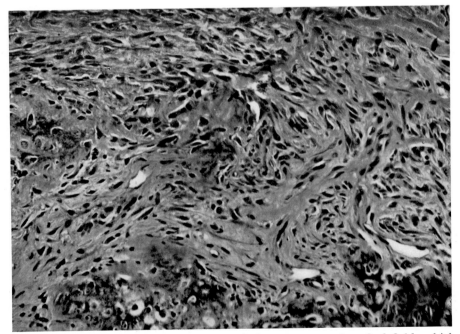

FIG. 281.   Parosteal sarcoma. Here and there one can often find fields which appear to be fibrosarcoma and elsewhere osteosarcoma. Or, as in this field, they appear to be mixed. (× 200.)

ance of the cells of the recurrence was quite obviously malignant. The same experience has been reported by Dwinell et al.

If future reported descriptions of parosteal sarcoma are consistent with the lesion as described above, the diagnosis to one who knows he is dealing with an extracortical lesion need not necessarily be difficult. The roentgenogram should help to rule out periosteal chondroma (see page 489). The cytologic pattern of osteochondroma is orderly and the cells mature. Periosteal fibrosarcoma usually has a characteristic cell pattern (see page 523), and the finding of neoplastic cartilage in some sections would make this diagnosis untenable. One may find it necessary to differentiate central osteosarcoma on the basis of the roentgenogram.

PROGNOSIS

Parosteal sarcoma should be held distinct from central osteosarcoma, if for no other reason than on the basis of its behavior. It is a slowly growing tumor. Evidence of its presence for many years before its diagnosis has been recorded. If the diagnosis is made reasonably early and the proper treatment carried out, one can expect a cure in the great majority of cases. Just what the proper treatment is, is not yet clearly apparent. One is tempted on the basis of the initial biopsy material to treat the lesion conservatively. The incidence of recurrence after local resection (nine out of ten in the series of Dwinell et al.) makes it appear that conservative measures are not enough. The change in the microscopy as shown by the recurrence following surgical intervention may be due to the manipulation or it may represent the natural behavior of the lesion.

In the tumors which have recurred there is a fairly high incidence of pulmonary metastasis. Unlike osteosarcoma, however, these metastases may occur several years after ablation of the recurrent tumor, and some of them have grown much more slowly than one would expect of the osteosarcoma secondary. Only the accumulation of data on large numbers of these cases will serve to enlighten us as to how the parosteal sarcoma may be expected to behave and therefrom how it should be treated.

REFERENCES

BENIGN OSTEOBLASTOMA

1. Lichtenstein, L.: Cancer, *9*:1044, 1956.
2. Jaffe, H. L., and Mayer, L.: Arch. Surg., *24*:550, 1932.
3. Golding, J. S. R., and Sissons, H. A.: J. Bone & Joint Surg., *36B*:428, 1954
4. Dahlin, D. C., and Johnson, E. W.: J. Bone & Joint Surg., *36A*:559, 1954.

OSTEOSARCOMA

5. Moseley, J. E., and Bass, M. H.: Radiology, *66*:41, 1956.
6. Fine, G., and Stout, A. P.: Cancer, *9*:1027, 1956.
7. Thomson, A. D., and Turner-Warwick, R. T.: J. Bone & Joint Surg., *37B*:266, 1955.
8. Perkinson, N. G., and Higginbotham, N. L.: Cancer, *8*:396, 1955.
9. Hatcher, C. H.: J. Bone & Joint Surg., *27*:179, 1945.
10. Martland, H. S.: Am. J. Cancer, *15*:2435, 1931.
11. Janes, J. M., Higgens, G. M., and Herrick, J. F.: J. Bone & Joint Surg., *38A*:809. 1956.
12. Woodward, H. Q., and Higginbotham, N. L.: Am. J. Cancer, *13*:221, 1937.
13. Price, C. H. G.: J. Faculty Radiologists (London), *7*:237, 1956.
14. Engfeldt, B.: Cancer, *7*:815, 1954.
15. Goldenberg, R. R.: Bull. Hosp. Joint Dis., *15*:67, 1954.

PAROSTEAL SARCOMA

16. Geschickter, C. F., and Copeland, M. M.: Ann. Surg., *133*:790, 1951.
17. Dwinell, L. A., Dahlin, D. C., and Ghormley, R. K.: J. Bone & Joint Surg., *36A*: 732, 1954.
18. Lichtenstein, L.: Cancer, *8*:1060, 1955.

19

Chondrogenic Tumors

BENIGN CHONDROBLASTOMA

The benign chondroblastoma is a neoplasm of chondroblastic cytogenesis occurring predominantly in the epiphyses of adolescents with a somewhat greater frequency in males.

Because the lesion has a predilection for the ends of large, long bones and because giant cells often appear rather prominently in its cytology, it was classified as a calcifying giant cell tumor[1] and as a chondromatous giant cell tumor[2] until the paper of Jaffe and Lichtenstein in 1942.[3] These writers described the lesion as a distinct entity, stated that it was chondroblastic in origin and gave it the name by which it is now generally known.

Benign chondroblastoma is a rather rare tumor. To date, somewhat less than 60 cases have been reported, the largest series being 16.[4] Because of its peculiar microscopy it unquestionably has been misdiagnosed as chondrosarcoma, osteosarcoma and giant cell tumor with therapeutic tragedy as a consequence. Though it is an uncommon lesion all clinicians, radiologists and pathologists must be cognizant of its features in order that overtreatment may be avoided.

Until recently, the chondroblastoma was always reported arising in relation to the enchondral plate of a large cylindrical bone of an extremity, with the exception of one lesion in the talus.[5] In Codman's early series of 9 cases, all the lesions were in the proximal epiphysis of the humerus in patients between the ages of 12 and 24. In the early series of Jaffe and Lichtenstein there were 9 patients, all in the age group 12 to 24, in the later series by Lichtenstein and Kaplan there were 6 patients, all between the ages of 10 and 20, in the series of Valls et al. there were 8 patients, 13 to 18, and in that of Hatcher and Campbell, 6 patients, 13 to 19. In the 1956 series of Kunkel et al.

there were 16 patients. In 10 of these, all 21 or younger, the chondroblastoma apparently arose in relation to the enchondral plate of a large long bone, in 6 others a flat bone was involved. It is interesting that 5 of these 6 were patients over the age of 20 years.

It is obvious that the available material on chondroblastoma at present is insufficient on which to base final conclusions. Nevertheless, we must recognize it as a distinct entity of chondroblastic origin different from all other known tumors with the possible exception of chondromyxoid fibroma. It is most apt to affect adolescents. Certainly it is likely to involve the epiphysis in the great majority and in a few there will be secondary invasion of the metaphysis. These features, if they hold true in the future, set the chondroblastoma apart from all other bone tumors. Only the giant cell tumor characteristically involves the epiphysis, and this only after the epiphysis has ossified.

The only characteristic symptom of chondroblastoma is pain. Because the lesion is apt to be in the epiphysis, the pain is usually referred to a joint and therefore misinterpreted as a type of monarticular arthritis. The pain is insidious in onset and usually not severe at first. It may be of considerable duration, often two years or longer, suggesting that the lesion grows very slowly. A firm enlargement may be palpated in perhaps one third of the cases. There may be muscle stiffness and wasting secondary to interference with function.

ROENTGENOGRAPHIC MANIFESTATIONS

The cartilaginous nature of the benign chondroblastoma is responsible for a radiolucent defect. Since the lesion arises from young chondroblasts in the enchondral plate, the initial involvement is located in the center of ossification. The lesion subsequently may grow to involve the metaphysis and even the adjacent diaphysis. The lesion tends to be round or ovoid and fairly well demarcated by a thin zone of sclerotic bone; this is probably the result of the slow growth of the neoplasm. Tiny areas of calcification within the cartilage often produce a mottled appearance that may obscure its outline in some areas. When it extends into the diaphysis, erosion of the cortex results in the production of periosteal bone and widening of the involved segment of the shaft.

The epiphyseal location of this neoplasm in an adolescent patient is quite characteristic and should strongly suggest the diagnosis.

MORBID ANATOMY

It appears, from available evidence, that the benign chondroblastoma usually or always arises from the young chondroblasts in the deep portion of the enchondral plate. It almost always begins to manifest itself soon after puberty; the youngest reported patient was eight years. It usually invades the bony nucleus of the adolescent epiphysis to produce a mass from 1 to 3 or 4 cm. in diameter. It may erode the articular plate and protrude into the joint space. Less often it progresses toward the metaphysis and in a few instances it seems to lie wholly within the metaphysis but always abutting on the epiphyseal line, suggesting an enchondral origin.

Its gross description is nondescript. It is usually more pale than red or brown. Areas of degeneration are common as one would expect in any cartilaginous neoplasm. Irregular deposits of calcium salts are usual and may give the tissue a gritty consistency. When it impinges on the metaphysis its slow growth allows a bony reaction in the surrounding cancellous tissue. This may produce a narrow sclerotic zone. It may erode the overlying compacta and cause the periosteum to deposit a layer of bone on the outer surface, giving the appearance of cortical expansion.

The microscopic appearance of chondroblastoma is highly characteristic but unless the pathologist is familiar with its features he is

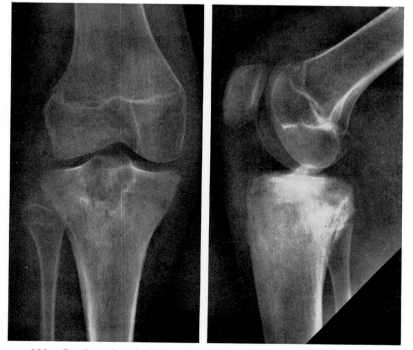

FIG. 282.   Benign chondroblastoma. The radiolucent lesion is evident in the proximal end of the tibia. The epiphysis is primarily involved but there is extension to the metaphysis. A fine line of sclerosis can be seen in relation to the tumor, particularly on its medial aspect; laterally the outline of the tumor is indistinct.

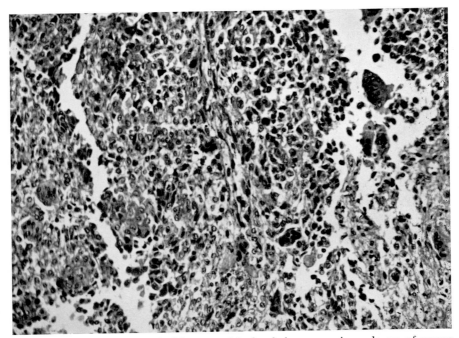

FIG. 283.   Benign chondroblastoma. Much of the tumor is made up of young chondroblasts. There is little or no hyalin production in these fields. Note the numerous giant cells. (× 200.)

apt to misinterpret it as an undifferentiated type of bone sarcoma. The characteristic cell is the young chondroblast (Fig. 283), somewhat larger than the normal and with a cytoplasm which is more durable to the rigors of processing than the normal chondroblast. It is spheroid, or nearly so, and its cytoplasmic membrane is usually obvious. It produces relatively little hyalin in most areas so that some fields appear very cellular. Because the morphology of these areas is quite uniform, this is apt to frighten the uninitiated into a diagnosis of malignant tumor. These cellular areas compose from one-third to one-half the tumor mass. They lie in a field of recognizable hyalin (Fig. 284), of myxoid material and of collagenized connective tissue. These intercellular substances almost always contain irregular masses of deeply staining calcium, much of which is in the amorphous state and, therefore, appears powdery or flocculated rather than like the crackled chips of calcified osteoid. Here and there some fragments of osteoid may be recognized but it is immature and never prominent. Giant cells (Fig. 285) are usual but they rarely if ever dominate the picture as they may in giant cell tumor. Since the lesion grows slowly, one does not expect to find mitotic figures except rarely.

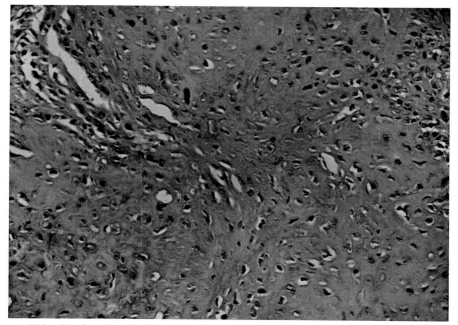

FIG. 284. Benign chondroblastoma. In some fields the cartilage is more adult. Here a hyalin matrix is formed. (× 200.)

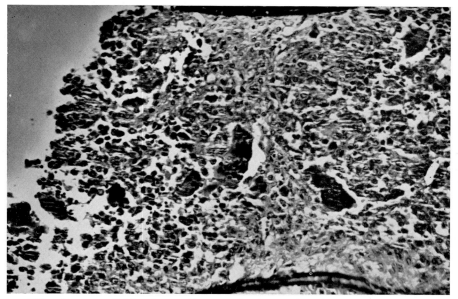

FIG. 285. In some fields giant cells may dominate the picture. Benign chondro-blastoma was originally called "cartilaginous variant of giant cell tumor." (× 200.)

PROGNOSIS

When Codman collected his original series from the Bone Tumor Registry he was surprised to find so many survivals with treatment which would be considered inadequate for malignant tumor. He concluded that the lesion is benign. Subsequent observation has proved this conclusion correct. Some cases have healed with curettage which was known to be incomplete. Most writers consider the chondroblastoma to be a completely benign tumor. In only one series, that of Copeland and Geschickter, is a malignant behavior considered unexceptional. In another series, one case underwent obvious cytologic and clinical change to a chondrosarcoma three and one-half years after irradiation. It seems safe to consider the chondroblastoma a benign tumor. Since simple, conservative surgery has resulted in cure in all or most proven cases, it would seem to be the treatment of choice.

CHONDROMYXOID FIBROMA

The chondromyxoid fibroma is a slowly growing, benign neoplasm of chondroblastic origin. It usually occurs in the metaphysis of cylindrical bones, most often the large, long bones of the extremities, but it has been reported in the ribs, the ilium, the metatarsals, a vertebra, and the writer has seen one in the clavicle. Since the lesion is not a fibroma the name is inappropriate. If the constituents of the lesion are to be expressed in the title it would be better to call it a fibromyxoid chondroma.

There is no account of this entity in the literature until the paper of Jaffe and Lichtenstein[6] in 1948. They reported a series of 8 cases, very clearly defining the clinical, radiologic and pathologic features and suggesting the name. Since that time less than 40 cases have been reported, the largest series of 11 cases by Dahlin.[7] There are only five cases in the material of the writer. It is obvious that the lesion is rather rare and that the data collected are as yet too scant to amply describe any but the common types.

In the earlier reports most of the lesions were found in patients between the ages of 12 and 30. As more cases are described it becomes apparent that any age may be afflicted with only a moderate preponderance in the younger group.

In the large bones the chondromyxoid fibroma has always been reported in the metaphysis. In the short cylindrical bones of the hands and feet it may begin in the metaphysis but ultimately involves the entire shaft. The lesion is usually small, averaging 2 to 3 cm. in diameter, but lesions of 8 cm. have been reported. In the metaphysis of large bones it is usually eccentric, growing slowly and often producing a thin line of reactive sclerosis along the margin in contact with cancellous tissue. It may erode the compacta from within and cause the overlying periosteum to lay down a shell of bone, resulting in the appearance of cortical expansion. At times there is no reactive bone formation and then the tumor may perforate the cortex and produce a mass on the outer cortical surface, lifting the periosteum over it without invading or penetrating it. The cortex may be thinned to the point of fracture and then the resulting callus formation mixed in with the expanding cartilaginous tumor presents a most confusing picture. In the metaphysis there is usually a centimeter or more of normal spongiosa between the distal pole of the lesion and the epiphyseal line, but it may abut directly upon the epiphysis. When such is the case it becomes exceedingly difficult to be sure whether one is dealing with a chondromyxoid fibroma or a benign chondroblastoma. Since the histologic elements of the two lesions are so nearly the same, one might ask if a differentiation is justifiable. This has caused some, including the writer, to suspect that benign chondroblastoma and chondromyxoid fibroma are the same neoplastic process, the peculiar features of each lesion arising from the environmental difference of its location, the one in the epiphysis and the other in the shaft.

Both lesions are chondroblastic in genesis. Both produce slowly growing, lobulated masses of embryonic cartilage cells which may mature to the status of hyalin production and lacuna formation. Myxomatous tissue is highly characteristic of all cartilaginous tumors; it is more abundant in the chondromyxoid fibroma than in the chondroblastoma. The disparity in the age incidence is the most outstanding difference in the two lesions. The chondroblastoma usually occurs between puberty and ossification of the epiphysis, the period when young chondroblasts are present in this region. If it occurs after epiphyseal ossification it must arise from an immature rest of chondroblasts. The chondromyxoid fibroma may occur at any age at which a group of chondroblasts, left behind in the metaphysis by the advancing epiphyseal frontier, develops the ability to proliferate. Thus the location may also explain the age incidence.

The symptoms of chondromyxoid fibroma are much like those of chondroblastoma except that the joints are not usually involved. Pain is the outstanding symptom but it is probably not very severe, since a history of a year's duration is not infrequent. If there is cortical expansion there may be a palpable mass. Tenderness is often found. In the author's five cases, fracture occurred at least twice.

ROENTGENOGRAPHIC MANIFESTATIONS

The lobulated masses of cartilage that characterize the chondro-myxoid fibroma cast a shadow of the density of soft tissue, as a result of which the lesion appears radiolucent in contrast with the surrounding bone. Its borders tend to be scalloped and well defined by a narrow band of opaque sclerotic bone. This neoplasm arises eccentrically in the spongiosa and erodes, thins and expands the overlying cortex as

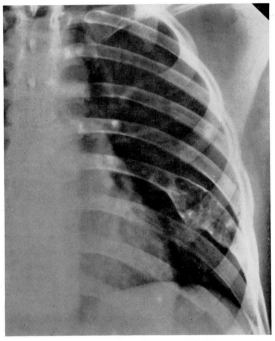

FIG. 286.   Roentgenogram of a chondromyxoid fibroma of the rib. A septate radiolucent area is seen in the rib. The lesion has caused expansion of the cortex. Chondromyxoid fibroma is more often seen in cylindrical bones.

it grows. The lobulated character of the neoplastic tissue produces a radiographic image suggesting the presence of septa within the lesion.

MORPHOLOGY

The chondromyxoid fibroma appears to be well circumscribed when sectioned and viewed grossly, unless it has penetrated the cortex. It is a pliable mass of soft tissue which separates rather easily from its surrounding bony walls. It has the appearance of a rather coarse, gray fibrous tissue. There may be some gritty fragments representing calcified hyalin.

The pathologist is apt to be surprised when he examines this tissue through the microscope. The tissue which appeared fibrous grossly is largely primitive cartilage, and moreover where the tumor tissue is pressed against the bony wall it often penetrates the interspicular spaces. The myxomatous character which may be quite dramatic on the section is not appreciable on gross examination. Often the sections give the impression that the technique of preparation has been poor. This is probably because the young chondroblast is a very fragile cell and collapses under the usual technical stresses.

The lesion is composed essentially of lobulated masses of cartilage cells of various ages. The center of the lobule may consist of rather tightly packed immature cells which are small, round and have a scanty but rather intensely pink cytoplasm (Fig. 287). In other areas the center may have a rather amorphous, deeply pink staining character with only shadow cells to suggest its origin. About the scalloped periphery the cells are much larger and more distinct. The nuclei may be uniformly round or bizarrely folded. The cytoplasmic outlines are apt to be intact, the cytoplasm clear or pale and the configuration that of highly cellular cartilage. There may be some hyalin production between the cells. Elsewhere there should be fields of recognizable hyalin, often with only sparsely scattered cells forming lacunae (Fig.

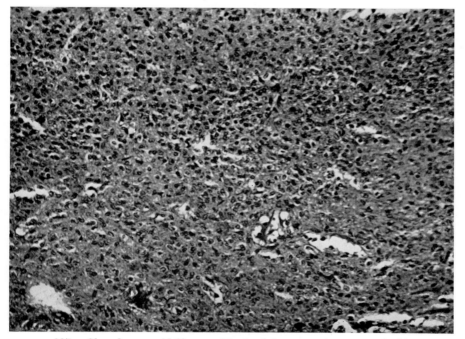

FIG. 287. Chondromyxoid fibroma. Much of the tumor is composed of immature chondroblasts. There is little hyalin formation in these areas. Note the similarity to chondroblastoma in Fig. 283. (× 200.)

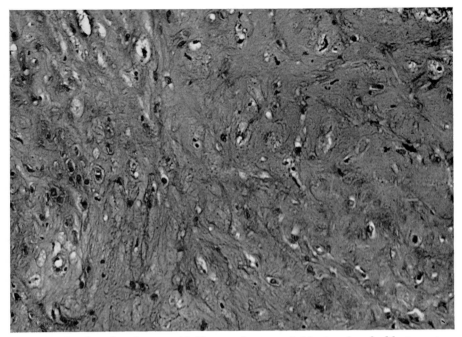

FIG. 288.   Benign chondromyxoid fibroma. In some fields the chondroblasts mature sufficiently to form recognizable hyalin. (× 200.)

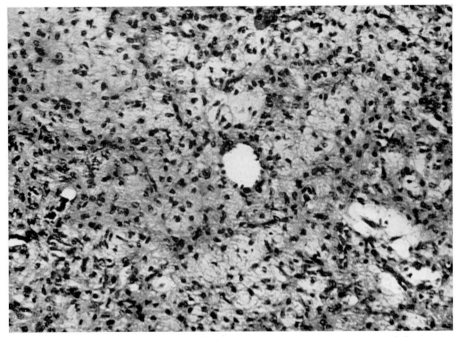

FIG. 289.   Benign chondromyxoid fibroma. The tumor is characterized by myxomatous areas made up of stellate cells in a pale mucinous matrix. (× 200.)

288). These constituents are embedded in a fibrous and myxomatous matrix. The fibrous tissue may be quite densely collagenized and it is this structure which presumably gives the gross appearance. The myxomatous fields are made up of spindled and less often multipolar cells loosely arranged in a pale background (Fig. 289). When very young chondroblasts are isolated in this matrix they are very small with a deep pink cytoplasm, vaguely suggesting plasmacytes. This material in the aspirate of one of the writer's cases led to the first suggestion of the correct diagnosis.

In the sclerosed bony margin one may find irregular masses of large, deeply blue staining cartilage cells with considerable pleomorphism of their nuclear morphology. The nature of these cells is hard to define, whether they belong to the tumor or to the reaction consequent to infractions in its overlying cortex. It is these cells and groups of the younger chondroblasts at the periphery of the lobules which may lead the pathologist to pronounce this lesion a chondrosarcoma. This danger becomes apparent when the biopsy is superficial.

There are other constituents which are less characteristic but often found. Giant cells are usual (Fig. 290). Their nuclei, varying from a few to over fifty, are small, deeply staining and scattered at random throughout the cytoplasm. Xanthoid cells are reported but have not

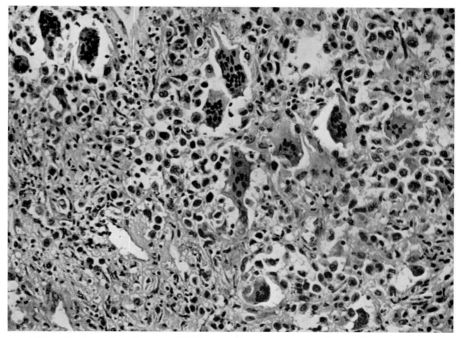

FIG. 290.   Benign chondromyxoid fibroma. In some areas giant cells are numerous.
(× 200.)

appeared in the author's material. Pigment granules can usually be found. In the original series of Jaffe and Lichtenstein they mention the presence of exudative inflammatory cells. Lymphocytes and neutrophils have been more prominent in the writer's sections than reported descriptions in other series suggest.

PROGNOSIS

The greatest danger which threatens the patient with a chondromyxoid fibroma is that it will be misdiagnosed and overtreated. Because the lesion is so recently described the index of suspicion is presumably low. Because every pathologist has had difficulty with the diagnosis of chondrosarcoma he is apt to lean toward the radical side. And because of the cellular pleomorphism of chondromyxoid fibroma the microscopist is apt to be led into the camp of malignancy.

Actually, there is no report of malignant behavior of this tumor, even in lesions which have been knowingly incompletely curetted. Two cases in one series recurred but with conservative treatment were cured. Analysis of the available data suggests that thorough curettage is adequate and the treatment of choice.

In the material of the writer there is one case in the rib of a 5 year old patient which is generally believed to be a chondrosarcoma by the pathologists who have studied it. Yet there are many unusual features about the sections which are suggestive of chondromyxoid fibroma. One cannot help but wonder whether this was a chondromyxoid fibroma on which was superimposed a chondrosarcoma. Since our knowledge of the former is based on so few lesions, the writer prefers to wait for a greater experience to define the ultimate behavior of chondromyxoid fibroma.

CHONDROMA

In considering the chondrogenic tumors and tumor-like processes, if one removes the enchondromas which are hamartomas, the benign chondroblastomas and chondromyxoid fibromas which are specific entities of chondroblastic cytogenesis, and the chondrosarcomas, there still remains a small group of progressively growing tumors, the chondromas, which arise either within the shaft or from the outer surface, usually where cartilage and bone are approximated. Cytologically, they are identical with the enchondroma, but the central chondromas, unlike the enchondromas, may arise anywhere within the diaphysis rather than only in the subchondral metaphysis, and more important they may produce immense tumors since they do not cease to grow with ossification of the epiphyses. Even if one refuses to admit the separate identities of enchondroma and central chondroma, those tumors which grow from the outer surfaces of bone, the ecchondromas, must still be considered.

We prefer to classify under the heading of chondroma the ecchondromas and central chondromas, on the basis that their behavior is different from that of other chondrogenic lesions. Some writers refuse to admit the existence of any cartilaginous tumors growing from the outer bone surfaces except those which spring from previously existing osteochondromas. This position may be valid because certainly many chondrosarcomas do arise in the cartilaginous caps of osteochondromas, but in the author's material there are 11 ecchondromas without any evidence whatsoever that they occupied the sites of previously existing osteochondromas. Occasionally, one may find a chondroma apparently arising from the periosteum and these have been called periosteal chondromas.[8] Usually these tumors will include considerable amounts of osteoid and collagenizing fibrous tissue and these that do, we feel, should be classified as parosteal sarcomas. If they

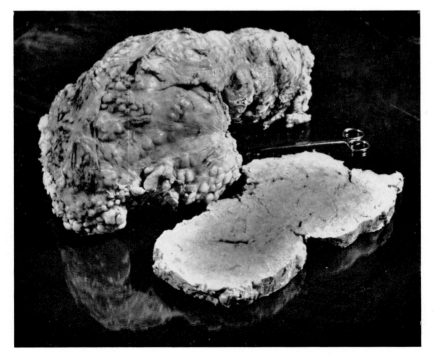

FIG. 291.   This huge chondroma weighed 23 pounds. Note the lobulated surfaces. Within the substance of the tumor there are many areas of myxomatous "degeneration."

are purely cartilaginous and cytologically benign, we prefer to call them ecchondromas.

The chondroma grows very slowly but it is progressive and eventually it may produce a huge mass. In the material of the writer there is one which grew over a period of many years from the lateral surface of the ilium, achieving the size of a large watermelon and a weight of 23 pounds (Fig. 291). Blocks taken from many areas failed to reveal any evidence of the criteria for malignancy. The tumor was successfully removed and the patient lived for many years without evidence of recurrence. Some writers feel that these massive cartilaginous tumors are all slowly growing chondrosarcomas and doubtless some of them are, but a few at least fail to show any capacity for malignant activity over extended periods of observation.

The chondroma may occur at any age. We have seen one in a child of 10 and another in a patient aged 67. Preponderantly, however, they are found in those over 35. They may involve any bone, flat bones as often as cylindrical bones. The bones of the thorax, ribs, sternum, clavicles and vertebrae are probably the most commonly affected, perhaps because of the considerable amounts of cartilage that normally persist here throughout life.

The symptoms of chondroma depend upon its site. Central chondromas may replace the medullary tissues of an entire shaft or erode the cortex from within and eventually cause pathologic fracture. Ecchondromas press upon nerve roots or upon the spinal cord itself if they arise in the costovertebral area or the vertebrae. Because they grow very slowly, pain does not usually become evident until the complications of fracture or nerve pressure occur.

ROENTGENOGRAPHIC MANIFESTATIONS

The central chondroma appears radiographically as a radiolucent defect within the spongiosa of the diaphysis of a cylindrical bone. In some instances the neoplasm is eccentrically located. Speckled opacity within the lesion is often present and reflects calcification of the cartilage. As the neoplasm grows, the cortex is thinned and the overlying bone is expanded. At times, however, slow growth of the tumor may be associated with periosteal new bone formation as a result of which the cortex over the involved area becomes appreciably thickened. More frequently, periosteal formation of new bone occurs secondary to cortical infraction. The central chondroma may be delineated by a thin, opaque margin of bone.

The ecchondroma arises from the outer surface of a bone and produces very little abnormality of the underlying cortex. The neo-

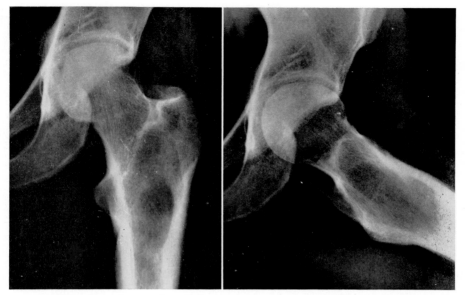

FIG. 292. Chondroma. A radiolucent lesion involves the proximal shaft of the femur and the greater trochanter. Its outlines are smooth. Probably as a manifestation of its slow growth, periosteal new bone has thickened the overlying cortex which shows erosion of its inner aspect.

plasm is of the density of soft tissue but usually contains irregular areas of opacity which reflect calcification.

GROSS AND MICROSCOPIC APPEARANCE

Neoplastic cartilage resembles normal hyalin cartilage to some extent. It produces masses of bluish white, resilient, glistening tissue (Fig. 293). There are two features which are characteristic enough to be helpful. Neoplastic cartilage, if uninhibited, grows in lobules, producing a bosselated outer surface and a cut surface with a lobulated pattern. Almost always associated with the formation of hyalin there is the production of a clear, slippery, liquid or gelatinous material which has much the same appearance and consistency as egg white. This substance has a chemical constituency very similar to that of hyalin cartilage but its physical properties are obviously quite different. Some authors consider it to be the product of cartilage degeneration. A more plausible explanation is that it represents the product of the metabolic activity of the chondrocytes. These cells normally produce hyalin but because their metabolism is perverted by neoplastic alteration, this myxomatous substance is the result of their activity. This material collects in smooth-walled spaces which sometimes have the appearance of blue-domed cysts.

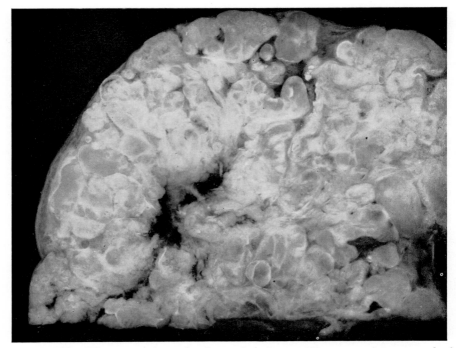

FIG. 293.   The cut surface of a large chondroma. The tumor is composed of lobules of glistening blue-white, translucent tissue. Myxomatous areas are found throughout.

When sectioned, the chondroma is found to consist of aggregates of cartilage cells of varying age and size. The majority will be sufficiently mature to produce hyalin and form lacunae within it. Elsewhere the cells are less mature, the cells being smaller, ovoid or spindled, and there is no evidence of hyalin formation. The cartilage cell is difficult to process without causing great distortion. It is not often that one is able to get a preparation in which the cell fills its lacuna as it must in life, and in which the cytoplasm is intact and homogeneous and the nucleus and nucleolus clearly discernible (Fig. 294). Usually, one must form opinions upon badly shrunken cells in which it is difficult to distinguish the nucleus from the cytoplasm. It is small wonder that the chondroma and chondrosarcoma are often difficult to diagnose and prognose. Lichtenstein and Jaffe[9] have set up the most reliable criteria for this distinction. They point out that only the fields of cells which are producing hyalin should be judged. In chondroma, the lacunae should rarely contain more than one cell, the cells should be small and rather uniform, the nuclei round and darkly staining (Fig. 295). Mitoses should be rare. Multiple large irregular nuclei with coarse, rough masses of chromatin and prominent nucleoli denote malignant character. Multiple blocks should be selected from different

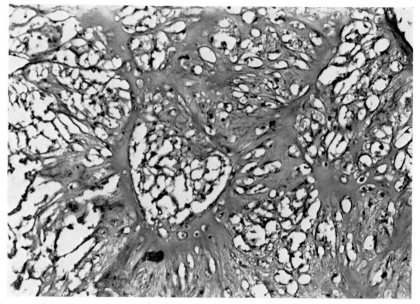

FIG. 294.   Section of a chondroma. Many of the lacunae appear to be empty. In others the cells are shrunken and distorted, making it difficult to evaluate their character. Numerous sections should be cut and a search made for an area in which the cells are better preserved. (× 130.)

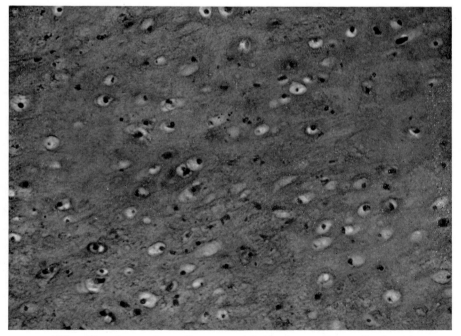

FIG. 295.   Chondroma. In well preserved fields the cartilage cells should appear uniform in size. There should be few lacunae containing more than one cell. The nuclei are small, the borders are regular, the chromatin not too great in amount and the nucleoli inconspicuous. (× 200.)

levels of every cartilaginous tumor. In any case in which the microscopy is dubious, a firm diagnosis should be made only after consultation with the clinician and radiologist.

PROGNOSIS

The difficulties in accurate prognosis of cartilaginous tumors are many. Some diagnosed as chondromas are probably slowly growing chondrosarcomas. It is also likely that many chondromas undergo a change to sarcomatous behavior late in their existence, especially if they have been surgically manipulated or irradiated. A central tumor of the small bones of the hands and feet is almost certainly benign, though the author has one chondrosarcoma of this area in his material. One must be more cautious with central tumors of large cylindrical and flat bones. If a tumor arises in the mid-shaft area of a large cylindrical bone, it is more apt to be chondrosarcoma than chondroma. Cartilaginous tumors arising from the outer aspects of bones should be regarded as malignant until proven otherwise, with the exception of the periosteal chondroma. These occur in the periosteum of the diaphyses of the cylindrical bones of the hands and feet and two have been reported in relation to large long bones.[8] Too little is known as yet about this particular entity but it appears that it runs a completely benign course.

CHONDROSARCOMA

The chondrosarcoma is the only tumor of chondrogenic origin with an expected malignant behavior. For nearly a century it was classified as a primary osteogenic neoplasm and only in the past twenty-five years has it been recognized as a distinct entity. In a paper by Phemister[10] in 1930, it was pointed out that the clinical behavior of chondrosarcoma is quite different from that of osteosarcoma. Since that time analysis of several series of "osteogenic sarcomas" has brought out differences in sites of involvement, age group, microscopy and prognosis. Though the differentiation of chondrosarcoma and osteosarcoma is often more difficult than that of osteosarcoma and myeloma, it is, nevertheless, just as important.

The osteosarcoma arises from osteoblasts and primitive fibrous tissue with the potential of forming osteoid, hyalin and collagen. It is made up of tumor cells resembling osteoblasts, chondroblasts and fibroblasts and the intercellular products of these cells. The chondrosarcoma arises only from chondroblasts, can produce only hyalin and hyalin-like myxoid substance. The osteoid and collagenous tissue found in sections of the chondrosarcoma are incidental and play no role in the tumor process. In brief, the osteosarcoma often contains neoplastic elements of all the tissues involved in normal enchondral bone formation; the chondrosarcoma is wholly cartilaginous.

Chondrosarcoma is about one-half as common as osteosarcoma. It affects males somewhat more frequently than females just as do all malignant tumors with the exception of those of the genitalia, but this difference is not great enough to be helpful in diagnosis. In the largest series published to date, by Dahlin and Henderson,[11] over three quarters of the cases affected the bones of the trunk and the upper ends of the humerus and femur. In a smaller group from the author's series, about one-half involved these areas and the next commonest site was the tibia. Excluding the myelomas, the chondrosarcoma is the most common tumor involving the bones of the trunk, shoulder and hip. It has been said that though chondrosarcoma may affect any bone, the nearer a cartilaginous tumor occurs to the trunk the more apt it is to be malignant. Chondrosarcomas of the small bones of the hands and feet are rare but they do occur. There were only four in the series of 212 cases of Dahlin and Henderson. The author has seen but one.

The age incidence of chondrosarcoma is interesting. It is quite unusual in patients under 30. After 35 the incidence rises progressively and the curve is very similar to that of carcinoma. This is in contrast to the incidence curve of osteosarcoma in which the greater elevation is on the left. Chondrosarcoma is a very slowly growing tumor and the question arises whether it may begin in youth, like most other bone tumors, but require several years to manifest itself. There are very few facts to support this thesis though a history of symptoms of five years' duration is not unusual.

Chondrosarcoma, like chondroma, can be divided into those which occur within bone and those which arise from the outer bone and cartilage surfaces. The former is usually called central and the latter peripheral chondrosarcoma. Some authors have stated that most central chondrosarcomas represent secondary changes in enchondromas and all or most peripheral chondrosarcomas arise in osteochondromas. In the series of Lichtenstein and Jaffe,[12] 5 of their 15 cases were peripheral and all are stated to be secondary to osteochondromas. In the series of Dahlin and Henderson, only 19 of their total 212 cases (they were not always able to distinguish between central and peripheral tumors) were secondary. In the author's material (29 cases) there was evidence that 5 were in areas where osteochondromas had previously existed. Four of these were cases of hereditary multiple exostoses and one was a solitary osteochondroma. One of our central lesions developed in a

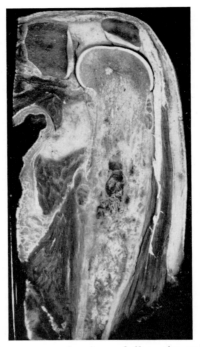

FIG. 296.   When chondrosarcoma arises in medullary tissues it may infiltrate a considerable proportion of the shaft before it penetrates the cortex.

patient with enchondromatosis. In Lichtenstein's[13] 10 central lesions, 5 are said to have arisen in enchondromas; in the writer's material there was but one in which this fact could be established, a case of enchondromatosis.

Central chondrosarcomas in cylindrical bones usually begin in the metaphyseal region, but to a greater extent than osteosarcoma they may start in other portions of the shaft. They usually replace a good proportion of the cancellous and medullary tissue before they break through the cortex (Fig. 296). The more slowly growing type erodes the compacta from within and causes the periosteum to lay down new bone over it. A biopsy through this area containing new bone and neoplastic cartilage is apt to result in a microscopist's diagnosis of osteosarcoma. More characteristically the central chondrosarcoma infiltrates the medullary tissue and then perforates the cortex, frequently at a single small area. Then producing a large, soft-tissue mass it develops a "collar button" silhouette (Fig. 297). Thinning of the cortex to the point of pathologic fracture is unusual.

The peripheral chondrosarcoma grows from the cartilaginous cap of an osteochondroma or from any area where cartilage normally persists. The tumors which arise from periosteum are usually mixed, containing not only cartilage but osteoid and collagenous tissue. These are probably better designated "parosteal sarcomas" than periosteal chondrosarcomas. Often there is surprisingly little bone erosion produced by the peripheral tumors, even though they become massive as they often do. Several reports have described peripheral chondrosarcoma penetrating the walls of veins and producing a continuous column of tumor along the course of the lumen. One of these eventually grew through the right heart and into the pulmonary vasculature very much as hypernephromas are apt to do. Peripheral chondrosarcoma may be superimposed on Paget's disease of bone.

The symptoms of chondrosarcoma depend upon the area affected and whether it is central or peripheral. Because it is slow growing, both types may be silent until a considerable tumor mass is produced. The only consistent symptom of chondrosarcoma is pain. This pain may be insidious at outset but it gradually becomes persistent and severe. Eventually, a palpable firm mass may be produced. Sometimes a history of osteochondroma may be obtainable. When so, a history of trauma is probably pertinent since presumably a fracture of an osteochondroma may activate growth in the cartilaginous cap and conceivably the young chondroblasts may develop neoplastic propensities.

The expected growth rate of chondrosarcoma is much slower than that of osteosarcoma. Symptoms may persist over a period of from

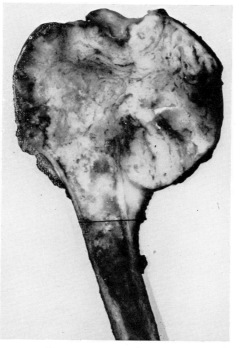

FIG. 297.   Chondrosarcoma often penetrates the cortex at a single point and then mushrooms into a soft tissue tumor to produce a "collar-button" lesion.

one to three years before a diagnosis is established. If treatment is inadequate, recurrence at the original site is the rule and this may not be manifest for several years after the original intervention. Surgical manipulation appears to speed up the growth process and often the character of a smoldering and mildly aggressive tumor will change to that of an explosively metastasizing malignant growth. In some of these, osteoid formation will be noted in the metastatic deposits and one wonders if they have not undergone metaplasia into an osteosarcoma. Chondrosarcoma has also been reported to seed itself in the soft tissues of the surgical wound. Precautions in technique should be observed in its removal.

ROENTGENOGRAPHIC MANIFESTATIONS

Roentgenographically, the chondrosarcoma usually appears as a bulky mass, with the density of soft tissue, containing scattered irregular opacities. This reflects the cartilaginous nature of the neoplasm and the calcification of the neoplastic tissue that so frequently occurs. The effect of the tumor on the osseous structures depends on the site of origin. Those tumors that originate within the bone destroy the trabeculae of the medullary canal, so that early a radiolucent defect in the bone may be evident. Periosteal new bone may be apparent

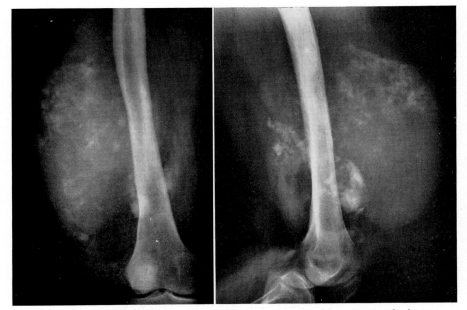

FIG. 298.   Chondrosarcoma. The neoplasm has resulted in a large soft tissue mass containing irregular patches and streaks of calcification. The cortex underlying the lesion is eroded both on its inner and outer aspects.

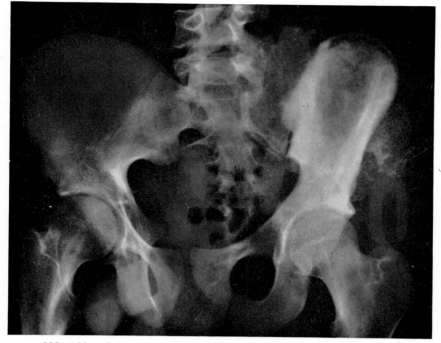

FIG. 299.   Chondrosarcoma. Destruction of the left lateral aspect of the sacrum and ilium is evident as well as a soft tissue within which there are irregular scattered areas of calcification.

when the inner surface of the cortex is eroded, so that the cortex may be somewhat thickened. This new bone formation is a reflection of the slow growth of the neoplasm. As enlargement of the tumor continues a portion of the cortex becomes indistinct, and later a mass will be evident in the adjacent soft tissues.

Peripheral chondrosarcomas are bulky masses of tissue that displace more radiolucent muscle planes. The underlying cortex may show very little alteration from the normal or there may be evidence of destruction from without.

PATHOLOGY

The chondrosarcoma usually produces a tissue which is grossly recognizable as cartilage. A white or bluish mass of glistening, moderately firm consistency is found. Though malignant, it is often quite well delineated by a capsule of compressed normal tissue or a subperiosteal lamina of bone. The lobular pattern is less conspicuous than in chondroma and there is apt to be more discoloration from degeneration and old hemorrhage. Two features are helpful. Areas of myxomatous change are usual and sometimes the major portion of the tumor

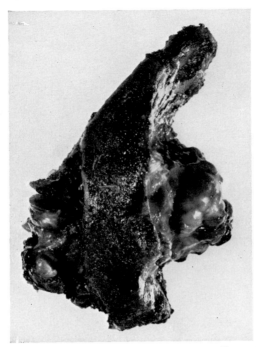

FIG. 300.   This chondrosarcoma arose within the cancellous tissue of the ilium. It penetrated both the inner and outer tables. Cartilaginous tumors of flat bones are apt to be malignant. Penetration of the cortex and the formation of a soft tissue tumor make the diagnosis of malignancy almost certain.

may consist of a slimy mass. The second feature is calcification. Irregular areas of chalky white, never very large, may be grossly obvious. The chondrosarcoma is apt to be a large tumor. Any abnormal cartilaginous mass larger than 3 cm. in diameter should be regarded with suspicion. Destruction and perforation of bone are incriminating evidence of malignant character (Fig. 300).

The diagnosis of chondrosarcoma by microscopy alone is often not an easy task. Lichtenstein and Jaffe[12] and Lichtenstein[13] carefully listed the features to be evaluated in making the distinction between chondroma, chondrosarcoma and osteosarcoma. The last is usually easy to rule out by the paucity of cartilage and the presence of neoplastic osteoid. The differentiation between actively growing chondroma, and sometimes cartilaginous callus, and chondrosarcoma is not as simple. These authors point out that only viable, non-calcified areas should be judged. If, here, more than a few lacunae per field contain more than one cell (Fig. 301) and if there are cells with more than one nucleus, the pathologist should seriously consider chondrosarcoma. If the nuclei are large and heavily chromatized this is added evidence (Fig. 302). The author has found irregularity in nuclear outline and the presence of prominent nucleoli helpful. Areas of calcification and myxomatous change are usual but not very valuable since they occur in chondromas, though the latter should not be found in healthy callus. Mitotic figures need not be common in chondrosarcoma, but when they are abundant they are very significant.

Very clearly etched in the memory of the writer are three cases, a brief account of which may be informative to those who deal with the problem of cytologic diagnosis of chondrosarcoma. All were males whose ages were 40, 52 and 59. All had pain of long standing in the region of the hip. Two had x-ray-discernible lesions of the ilium in relation to the acetabulum, the third a lesion in the neck of the femur. On clinical and radiologic evidence the diagnoses in all were chronic inflammatory or degenerative disease. In each a series of four biopsies was done before a correct diagnosis was achieved. The earlier diagnoses were consistently "chronic osteomyelitis, degenerating bone and cartilage with necrosis and calcification." All three patients eventually died of metastatic chondrosarcoma. In reviewing these cases it was established that a correct diagnosis might have been made at least a year earlier if all the facets of the cases had been known and all the features of the microscopy sections had been properly evaluated. It is true that the earlier biopsy material in all cases consisted almost entirely of myxomatous tissue, calcium deposits, necrotic cartilage and bone and other products of degenerative inflammation. But on hindsight one

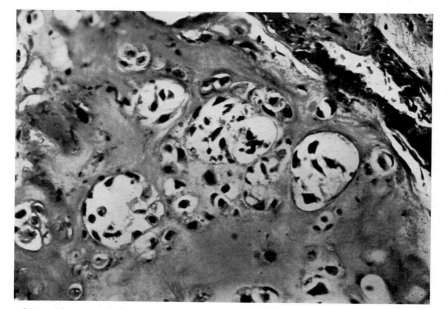

FIG. 301.   If many of the lacunae contain more than one cell, the tumor is probably malignant. (× 300.)

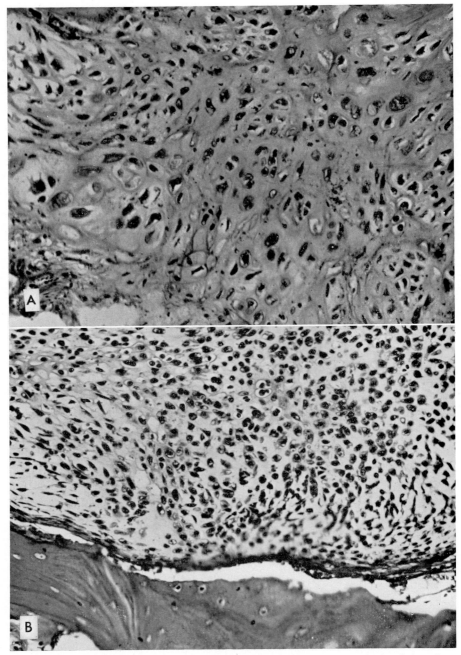

FIG. 302.   Chondrosarcoma. *A,* Variation in cell size, irregularity in nuclear borders and hyperchromatism are important features of malignancy. *B,* Sometimes the cells are small and rather uniform but one can still find more than one cell in a lacuna and there is usually hyperchromatism. ($\times$ 200.)

could find viable cartilage cells, some singly and some in small groups, some embryonic and others more mature, whose presence should have been weighed more seriously. This experience has allowed the author to make the diagnosis of chondrosarcoma in a fourth case, again a male, aged 64, and again in the hip region on material which casually treated is no more informative than that of the earlier three.

Most pathologists see too few chondrosarcomas to feel comfortable in evaluating these quantitative differences. It is a trying experience to place a tumor with such minimal evidence of malignancy in a category which will necessitate mutilating surgery. This is probably the reason why chondrosarcoma, more than any other tumor, has the reputation of developing from a benign forerunner. It is probable that the primary lesion in many instances was chondrosarcoma from the start and only behavior following the initial investigation made the final diagnosis apparent. A careful evaluation of all the available criteria and comparison with sections of known lesions, both benign and malignant, will help to better the diagnostic acumen but there will still be border cases where technique, notably poor in cartilaginous lesions, and inadequate biopsy material will give the sincerest microscopist trouble. And, if the general pathologist seeks solace he may be assured that not even many years of experience are a guarantee of accurate prognosis.

PROGNOSIS

The typical chondrosarcoma grows slowly and metastasizes late. Only an occasional tumor will run a rapid and fatal course and one may suspect that these are actually osteosarcomas in which the biopsy sections failed to reveal osteoid tissue. Chondrosarcoma is much more apt to recur at the site of operation than osteosarcoma, and even after recurrence a cure is often obtained if adequate excision is still possible. But repeated surgery may cause a change in the degree of malignancy of a chondrosarcoma. Every effort should be made to secure a firm diagnosis and once the diagnosis of chondrosarcoma is made the surgeon should proceed with the courage of his convictions. The rule is "all neoplastic tissue must be removed widely enough to give assurance that none remains." In a large percentage of cases this means amputation through the proximal bone, since chondrosarcoma may infiltrate through the medullary tissues farther than the eye or the microscope will discern. If there is recurrence excision should be repeated. If there is metastasis, even pulmonary metastasis, excision should be considered. The value of persistent vigilance and determined surgery is nowhere so great in bone tumors as in chondrosarcoma.

REFERENCES

BENIGN CHONDROBLASTOMA

1. Ewing, J.: Report International Conference on Cancer. John Wright and Sons, Ltd., Bristol, 1928.
2. Codman, E. A.: Surg. Gynec., & Obst., *52*:543, 1931.
3. Jaffe, H. L., and Lichtenstein, L.: Am. J. Path., *18*:969, 1942.
4. Kunkel, M. C., Dahlin, D. C., and Young, H. H.: J. Bone & Joint Surg., *38A*:817, 1956.
5. Valls, J., Ottolenghi, C. E., and Schajowicz, F.: J. Bone & Joint Surg., *33A*:997, 1951.

CHRONDROMYXOID FIBROMA

6. Jaffe, H. L., and Lichtenstein, L.: Arch. Path., *45*:541, 1948.
7. Dahlin, D. C.: Cancer, *9*:195, 1956.

CHRONDROMA

8. Lichtenstein, L., and Hall, J. E.: J. Bone & Joint Surg., *34A*:691, 1952.
9. Lichtenstein, L., and Jaffe, H. L.: Am. J. Path., *19*:553, 1943.

CHONDROSARCOMA

10. Phemister, D. B.: Surg., Gynec., & Obst., *50*:216, 1930.
11. Dahlin, D. C., and Henderson. E. D.: J. Bone & Joint Surg., *38A*:1025, 1956.
12. Lichtenstein, L., and Jaffe, H. L.: Am. J. Path., *19*:553, 1943.
13. Lichtenstein, L.: Bone Tumors. C. V. Mosby Co., St. Louis, 1952.

Collagenic Tumors

GIANT CELL TUMOR OF BONE

Giant cell tumor of bone has been recognized as a neoplastic entity for slightly over a century. It is a tumor composed of a fibroblastic stroma interspersed with multinucleated giant cells. It usually occurs at or near the ossified epiphyseal line of a long bone in which enchondral growth has been completed. It is progressive, aggressive, and in rare instances may display all the characteristics of malignant behavior including metastasis. This is about all that can be said of giant cell tumor of bone without provoking controversy, for it has been responsible for more argument than any other neoplasm of bone. Even today, each new paper usually presents some new hypothesis concerning its genesis or an explanation for its behavior. This account will be no exception.

The cause for all this controversy is understandable. The tumor is composed of two types of cells, the origins of neither of which are known. The giant cells resemble and may be related to osteoclasts. The origin and the function of the osteoclast are not known. The combination of a spindle cell matrix with multinucleated giant cells is commonly produced in a number of bone lesions, both neoplastic and non-neoplastic. Many of these lesions have been diagnosed in the past and probably still are being diagnosed as giant cell tumors. In order to establish a clearly defined concept of this curious entity it may be profitable to examine this controversial material in more detail. Nothing herein may change the concept of the reader but if it provokes thinking on the subject, it will be worth while.

The hallmark of the giant cell tumor is its giant cell. Most British and some American writers have expressed the opinion that it is a form of osteoclast, hence the term "osteoclastoma." The origin and function of the normal osteoclast is an enigma. Many theories of its genesis have prevailed and the one in vogue is that it is a transitory form of the osteoblast. In birds the osteoclast is said to form from combining osteoblasts, and when the bone lysis which precedes shell mineralization is completed the osteoclast returns to its osteoblastic form. Such conclusions are hazardous when they are based on the morphology of cells as they appear in fixed, stained sections. To date no one has observed the transition of osteoblasts into osteoclasts in living human tissue.

The function of the osteoclast is even more enigmatic. Since it is found in Howship's lacunae and in areas where bone is undergoing lysis, it has been presumed that it is responsible for bone destruction. Actually, there is very little fact to support this presumption. Bone is formed by the deposition of mineral in a preformed matrix of osteoid. The mechanism is still incompletely understood but a "local tissue factor" appears to be necessary. This factor is probably concerned with a chemical change in the matrix. Lysis of bone is apparently not the reverse of this process since in life an organic matrix never remains when the mineral salts have been released. This suggests that the matrix "dissolves," freeing the salts which are taken into solution by the local fluids. Crystalline salts have been found in this fluid and in macrophages of the area, suggesting that when the fluids are saturated the salts may precipitate. Thus to accomplish bone lysis the osteoclast must be endowed with the ability to cause mineral salts to go into solution and to lyse the components of collagen, that is, it must contain collagenase and hyaluronidase or enzymes that accomplish the same end. None of these properties has been found in the osteoclast. Moreover, there are factors such as the lack of stress stimulus and high parathormone levels which are known to cause bone lysis. Unless these act by stimulating the proliferation of osteoclasts the latter must be, at best, of secondary importance. Yet the osteoclast is always seen in the presence of bone lysis and the most informed sources insist that its presence is more than coincidental. Some writers have contended that it is a phagocyte, that bone lysis is accomplished and the osteoclast is called in like the mononuclear phagocytes to clear away the debris. Against this hypothesis is the lack of evidence of phagocytic activity. Bone particles have not been found in the cytoplasm and bone salts are not consistently seen. No one has shown, however, that demineralized organic matrix or the breakdown products of such may not stimulate the proliferation of this curious cell. Whether the osteoclast phagocytizes the degenerating organic matrix has never been shown. It might be worth while to tag the polysaccharide or amino building blocks of this matrix and trace them through disintegration.

The giant cells which accumulate in the vicinity of non-specific bone destruction and reparative reaction are often indistinguishable from osteoclasts. One might contend that in such areas one finds a mixture of giant cells and osteoclasts. If such is the case we, as yet, have no technical means of distinguishing the two.

Empirically, there are three known mechanisms in the formation of pathologic bone lesions: (1) There may be a failure in production of organic bone matrix such as that seen in osteoporosis and scurvy. Here giant cells are scarce or entirely lacking. (2) The matrix may be normally formed but there is an inability to mineralize it. This type of lesion is exemplified by rickets and osteomalacia. Giant cells are usually present and sometimes numerous but they are never seen in large aggregates. (3) The third mechanism is that of lysis or destruction of formed bone. This may come about by (a) alteration of the stress trajectories. The process is slow and giant cells are found in about the same amount as one would expect to find osteoclasts. (b) Bone may be destroyed by pressure or interference with blood supply as exemplified in bone which is the site of metastatic tumor growth. Here again giant cells are found in the proportion of osteoclasts. (c) There is widespread deossification in hyperparathyroidism. Giant cells are quite numerous throughout but in focal areas they may produce masses which actually suggest neoplasm. In these areas there may be little or no osteoid apparent. The giant cells are morphologically identical with those found in some lesions classified as giant cell tumors and it is only by careful evaluation of the stromal cells that true neoplasm can be excluded.

Hemorrhage into bone and related tissue is often accompanied by the presence of large numbers of giant cells. Again there may be little evidence of osteoid in the lesion and it may closely resemble the brown tumor of hyperparathyroidism. This phenomenon poses the question: is there some agent in extravasated blood which is similar in action to parathormone or in hyperparathyroidism are the brown tumors actually hematomas? The giant cell reaction to hemorrhage is also dramatically demonstrated in the large aneurysmal bone cysts which have undergone fracture with spillage of blood. In a recent report[1] six of seven aneurysmal bone cysts were diagnosed on histologic sections as giant cell tumors. In the author's material there is an aneurysmal bone cyst, classic in every respect, clinically, radiologically and pathologically, which has a giant cell reaction to complicating hemorrhage. Biopsy material from one of these areas was diagnosed by one of the leading pathologists in this country as giant cell tumor. Though he is cognizant of all the findings and of the conflicting diagnosis of other authorities, including pathologists, he still insists that this is the micros-

copy of giant cell tumor. Large numbers of giant cells are characteristic of still another lesion, the so-called "benign synovioma." Since
there is evidence of extravascular blood in these lesions, hemosiderin
granules and xanthoid cells, one might ask if this is the same type of
reaction. It would be immensely helpful to know whether the giant
cells in these various lesions, brown tumor of parathyroid adenoma,
hemorrhage in bone and related tissues and benign synovioma, are
related to the normal osteoclasts.

The giant cells of the above enumerated conditions may be very
similar to or identical with those seen in certain lesions classified as
benign (Grade I) giant cell tumor of bone. If one cannot distinguish
reaction from neoplasm by the appearance of the giant cells, then one
must rely upon the stroma to make the differentiation. It is highly unfortunate that the tumor fibroblast does not carry a flag to designate its
neoplastic potentialities. The microscopy of the fibromatoses is notably
untrustworthy in predicting their behavior. It is the contention of the
author that many simple reactive processes in bone, characterized by
a fibrous stroma and giant cells, are still diagnosed as giant cell tumors.
It is this unfortunate situation which has made the literature on the
subject so chaotic. The writer has seen more than one instance in
which a malignant bone tumor has produced a giant cell reaction.
Biopsy of the latter has resulted in a diagnosis of benign giant cell
tumor. Progression and even metastasis of the primary lesion have
astonished the clinician and confounded the pathologist. Thus, accurate prognosis on the basis of recorded descriptions may be completely futile.

In summary, neither the giant cell nor the stromal cell is an
infallible guide in distinguishing reaction to injury and true neoplasia
since they occur in both processes. Because of this situation we have
probably included numerous non-neoplastic lesions in the category of
giant cell tumor. Descriptions and conclusions based on series with
such inclusions are obviously unsound and probably account in part,
at least, for the seemingly erratic behavior of this group of tumors.

CLINICAL ASPECTS

In some series, the occurrence of giant cell tumors has been
greater in males than females. If this difference is real it is probably not
great enough to be of diagnostic value. About half of these tumors
occur in the age group between 20 and 35. Giant cell tumor of bone
occasionally occurs in patients under the age of 20. When it does,
however, it probably always occurs in a cylindrical bone at an epiphyseal line which has normally ossified. Thus it is possible for a

tumor to occur at the epiphyseal line of a metacarpal bone in a patient aged 14 because this is the lower limit of normal ossification at this site. In general these limits are at a slightly younger age in females than in males. It has been said that giant cell tumor never occurs in children. It is probably more accurate to state that it never occurs in a growth center which is still active. Over the age of 35 the age distribution is fairly even throughout the remaining life span.

The tumor is characteristically found in cylindrical bones. This prevalance is so constant that if a suspected giant cell tumor is found in a flat bone, the diagnosis should be questioned. However, in most reported series of 15 or more lesions there is at least one involving a flat bone and the correctness of these reports cannot be denied. There is a rather common lesion occurring in the jaws, usually the mandible, which is often misdiagnosed as giant cell tumor. Jaffe[2] has called these "giant cell reparative granulomas." They consist of a vascular fibroblastic stroma with numerous giant cells and are simply a manifestation of reaction to injury within bone. The giant cell epulis which arises from the periosteal and contiguous tissues of the jaws is likewise a non-neoplastic lesion, usually a proliferative reaction to trauma. Indeed, these giant cell reactions are so common within and without the jaw bones that one is tempted to regard any diagnosis of true giant cell tumor of this area as false. If a tissue diagnosis of giant cell tumor is made on any lesion of the vertebrae, the jaws or indeed any other flat bone, this diagnosis should be withheld until the clinical and radiologic aspects are thoroughly investigated.

Giant cell tumor characteristically arises in the site of a former epiphyseal line after the enchondral plate has ossified. In the opinion of some experienced workers, giant cell tumor of bone never occurs elsewhere and all lesions so designated have been misdiagnosed. We are not yet ready to go to this extreme but we admit that we do not have uncontroversial evidence which will disprove this statement. It is certainly true that the great majority of authentic giant cell tumors do occur in the ends of long bones at the site of the old epiphyseal line.

The femur is the bone selected in from one third to one half of the cases. The distal end of this bone is somewhat oftener involved than the proximal end. The remainder of the tumors are about equally divided among the other cylindrical bones of the skeleton. The short cylindrical bones of the hands and feet may be involved, a feature which helps to differentiate giant cell tumor and osteosarcoma. From the site of the old epiphyseal line the tumor invades both ways, into the metaphysis and less extensively into the ossified epiphysis.

Most giant cell tumors grow rather slowly but the growth rate

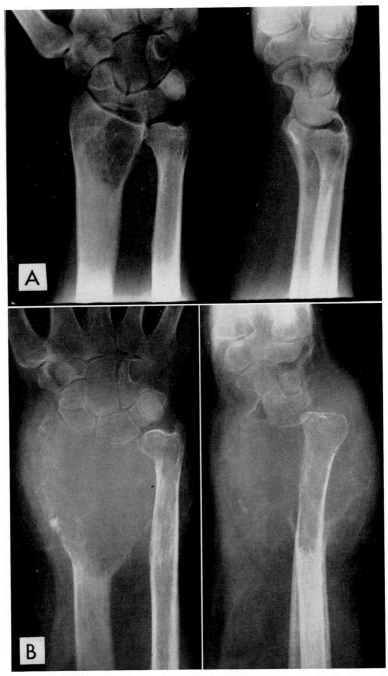

FIG. 303.   Giant cell tumor of bone. *A,* The lesion is eccentrically located in the
distal end of the radius. It is radiolucent and has thinned the cortex medially. *B* illustrates this same lesion two years later. A very thin shell surrounds this huge neoplasm
which has resulted in a dislocation at the wrist.

during the prediagnostic period is difficult to evaluate because the literature is so cluttered with non-neoplastic lesions under this heading. The duration of symptoms varies from a few weeks to several months. Lesions with a symptomatic history of six months or longer are not apt to be giant cell tumors. The tumor invades, weakens and destroys the cancellous bone of the metaphysis and ossified epiphysis and its overlying compact bone. The pain is deep and eventually progressive and intense. Pathologic fracture may occur but it is not characteristic. Giant cell tumor is destructive and there may or may not be a covering shell of apposed bone laid down by the lifted periosteum. If allowed to progress, most giant cell tumors will eventually produce a palpable tumor mass. When the epiphysis is invaded, maximum pain may be experienced in the joint. This may lead to lameness, disability and eventually disuse atrophy of muscle and bone.

ROENTGENOGRAPHIC MANIFESTATIONS

Roentgenographically, the giant cell tumor of bone is a radiolucent lesion as a reflection of the soft tissue, solid or semiliquid, of which it is composed. Incomplete septa are often evident within the substance of the tumor; these do not represent newly formed trabeculae of bone but rather residual normal trabeculae. When located at the

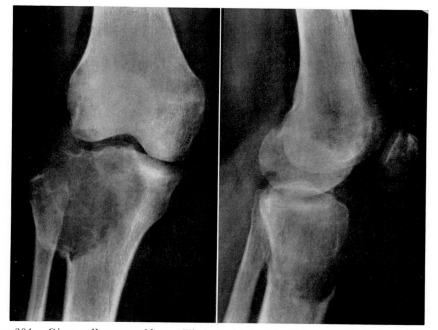

FIG. 304.   Giant cell tumor of bone. The proximal tibia is the site of the tumor. There is no evidence for bone reaction.

end of a long bone, the neoplasm is often eccentrically situated. The cortex may be expanded and quite thin, but periosteal new bone formation is not a feature of this tumor. Similarly, sclerosis of its margins as a result of reactive new bone formations is not apparent. The ossified epiphysis in which the neoplasm arises is involved but only rarely is the articular plate destroyed.

GROSS PATHOLOGY

Giant cell tumor of bone is a highly vascular tumor. It usually has a deep red, red-purple or brown color due to considerable amounts of blood pigment. Most of the tumor is soft and where gritty areas are encountered these particles are fragments of distintegrating bone rather than newly formed, mineralized osteoid deposits. Large irregular areas of degenerating tumor tissue are common and often these go on to cyst formation. The cysts are filled with amorphous, brown, granular or semifluid material. In a resected specimen which has been frozen and band-sawed the amount of bone destruction is often quite remarkable. Sometimes the entire epiphysis has been invaded by tumor, the cortex expanded and the articular plate lifted. The latter usually resists infiltration but its supporting arches may be destroyed so that it eventually collapses and fragments. In rare instances the tumor may grow into the joint structure. The metaphysis is almost always extensively destroyed. The compacta on one or more sides may disappear completely and there may or may not be a thin layer of bone laid down by the expanding periosteum. At times the entire end of the bone is converted to a huge, bulbous, club-shaped enlargement. There is rarely gross evidence of invasion into the surrounding soft tissues.

MICROSCOPIC PATHOLOGY

Giant cell tumor of bone is composed of a matrix of spindled tumor cells in which are embedded numerous giant cells. One can do no better than read the now classic description of the microscopy by Jaffe, Lichtenstein and Portis.[3] After a careful analysis of 28 lesions which had been diagnosed as giant cell tumors of bone, they found that only 14 could be accepted as unquestionable examples of this tumor. On the basis of their microscopy they divided these into three groups. In the Grade I group they placed those tumors with a moderately loose stroma of spindled or ovoid cells showing few or no mitotic figures. The stroma was quite vascular and giant cells were numerous. There was little evidence of collagen formation and osteoid was very scarce or completely lacking. In the Grade III group the stroma was much more cellular and compact, the cells were pleomorphic, the nuclei were variable in size and staining quality and mitotic figures were common. The Grade I tumors (Fig. 305) they designated as obviously benign and those of the Grade III group frankly malignant. Between these two types they placed a third group, the Grade II tumors which were neither obviously benign nor frankly malignant. They stated that the character of the tumor must be judged by the morphology of the stromal cells; the giant cells were considered of little importance in this regard.

For the past decade and a half their criteria and classification have been quite generally used by most pathologists. This usage has resulted in a certain amount of disillusion on the part of the author. Those cases of Grade III, being considered malignant, were widely resected or amputated and the patients cured. Those lesions falling in the Grade I or Grade II groups have not always behaved as they were supposed to. These results may have been the consequence of improper interpretation and application of the criteria, or because the Grade II tumors were more aggressive than their microscopy indicated, or because in the Grade I group some non-neoplastic entities were unwittingly included. The author suspects that all of the above conditions may apply.

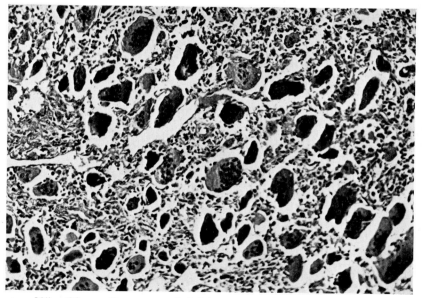

FIG. 305.   Giant cell tumor grade I. The matrix consists of a loose arrangement of vaguely spindled cells. They are moderately mature and mitotic figures are lacking or scarce. Giant cells are numerous. They are large and tend to be separated from the matrix cells by a clear space. The nuclei are multiple and uniform in size and staining quality. It is often difficult to be sure that this is a true neoplasm. ($\times$ 130.)

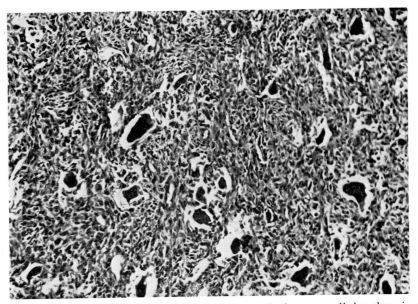

FIG. 306.   Giant cell tumor Grade II. The matrix is more cellular than in the Grade I type (Fig. 305). Its cells demonstrate more pleomorphism. Giant cells are fewer, smaller and their nuclei are less numerous. The matrix suggests neoplasm, probably benign. (× 130.)

A very small number, perhaps 10 per cent, of these lesions will show all the microscopic characteristics of malignant tumor. How they will behave is not known and perhaps never will be known, since the only reasonable treatment is ablation and this is curative if the lesion is a giant cell tumor. If metastasis occurs later the tumor was probably a giant cell osteosarcoma and would have metastasized whatever treatment was instituted.

There is almost certainly a percentage of tumors, most of them in the Class I group, which are giant cell reaction and not true tumors. When such lesions are encountered every effort should be made to find a cause for a giant cell reaction. If the lesion involves an unossified epiphysis, the diagnosis of giant cell tumor can probably be discarded. If the site is a vertebra, aneurysmal bone cyst must be ruled out. If the lesion occurs at the end of a mature cylindrical bone the biopsy should be repeated, taking samples of various levels of the lesion with the hope of finding a process which has caused the reaction. When the diagnosis of giant cell tumor Grade I is viewed with healthy skepticism this group will inevitably shrink in number. But almost certainly a hard core of bona fide giant cell tumors will remain, since like other fibroblastic tumors the exact character and potentialities cannot always be judged by the morphology of its constituent parts.

Those lesions whose stromal cells are unquestionably of neoplastic type but lack the significant features of malignancy fall in the Grade II group (Fig. 306). There is no doubt as to their authenticity as giant cell tumors. There is considerable doubt in the mind of the writer that their behavior can be predicted. About one third of these will recur if treated by curettage and about half of these will display frank evidence of malignant aggression if they are not radically treated. For this group, complete removal even though it means amputation is probably justifiable.

The diagnosis of giant cell tumor on histologic evidence alone is a difficult task. Though it is often impossible to tell by the appearance of the giant cells whether the lesion is true tumor or mere reaction,[4] these cells are helpful, if the lesion has been designated as tumor on the basis of its stroma, in deciding whether it is malignant. In general, the giant cells of a malignant tumor (Fig. 307) are smaller and fewer than those of the benign group. The cytoplasm-nucleus ratio is apt to be smaller and the cell outline less regular. The cell often appears to be incompletely divided from the surrounding stromal cells, some of the latter appearing to merge with the cytoplasm of the giant cell. The nuclei are fewer in number, more hyperchromatic, larger and less regular in shape. Rarely a mitotic figure can be found. Recently there has been a tendency to discount the appearance of the giant cell in

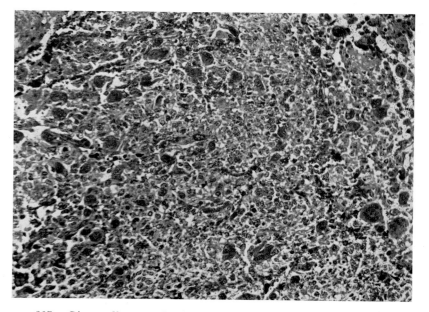

FIG. 307.   Giant cell tumor Grade III. The matrix is cellular. The cells are pleomorphic, some spindled and other polyhedral. Mitotic figures are in evidence. Giant cells are small and usually contain few nuclei. The latter often show irregularities in size, shape and staining quality. The giant cells often appear to merge with the surrounding matrix cells. (× 130.)

judging these tumors. The older experience of Kolodny and others should not be so casually discarded.

It is true that the character and pattern of the stromal cells are the most important guides leading to a correct diagnosis of the giant cell tumor. When the arrangement of the stromal cells is crowded and compact and the nuclei are young, there is usually no question about the nature of the lesion. A loose pattern of cells, arranged without regard to alignment of their axes, is more suggestive of reaction than of tumor. The formation of collagen is against tumor, though conceivably some slowly growing giant cell tumors may mature sufficiently to produce small amounts.

The tumor cells of giant cell tumor probably never produce osteoid. If osteoid is found in a matrix of malignant tumor cells, the process is probably a giant cell type of osteosarcoma. If the matrix cells are benign in appearance, the lesion is either reactive hyperplasia or an area of reactive bone formation which is being stimulated by tumor.

The matrix of the giant cell tumor is usually quite vascular and there may be extravasation of blood among the tumor cells. Hemorrhage, however, is not characteristic and should always suggest giant cell reaction rather than tumor. Along with hemorrhage one usually finds aggregates of xanthoid cells and scattered clumps of hemosiderin pigment. These are features which should dampen one's enthusiasm for a diagnosis of giant cell tumor. In reactive processes due to hemorrhage the giant cells may be as numerous as in a giant cell tumor, but they tend to aggregate about lakes of blood and resultant tissue damage rather than have an even dispersion throughout the lesion. Indeed, if one finds large fields in which there are no giant cells, these areas at least are probably not part of a giant cell tumor.

In the giant cell reactions about a hematoma, the stromal proliferation may be young and vigorous, the giant cells numerous and evenly disseminated. But here one is apt to find at least a few exudative inflammatory cells in the stroma and the giant cells are usually large and have thirty or more rather small nuclei, sometimes arranged about the periphery of the cell. In brown tumor of parathyroid adenoma the giant cells may be identical with those of giant cell tumor of benign appearance, but the stromal cells are less compactly arranged and there is usually more evidence of hemorrhage.

PROGNOSIS

The prognosis of giant cell tumor depends upon treatment and treatment of course depends upon the diagnosis and grading. During

the past decade many workers who felt they had mastered the difficulties of the last have been disappointed in the results of their
therapy. Occasional disappointments will continue to occur because as
yet we must candidly admit that the criteria for precisely accurate
diagnoses have not been defined. Until the time when these lesions
can be definitively classified, several facts should be kept in mind when
dealing with a possible giant cell tumor.

1. The incidence of giant cell tumor is actually quite low. In
frequency it does not compare with myeloma or osteosarcoma.

2. A considerable number of the lesions thought to be giant cell
tumors on the basis of clinical and radiologic evidence will eventually
be proved to be other conditions if the investigation is relentlessly
pursued.

3. Only a fraction of giant cell tumors, probably less than 10 per
cent, will run a forthrightly malignant course. If all types of malignant
tumors with an accompanying giant cell reaction are excluded, this
number is doubtless very small.

4. A high degree of skepticism should be maintained about all
lesions diagnosed as giant cell tumor Grade I. Every effort should be
made to uncover another type of lesion which might cause a giant cell
reaction.

5. All lesions with a firm diagnosis of giant cell tumor should be
treated by complete resection. Curettage will certainly cure a giant cell
reaction provided the cause is no longer active. It may cure a majority
of the histologically benign tumors but not all of them, and there is
no way of knowing which ones will recur. Recurrence is a serious complication since a good proportion of giant cell tumors which recur
eventually metastasize. It has been assumed that surgical manipulation
predisposes to a change in the character of the tumor. Sections of
recurrent tumors frequently reveal features of malignancy. In several
instances the giant cell tumor has recurred as a frank fibrosarcoma.

The efficacy of modern x-ray therapy in giant cell tumor of bone
has not been fully evaluated.[5] In the years from 1930 to 1940, it was
customary in many centers to treat lesions so diagnosed by this method.
There have since been several reports of these lesions developing into
malignant giant cell tumors, osteosarcomas or fibrosarcomas (Fig. 308).
In the author's material of 35 cases a lesion in the upper end of the
radius diagnosed as "giant cell tumor, probably grade III" was treated
with a cancericidal dose of x-ray. There was recurrence three years
later which necessitated amputation. A second patient was given approximately 1000 r of roentgen therapy for a lesion in the distal femur
diagnosed as benign giant cell tumor on the roentgenograms. Twenty-

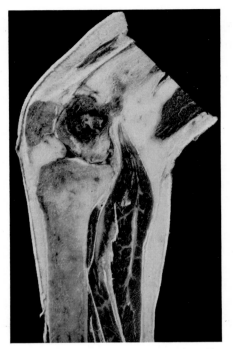

FIG. 308.   Malignant giant cell tumor at the site of a lesion diagnosed as benign giant cell tumor 21 years previously and given 1000 r roentgen therapy.

one years later he developed a malignant giant cell tumor (tissue diagnosis) in the same site. It would be unjust to condemn irradiation therapy on the basis of the reported series. In most instances diagnoses were unconfirmed by tissue examination and, in the light of our present knowledge of giant cell tumors, many of these lesions represented other conditions. The possibility of inducing primary bone tumor by large amounts of irradiation must always be considered.[6]

CYTOGENESIS

The cell genesis of neither the stromal cell nor the giant cell of giant cell tumor is known with certainty. Today most writers have adopted the conclusion of Jaffe, Lichtenstein and Portis that the tumor is essentially a type of fibroma or fibrosarcoma and that the giant cells represent a fusion or a failure of division of the stromal cells. There is much to be said for this theory but it still lacks proof. Most British writers and some Americans adhere to the term "osteoclastoma" and thereby imply that the tumor is a neoplastic proliferation of osteoclasts. Though this theory has fallen into disrepute in the United States it has many attractive features. If one considers the stromal cells as immature osteoclasts, the objection that "the fibroblastic stromal cells and not the giant cells are the essential neoplastic element" can be refuted. One must consider the giant cell tumor as an osteolytic and destructive type of neoplasm, and if the osteoclast is capable of causing bone lysis this character might be expected in its tumor analogue. Moreover, no good reason has been offered why the giant cell tumor probably always occurs at an ossified epiphyseal line of a long bone in which enchondral growth has been completed.

The entire problem would be greatly simplified if we knew the origin and function of the normal osteoclast.

FIBROSARCOMA OF BONE

Fibrosarcoma of bone is one of the most poorly defined and poorly described of the primary tumors of the skeleton. Like giant cell tumor of bone it has been confused with many other lesions, some non-neoplastic such as the reticuloendothelioses, non-osteogenic fibroma, subperiosteal cortical defect and Paget's disease, and some highly malignant such as Class IV osteosarcoma. As a result most accounts portray the fibrosarcoma of bone as a tumor of highly variable morphology and behavior.

Some authors[7] deny the existence of a primary intracortical fibrosarcoma. They believe that the lesions so diagnosed are all either osteosarcomas or chondrosarcomas which are too undifferentiated to produce their intercellular osteoid or hyalin. That many highly undifferentiated osteosarcomas are diagnosed as fibrosarcomas cannot be denied. However, to state that intracortical fibrosarcoma does not exist, appears to the author to be a stand which is difficult to defend. Occasionally, one encounters a tumor of the metaphyseal or medullary tissues which has the microscopic features of the fibrosarcoma of soft tissues; it grows slowly and metastasizes late if at all, just as do fibrosarcomas elsewhere in the body. Its behavior is quite different from the rapidly growing, early metastasizing, undifferentiated Class IV osteosarcoma (see page 465). To classify this tumor with the osteosarcomas because it grows within bone is to confuse and complicate the characteristics of both tumor types. That this is quite generally done is granted but not condoned.

Fibrosarcoma is the least common of the primary malignant tumors of bone, excluding parosteal sarcoma and reticulum cell sarcoma. Batts[8] described 27 cases in 200 primary bone tumors but this proportion is much higher than reported in any other series. In some series there is a preponderance in males, in others the sex incidence

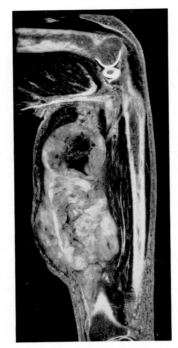

FIG. 309.   A periosteal fibrosarcoma involving the fibula. It forms a bulky, firm, pale soft tissue tumor mass which erodes the bone from without.

appears to be fairly equal. It is said that fibrosarcoma of bone has a predilection for those in the second and third decades of life. In the author's series of 26 cases the greatest number occurred in young adults, but there was a wide age distribution, the youngest being 11 and the oldest 61.

Bone fibrosarcoma is of two types, those arising in the metaphyseal and medullary tissues—central fibrosarcoma—and those which spring from the periosteum. The periosteal fibrosarcoma is probably considerably the more common (Fig. 309). Both cylindrical and flat bones are involved. If those of the jaws are included the incidence in flat and cylindrical bones is about equal. When fibrosarcoma affects the bones of the skull or those of the pelvis, one should look for concomitant Paget's disease.

Fibrosarcoma grows slowly. In Batt's series of periosteal fibrosarcomas the average duration of symptoms before diagnosis was twenty months. Pain is the principal symptom of central fibrosarcoma. It is usually not as severe or persistent as that of osteosarcoma and pathologic fracture is much less characteristic. Periosteal fibrosarcoma produces a palpable tumor mass (Fig. 310). It is sometimes present for years before the onset of pain causes the patient to consult his physi-

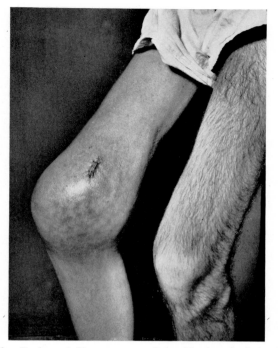

FIG. 310. Periosteal fibrosarcoma of the distal end of the femur.

cian. The periosteal type rarely causes pathologic fracture. Though both central and periosteal fibrosarcomas are aggressive and invasive they do not metastasize until late, often not until after there has been inadequate surgical intervention. Recurrence at the site of original resection is much more common. There may be multiple recurrences before metastasis occurs.

ROENTGENOGRAPHIC MANIFESTATIONS

The roentgenographic manifestations of fibrosarcoma of bone depend upon the site of the tumor. The periosteal fibrosarcoma may present as a large soft tissue mass which is visualized radiographically only because of distortion of more radiolucent muscle planes. Although no evidence of underlying bony abnormality may be present in some instances, in others there is frank destruction of bone ranging from irregular cortical roughening to frank destruction of cortical bone and spongiosa. The central fibrosarcoma is apparent when there is macroscopic destruction of trabeculae. The tumor casts a shadow of the density of soft tissue. As it grows, the spongiosa and later the cortex are destroyed. Since there is no bone reaction, the margins of the tumor are poorly defined. When the cortex is destroyed, however,

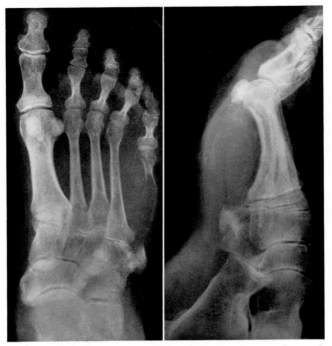

FIG. 311. Fibrosarcoma of bone. The tumor has involved almost the entire fifth metatarsal. The cortex has been thinned and perforated so that a soft tissue mass is present.

periosteal new bone may be evident, but this is subsequently destroyed as the tumor grows and the soft tissues are involved.

GROSS ANATOMY

Central fibrosarcomas usually begin in the metaphysis but in some instances they appear to start in the tissues of the medulla. They may replace the cancellous and medullary tissues of a considerable portion of the bone before cortical erosion is noted. The edges of the tumor are generally poorly delineated and are apt to extend farther than the naked eye can discern. The central type is usually more vascular than the peripheral fibrosarcoma. Eventually, it penetrates the cortex (Fig. 312) and causes extensive lysis, producing a soft tissue tumor mass whose origin is hard to determine. The periosteal fibrosarcoma is firmly anchored to the host bone but usually can be dissected away, leaving a concavity with a roughened surface. It is unusual for the periosteal fibrosarcoma to perforate the compacta and continue its growth in the intracortical tissues but this has been observed. Usually it grows outward, sometimes completely surrounding the bone with a collar-like mass. Many of the peripheral type appear to be encapsu-

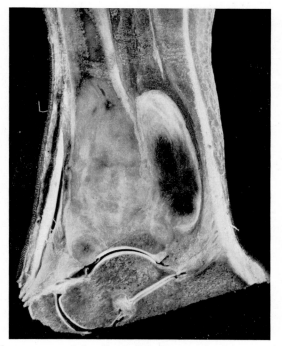

FIG. 312. Fibrosarcoma of the distal tibia. It arose in the metaphysis, perforated the cortex and produced an extramedullary soft tissue tumor. This behavior is similar to that of intramedullary chondrosarcoma.

lated, but this line of delineation is usually only a zone of compressed normal tissue which through the microscope is found to be infiltrated with advancing tumor cells. The periosteal fibrosarcoma is usually pale, sometimes white and glistening. Mineral deposits have been recorded but they are not characteristic as in chondrosarcoma.

MICROSCOPIC ANATOMY

The fibrosarcoma of bone has much the same microscopy as that of the fibrosarcoma of skin, viscera and the soft parts. The cells are fusiform or spindled. They course in fairly well organized trabeculae which weave irregularly through the substance of the tumor (Fig. 313). In central fibrosarcoma there is a tendency for whorl formation which is less frequently noted in the peripheral type. As a rule the cells are moderately mature and considerable amounts of collagen may be formed. When such is the case it may be exceedingly difficult to differentiate the fibrosarcoma from the non-osteogenic fibroma. To make the matter more difficult, when marrow and bone tissues have been destroyed there may be lipid-bearing macrophages and giant cells scattered through the sections. Prediction of the behavior of the fibro-

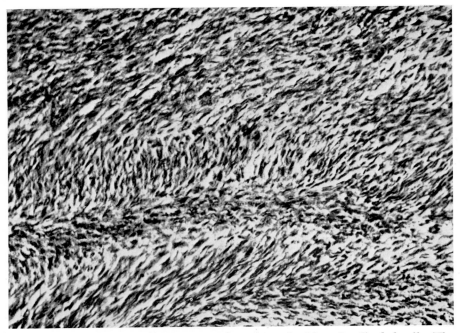

FIG. 313.   The periosteal fibrosarcoma often shows fascicles of palisaded cells. The nuclei may be quite mature in appearance. (× 200.)

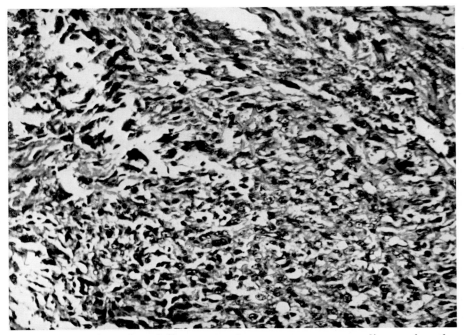

FIG. 314.   The endosteal fibrosarcoma is apt to appear more malignant than the periosteal variety; see Figure 313. In this section the cells are quite pleomorphic and there is almost no evidence of collagen. (× 200.)

genic lesions is more difficult than with any other class. Those composed of mature fibrocytes with abundant collagen production are obviously benign and those of pleomorphic cells with numerous mitotic figures (Fig. 314) and no collagen are just as obviously malignant. But the majority fall somewhere between and the line of distinction grows thinner and thinner until it may disappear altogether. The fibromatoses throughout the body, including those of the palmar and plantar fascias and the muscle desmoids, are notable prognostic hazards. The fibrous proliferations of bone share this characteristic. Silver stains may be done to demonstrate the reticulin fibrils which are woven about and between the cells, but they have not been of great help to the author. The clinician frequently becomes impatient when the pathologist admits that he cannot distinguish between a fibrosarcoma and an innocuous, non-neoplastic fibrosing process. He should be reminded that morphology is all the microscopist has to go by and one cannot always tell by its appearance what a cell is doing.

PROGNOSIS

The prognosis of bone fibrosarcoma is certainly better than that of osteosarcoma and probably somewhat better than that of chondrosarcoma. Its tendency to recur rather than metastasize usually gives the surgeon a second chance. Fibrosarcoma, like parosteal sarcoma, and chondrosarcoma, has been noted to change its cytologic characteristics toward the malignant side following surgical manipulation. Fibrosarcoma should be completely resected and often this necessitates amputation. If the diagnosis is firm and there is a question whether local resection will remove all of the tumor, then obviously amputation is the only course to be taken.

It has always been the dictum that fibrosarcomas do not respond well to irradiation therapy. Actually modern irradiation methods have been tried too infrequently to justify this statement.

The above prognosis holds for fibrosarcoma whether it be of soft tissue or bone, with one exception. The fibrosarcomas of the jaw appear to be more malignant than fibrosarcomas of other bones. This may be because mandibulectomy is attempted less often than limb amputation. Like the tumor elsewhere that in the jaw usually does not metastasize but destroys locally. Perhaps with more adequate facial surgery, the behavior of these tumors will prove to be no worse than those in other bones.

When bone fibrosarcoma eventually metastasizes it usually goes to the lungs. There is a somewhat greater incidence of lymph node metastasis than is found in osteosarcoma and chondrosarcoma.

REFERENCES

GIANT CELL TUMOR OF BONE

1. Beeler, J. W., Helman, C. H., and Campbell, J. A.: J.A.M.A., *163*:914, 1957.
2. Jaffe, H. L.: Oral Surg., Oral Med. & Oral Path., *6*:159, 1953.
3. Jaffe, H. L., Lichtenstein, L., and Portis, R. B.: Arch. Path., *30*:993, 1940.
4. Aegerter, E. E.: Am. J. Path., *23*:283, 1947.
5. Murphy, W. R., and Ackerman, L. V.: Cancer, *9*:317, 1956.
6. Cruz, M., Coley, B. L., and Stewart, F. W.: Cancer, *10*:72, 1957.

FIBROSARCOMA OF BONE

7. Stout, A. P.: Cancer, *1*:30, 1948.
8. Batts, M.: Arch. Surg., *42*:566, 1941.

Myelogenic Tumors

PLASMA CELL MYELOMA

The plasma cell myeloma is a malignant neoplasm arising from a reticulum derivative. Since reticulum, or derived cells which under certain conditions may revert to reticulum, are found in most body tissues, the tumor may be primary in many body sites. The great preponderance of these tumors arise from hematopoietic reticulum of the bone marrow and it is to this large group that the term plasma cell myeloma is applied. When, rarely, it is primary in the viscera or soft tissues it is called extramedullary plasmacytoma.

Other names for the plasma cell myeloma are multiple myeloma and myelomatosis. Since the tumor may be solitary, at least for a period of years, or since it may exist as numerous, probably multicentric focal deposits or involve the entire marrow, the above terms should be avoided except when referring to a specific type. The term solitary myeloma is permissible when referring to an early stage in which a single focus only is demonstrable, multiple myeloma when more than one focus is evident and diffuse myeloma or myelomatosis when all hematopoietic tissue is involved. The various types are not necessarily stages of the tumor process though most or all solitary myelomas may be expected eventually to develop into the multiple myeloma type, and some of the last may eventuate as diffuse myeloma in the terminal stage.

Until recently there has been valid argument as to whether the term "plasma cell" should be applied to these tumors. Though the tumor cells may closely resemble plasma cells, the precise cell of origin is not known and no one has answered the question why the tumor so consistently arises in bone marrow where the plasma cell is such an inconspicuous part of the normal cell population. Since we have learned more of the function of the plasma cell, i.e., its role in gamma globulin production, the disturbance in serum globulin levels in this neoplasm relates the cell in function as well as morphology.

Plasma cell myeloma is a tumor of the older age group, almost always occurring after the age of 40. It has been said that the chief incidence is between the ages of 40 and 60, but if one corrects the incidence with the life expectancy one finds no decline in the curve after the age of 60. The tumor is occasionally seen in the fourth decade and has been reported in adolescents[1] and even in childhood, but these are medical curiosities. It is somewhat more common in males than females but the difference is not great enough to be of diagnostic significance.

Multiple myeloma is the most common form of the tumor, though since the diffuse type has been more generally recognized[2] it can by no means be considered uncommon. Earlier and better clinical work-up and roentgenographic surveys are disclosing an increasing number of tumors in the solitary stage. All types included, plasma cell myeloma is the commonest primary malignant bone tumor.

In the solitary and multiple myeloma types the flat bones are the ones most commonly affected. In a series of 43 cases in the author's material, only two were initially found in cylindrical bones and both patients were under 40, one aged 32 and the other 16. This distribution might be expected since this is a tumor of red marrow and almost all of the hematopoietic tissue in the latter half of life is located in flat bones. The fatty marrow of cylindrical bones acts as a reserve tissue, undergoing conversion to red marrow only when the normal tissue is injured or replaced. This is probably the reason why cylindrical bones are involved in the advanced multicentric and diffuse types.

The vertebral bodies are the most commonly involved, and after them the bones of the pelvic and shoulder girdles and the skull. Plasma cell myeloma is rarely found in the bones distal to the elbows and knees.

Plasma cell myeloma is a neoplastic proliferation of the cells which normally produce gamma globulin. This substance and globulins which are more or less closely related to it are produced in excess quantities. These abnormal proteins are excreted through the kidney and interfere with its function. The symptoms and signs of plasma cell myeloma may, therefore, be divided into three groups: (1) those due to the presence of the tumor mass, its replacement of normal hematopoietic marrow and its lytic action upon bone; (2) those due to the excessive proteins; and finally (3) those secondary to impaired kidney function. They will be discussed in this order.

The most common symptom of plasma cell myeloma is pain. Depending upon the site of the lesion it may begin as back pain, pain in the thoracic cage or in the pelvic bones. Pain often precedes recognizable roentgenographic changes. In the early stages it may be intermittent or occur only on motion but eventually it may be intense, deep and constant. The symptom of back pain is so common in patients over 40 that it alone is of little diagnostic value.

Most plasma cell myelomas begin insidiously, the duration of symptoms before diagnosis is made averaging about nine months. The cells of this tumor apparently have a lytic action upon bone. Cancellous bone is melted away and eventually the cortex is eroded from within. The areas of deossification are usually quite sharply delineated. In thin flat bones such as those of the calvarium, the tumor may perforate both inner and outer tables to invade the contiguous soft tissues. Often the apparent metastatic deposits in the orbit, scalp, epidural and retroperitoneal regions are actually extensions of a tumor arising

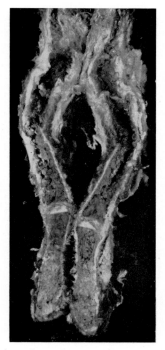

FIG. 315. Sagittal section through a sternum, the site of plasma cell myeloma. The cortices are thinned and expanded. The normal medullary tissues have been replaced by a mushy, reddish brown material representing the tumor. Fracture has occurred due to cortical thinning.

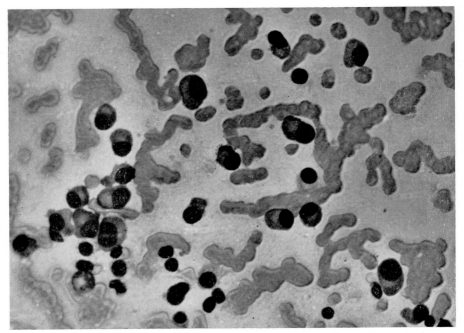

FIG. 316.   Marrow aspiration smear in plasma cell myeloma. Most of the cells pictured are obvious tumor plasma cells. These cells are often found in areas which give no evidence of bone involvement. Sternal or ilial aspiration should be done in all cases of suspected plasma cell myeloma. ($\times$ 440.)

in medullary tissue. Thinning of cortical bone causes weakening and eventual pathological fracture is common (Fig. 315). At times the tumor may be silent until this event. Compression fracture of a verte-bra may injure nerve roots and give rise to a wide range of symptoms of neurogenous origin. Sciatica is a not uncommon chief and some-times initial complaint.

When the tumor is multiple or diffuse, almost all of the bones of the skeleton excluding those of the distal portions of the extremities are involved. Huge amounts of calcium salts are freed; the serum calcium rises and spills out into the urine. The serum calcium level depends upon the extent of skeletal involvement. It is elevated at the time the diagnosis is made in about one-half the cases of plasma cell myeloma. Prolonged serum calcium levels above 12 mg. constitute a hazard because of metastatic calcification. The kidneys are most often affected and this insult compounds that caused by the excessive pro-teins. Pure nephrocalcinosis is rarely found as a serious complication of plasma cell myeloma.

In cases of myelomatosis the marrow may be so extensively re-placed by tumor that a serious anemia may result. Some degree of anemia is present in over one half of the patients with myeloma at the time of diagnosis, regardless of the extent of roentgenographically demonstrable lesions. This is because the marrow is more extensively involved than can be grossly appreciated. This fact makes marrow aspiration a very valuable diagnostic procedure. Tumor cells may be found in sternal marrow (Fig. 316) even though there is no evidence of a tumor mass or of bone destruction. The anemia may be enhanced by the bleeding which is such a common occurrence in plasma cell myeloma. This bleeding may be the result of a thrombocytopenia due to widespread destruction of the megakaryocytes, but another factor appears to play a part. The disturbance in protein formation apparently interferes with normal fibrinogen action though the exact mechanism is not known. The bleeding phenomenon is sometimes manifested by patients with normal platelet levels. Clot retraction time is often prolonged or retraction is sometimes completely lacking. Epistaxis is the commonest form of hemorrhage but melena and bleeding of the gums are also seen.

The total serum protein may rise to 10 mg. or higher. The excessive protein is in the globulin range and usually the albumin level is lowered. The curve obtained by the chromatographic method is illustrated in Figure 317. Though the contour of the curve varies considerably in different cases, the elevations are within a range which is highly diagnostic for plasma cell myeloma. The albumin curve is usually smaller than normal, the alpha$_1$ and alpha$_2$ waves are usually not altered, the beta wave may or may not be elevated and the gamma wave is usually many times its normal height. Protein diffraction has taught us that the kinds of globulin produced in plasma cell myeloma vary considerably from case to case. Some of these globulins are chem-

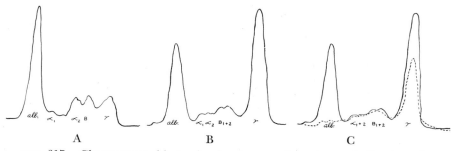

A   B   C

FIG. 317. Chromatographic tracing in plasma cell myeloma. *A*, Tracing of normal serum proteins. Note the relation of the curve representing albumin to those of alpha$_1$, alpha$_2$, beta and gamma globulins. *B*, Tracing in a case of multiple myeloma. The gamma globulin is greatly elevated. *C*, An extract of the tumor was made in the case represented in *B*. The tracing made with this extract is represented by the broken line showing that the tumor cells contain the protein which is elevated in the serum.

ically but not biologically normal. For example, though the gamma globulin level may be high, specific antibody formation may be seriously impaired. But new and abnormal globulin curves may appear in the diffraction pattern. A common variation is a peak between the beta and the gamma elevations which has been called the M (for myeloma) wave. That a variety of globulins are present should not surprise us. This material is produced by tumor cells whose metabolic activities have been greatly altered by the neoplastic process. Their function is no more normal than their shape and often considerably less so. The failure of normal antibody production makes the patient vulnerable to infection and this may be the important factor in causing death. The excessive and abnormal serum proteins may cause the erythrocytes to adhere so that rouleau formation is common. Clumping of red cells speeds the sedimentation rate. Abnormal serum proteins may also cause bizarre serologic reactions. The viscosity of the blood may be increased sufficiently to cause pulmonary and perhaps kidney embarrassment.

Henry Bence Jones in 1850 described a curious protein in the urine of patients with plasma cell myeloma. This protein was found to form a white precipitate when the urine was heated to a temperature around 50° C. which cleared when the temperature reached the neighborhood of 100° C. This protein acquired the name of its discoverer and today is considered a highly characteristic sign of plasma cell myeloma. Bence Jones protein occurs in the urine in probably less than one-half the patients with this tumor. In these cases it is usually intermittent and several analyses may be necessary to detect its presence. Since its molecular size (37,000) is about half that of albumin it passes the glomerular filter. Only rarely can it be found in the serum by ordinary methods but recently a precipitin test has been described[3] which is said to be helpful in the early diagnosis of the lesion. The protein has been extracted from the tumor cells. Bence Jones proteinuria is not pathognomonic for plasma cell myeloma since it has been found in carcinoma with extensive bone metastases and in certain types of leukemia. Liberal amounts of protein other than the Bence Jones type are almost constantly found in the urine in myeloma. Indeed, this finding has been the first indication of the tumor in some cases.

Excessive amounts of uric acid may sometimes be demonstrated in the serum. This is probably produced by the breakdown of nucleic acids which come from the degenerating tumor and normal marrow cells.

Amyloid may be demonstrated in the tissues of about one quarter of the patients dying of plasma cell myeloma (Fig. 318). Careful microscopic search must be made for it and rarely does it occur in sufficient amounts to be of diagnostic value. Amyloid is a sugar-linked protein which appears to be formed by the leakage of abnormal proteins out of the vascular channels. As it permeates the collagenous tissues it is transformed to a substance which is foreign to the normal tissue economy. Amyloidosis is usually divided into two types according to its distribution. In the primary or idiopathic type it is found predominantly in the skeletal, visceral (gastrointestinal) and cardiac muscles, lying in the supportive tissues between the muscle fibers. In the secondary type which usually follows longstanding infections the amyloid is found among the parenchymal cells of the viscera. A number of stains may be used to demonstrate amyloid, but because its chemical components are not constant its staining reaction is variable and sometimes it will take none of the usual stains. The distribution of the amyloid in plasma cell myeloma is characteristic of neither of the classic types though in general it is more apt to be like that of idiopathic amyloidosis. It is seen best in the tumor and medullary tissues, occasionally in muscles and sometimes it may be demonstrated in the viscera. Quite often it fails to take the amyloid stain. One must assume that the abnormal globulins formed by the tumor cells make up the protein moiety of the amyloid substance.

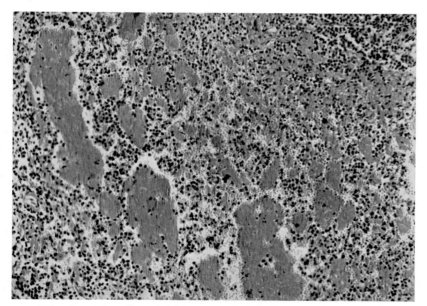

FIG. 318.   Deposits of amyloid in a lymph node of a patient with plasma cell myeloma. The amyloid appears as islands of homogeneous, acellular material. One of the amyloid stains may be helpful in demonstrating it since it stains much like collagen with hematoxylin and eosin stain. (× 130.)

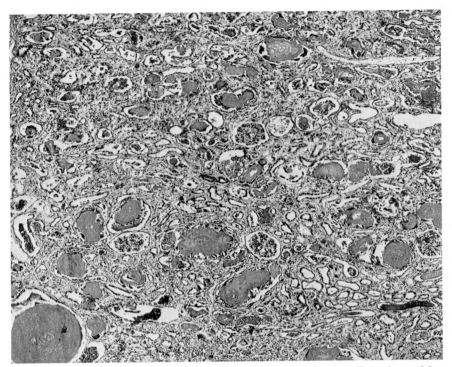

FIG. 319.   Section of a kidney of a patient dying with plasma cell myeloma. Many tubules are filled and distended with protein. In this case it is probably Bence Jones protein since this material was found in the urine. In other cases a protein which gives a negative Bence Jones test is found. (× 30.)

Evidence of kidney insufficiency occurs in about two thirds of the cases of plasma cell myeloma. The type of kidney disease is peculiar inasmuch as it is not associated with hypertension and alterations in kidney function are different from both diffuse glomerular nephritis and lipoid nephrosis.[4] The altered physiology of the kidney disease is not understood. Some authors believe that the Bence Jones protein acts as a toxic agent to the glomerular filter, others[5] contend that the Bence Jones and other proteins form casts in the distal tubules (Fig. 319) which obstruct the urine flow to cause what Ehrich has called an "internal hydronephrosis." This mechanism may play a role but not all cases demonstrate a decreased urinary output, which would of necessity be the outcome of massive tubule obstruction. Because some cases have developed severe renal damage in the absence of Bence Jones proteinuria, it has been postulated that the kidney disease may be due to the increased viscosity of the blood because of excessive amounts of a number of proteins in the serum. In any event nephritis is a serious complication and many patients die in uremia. Nephrocalcinosis secondary to the high serum calcium levels may contribute to the kidney inefficiency.

Some authors have attempted to establish the concept of solitary myeloma as a separate entity. It has been stated that early diagnosis and radical therapy in this type will result in a much better prognosis than that of multiple or diffuse myeloma.[6, 7] Others[8, 9] are of the opinion that the solitary myeloma is merely an early stage of the multi-centric form and that the patient with a single lesion will eventually develop the full-blown disease regardless of his treatment. The weight of evidence is with the latter group. Even in the solitary form one can sometimes find tumor cells scattered through the marrow in areas remote from the primary lesion.

The incidence of plasma cell myeloma in families is probably somewhat greater than is the average in the population at large. The tumor has been reported in a father, son and daughter[10] and the author has seen two brothers affected with the disease.

ROENTGENOGRAPHIC MANIFESTATIONS

The roentgenographic manifestations of plasma cell myeloma vary considerably and in approximately 25 per cent there are none. As with many bone lesions, one speaks of the classic picture, but variations are common. Flat bones, because they contain hematopoietic elements, are first involved. The process is a medullary destructive one and the radiographic appearance is dependent on the degree of local marrow involvement and the extent of the process. Thus, we speak of solitary myeloma or multiple myeloma.

Classically, one sees multiple areas of bone destruction, sharply defined areas of intermediate density involving the skull, vertebra, pelvis and shoulder girdle. This is often associated with a generalized decrease in bone density. There is no associated sclerosis. The cortex may be quite thin over a lesion and may bulge, and when the cortex is completely destroyed, a soft tissue mass is associated with the bony lesions. These destructive foci are manifestations of local proliferation of neoplastic cells within the medullary cavity.

The process may present radiographically as a less well defined destructive process with mottled areas in the bones. A diffuse osteoporotic variety may be recognized not accompanied by local destruction. Here, trabeculae are fine and sparse and the cortices thin, and pathologic fracture of the ribs or vertebra is not uncommon.

The radiographic manifestations then are secondary to proliferation of neoplastic cells within the medullary spaces. Marked local

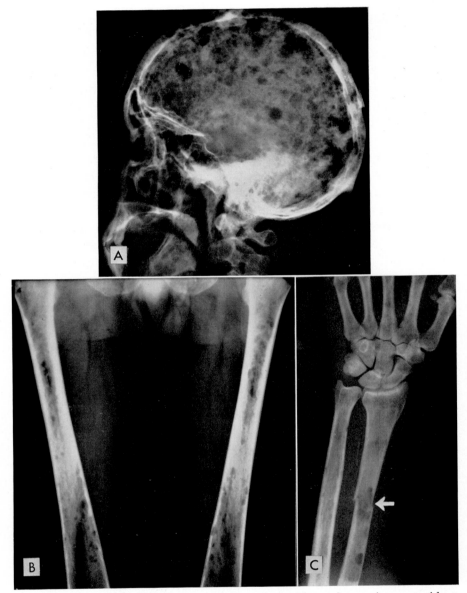

FIG. 320.   Plasma cell myeloma. Distinct areas of bone destruction are evident. There is no bone reaction to this diffuse process. A pathologic fracture of the left radius (arrow, C) is present.

proliferation causes focal bone destruction while diffuse involvement destroys the trabeculae and cortices uniformly to produce an osteoporotic-like appearance. When the process is seen early in its course, there may be no macroscopic evidence of its presence. One must be aware of the less classic manifestations of the disease to be suspicious of it radiographically.

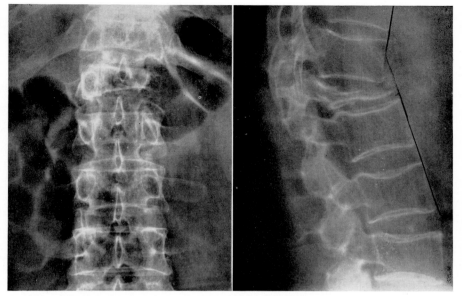

FIG. 321. Plasma cell myeloma. Involvement of the first lumbar vertebra has resulted in its collapse.

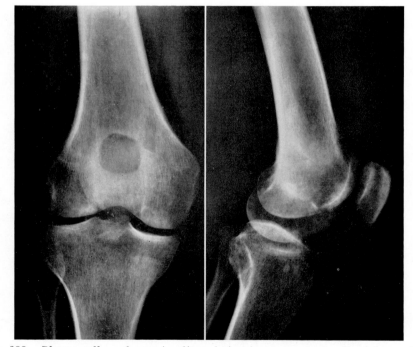

FIG. 322. Plasma cell myeloma. A solitary lesion is present in the distal femur. It is discrete with no surrounding sclerosis.

MORBID ANATOMY

The plasma cell myeloma usually has a red-gray color, often with the appearance and consistency of raspberry custard. This soft creamy mass oozes from the medullary area when the involved bone is opened. The tumor is often surrounded by a thin layer of cortical bone which may show multiple infractions. When the tumor perforates bone and forms a soft tissue mass it is frequently surrounded by a capsule of compressed fibrous connective tissue or muscle. The spleen is sometimes moderately enlarged,[11] and less often the liver and lymph nodes.

As a rule the diagnosis of plasma cell myeloma by microscopy is an easy matter. In most instances the tumor cells resemble plasma cells sufficiently to leave little doubt in the mind of the pathologist. Only rarely is the similarity so close that one may be concerned about whether the lesion is a chronic inflammatory reaction or a neoplasm. In the former one may expect to find other exudative inflammatory cells scattered among the plasmacytes. Also in the inflammatory reaction there is usually a more prominent fibroblastic reaction. In rare instances in which the mature type of myeloma has perforated bone and been involved in a secondary inflammatory reaction, the distinction on sections alone may be quite difficult.

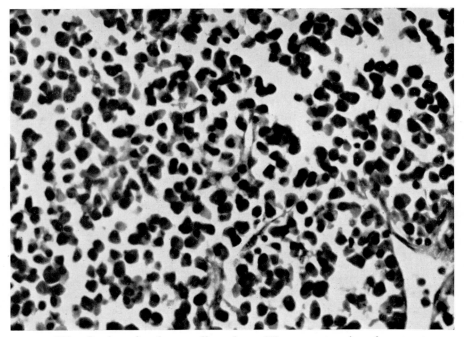

FIG. 323.   Section of a plasma cell myeloma. The tumor consists of a monotonous array of tumor cells resembling plasmacytes. The nuclei usually vary enough in size, shape and staining reaction to establish the diagnosis of tumor. (× 440.)

As a rule the tumor cells are round or ovoid (Fig. 323). The nucleus is often eccentrically placed just as it is in the normal plasmacyte. The cell membrane or at least its outline is usually discernible. The cytoplasm has much the same intense red-blue quality that is seen in the normal plasmacyte with hematoxylin-eosin technique. The nuclear chromatin is sometimes broken and clumped beneath the nuclear membrane in a peripheral distribution but more often this "clock-face" arrangement is lacking. Usually there is considerable disparity in nuclear size, shape and staining reaction and the cells are obviously neoplastic in character. There is great variation in the morphologic types, from those which are almost identical with plasma cells to those in which the resemblance is completely lacking (Fig. 324). In the latter the cells are larger, more irregular in outline and often contain two or more nuclei. At this end of the scale these cells may be difficult to distinguish from those of Ewing's tumor.

In a very small percentage of the cases tumor plasma cells may be found in the peripheral blood. Usually these are few in number but in rare instances they may dominate the blood smears. When this occurs it is usually encountered in the last few months of the disease and becomes in all respects a plasma cell leukemia.

In about 50 per cent of the autopsied cases one may find plasma

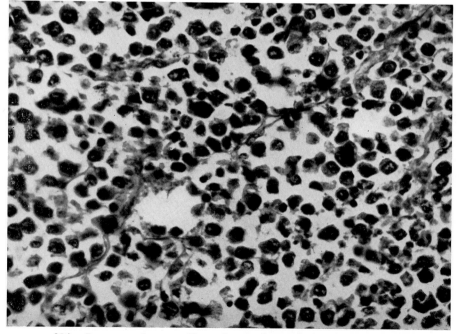

FIG. 324.   In some plasma cell myelomas the variation in cell morphology is considerable. Some typical tumor plasmacytes are found but other cells show little resemblance to the plasma cell. (× 440.)

cells infiltrating the spleen, liver, lymph nodes and less frequently the other viscera.[12] This aspect of myeloma leads to the concept that this is a systemic disease of the body reticulum. If such is the case, radical surgery (i.e., amputation) could not be conscientiously recommended for the solitary lesion. On the other hand, cures for as long as sixteen years have been reported following this method of treatment. Johnson and Meador[13] have described a lesion which they call "benign myeloma of bone." They claim that this may be mistaken for myeloma because it is a reticulum cell reaction and may be multiple. They believe it to be a type of inflammation which should be differentiated from myeloma by careful analysis of the microscopy.

The variation in cell morphology has led to an attempt to classify the plasma cell myelomas on this basis. They have been divided into four types: plasma cell myeloma, myelocytoma, erythroblastoma and lymphocytoma of bone. Since these types cannot be correlated with a characteristic clinical behavior and since all types almost certainly come from the same stem cell, such classification becomes a mere academic exercise of no practical importance. In recent years there has been an attempt to correlate the cell type with the kind of globulin found in the serum. Such association might prove to be of value if it is found to be related to prognosis. As yet our knowledge of the types of globulins involved is too superficial to construct such a classification. The protein chemistry of plasma cell myeloma needs much more extensive investigation.

The plasma cell tumors of soft tissues, extramedullary plasmacytomas, are still a mystifying group. About half of these occur in the upper respiratory passages, the nasal and oral pharynges, the larynx and the paranasal sinuses. Another quarter are encountered in the conjunctivae. The remainder involve the mucosal linings of the various body tracts and the soft tissues of the neck. Hellwig[14] reviewed 127 cases from the literature in 1943. In many of these cases accompanying myelomas are found in the bones; others go on to develop the picture of skeletal myelomatosis. Many of these cases, however, run a completely benign course. The microscopic appearance in these is apparently the same as that of plasma cell myeloma, yet one cannot help but feel that these are curious plasma cell inflammatory reactions which have been misdiagnosed as tumors.

PROGNOSIS

Plasma cell myeloma is a fatal disease. A few cases of cures have been reported following radical therapy of the solitary type, but one must always suspect the possibility of incorrect diagnoses in these cases.

The average survival time after the diagnosis of multiple myeloma is made is about two years. In a small percentage of cases, however, the process appears to advance much more slowly. Cases surviving ten years are not very unusual. The use of urethane is believed by many to prolong life for a year or longer.

In general, plasma cell myeloma must be regarded as a tumor with a prognosis similar to that of leukemia. Some patients will die in a few months, the average will survive about two years and an occasional case will run a course comparable to that of chronic lymphocytic leukemia in the older age group.

EWING'S TUMOR

Ewing's tumor is a malignant neoplasm which always arises in medullary tissue. It has several clinical characteristics which set it apart from other primary bone tumors. It almost always involves the bones of patients under the age of 30. It has a tendency to perforate the overlying cortex and form a soft tissue mass which is often larger than the intracortical lesion. It is usually accompanied by the systemic manifestations of fever and leukocytosis. It quite often metastasizes to other bones.

Ewing's tumor is the third most common malignant primary bone tumor, being surpassed in incidence only by plasma cell myeloma and osteosarcoma. It is surprising, therefore, that it was not delineated as an entity until 1921.[15] It was described in several earlier papers but was always grouped with other tumor entities and was usually thought of as a type of endothelioma. It was perhaps this precedent that caused James Ewing to consider it a tumor arising from the lining cells of the medullary blood or lymphatic channels. It was largely due to Ewing's three published discussions of the lesion that it was known as "endothelial sarcoma of bone." Oberling first published the opinion that this neoplasm came from the marrow stem cell, the reticulum, in 1928 and Stout,[16] Lichtenstein and Jaffe,[17] and McCormack, Dockerty and Ghormley[18] eventually subscribed to this theory of genesis. The term "endothelial sarcoma of bone" was abandoned when Ewing himself recanted his original thesis, and now to avoid cytogenic implication the term "Ewing's tumor" is widely used.

Since the hematopoietic cells of the marrow are derived from the reticulum it seems logical to classify the plasma cell tumor, Ewing's tumor and the reticulum cell sarcoma, if there be such an entity, together as tumors of marrow or myelomas. It seems odd to the writer that Lichtenstein categorizes Ewing's tumor separately as a neoplasm of "medullary fibrous connective tissue." It is in no sense a fibrosarcoma, and though it forms no recognizable blood cells there is as much reason to place its progenitive cells among the myelogenous or lymphogenous series as there is for plasma cell myeloma and reticulum cell sarcoma.

It is usually stated that Ewing's tumor is more common in the male. In the author's material there are 42 cases and the sexes are equally divided. The age incidence is diagnostically more helpful. It is usually stated that the chief incidence is in the age group of 10 to 25 years. Actually, if one extends the age limit to 30 years and includes the numerous cases in those younger than 10, one will rarely encounter a Ewing's tumor outside this group. In the author's material the oldest patient was 28, the youngest 3, and there were 11 patients under 10. Ewing's tumor, does occur over the age of 30, but rarely. When this diagnosis is contemplated in older patients the possibility of reticulum cell sarcoma, lipid reticuloendotheliosis, metastatic carcinoma or atypical plasma cell myeloma should always seriously be considered.

The skeletal location of Ewing's tumor is not as precise as with most other bone tumors. An epiphyseal primary location is exceedingly rare but other than that it may occur in almost any part of any bone. About two thirds of the cases begin in cylindrical bones and the younger the patient the more apt this is to be true. In the writer's material there were 40 cases in which the age at onset was known. Of those cases in patients under 20 years, 25 began in cylindrical bones and 5 in flat bones. Of the 10 cases in patients 20 or over, a flat bone was the primary site of involvement in all but one. This is another way of saying that the Ewing's tumor arises in hematopoietic tissue and after the age of skeletal maturity most of the red marrow is found in the cancellous tissue of flat bones. Most of the primary bone tumors which affect the shaft characteristically begin in the metaphysis. In contrast, Ewing's tumor may begin anywhere in cylindrical bones. For this reason a malignant tumor involving the middle third of the diaphysis of a cylindrical bone in a patient under 30 years of age is very apt to be Ewing's. Since it also occurs in the metaphysis, the anatomic position is often of little diagnostic aid.

Just as with most other bone tumors the femur is the most common bone affected and the tibia is second. The small bones of the feet, especially the os calcis, are frequently affected. Of the flat bones, those of the pelvic girdle are most commonly involved, but primary sites in the ribs and vertebrae are common.

The outstanding symptom of Ewing's tumor is pain. At first it may be vague and transient with quite long periods of remission. Eventually, it persists and becomes severe. As in most bone lesions the pain is often worse at night. More so than in most bone tumors, tenderness over the involved area may develop early. The explanation for the pain and tenderness is obvious when one examines a series of amputated specimens. Ewing's tumor has a strong propensity for the invasion and penetration of bone without destroying its contours. Very early it grows through the fine nutrient canals of the cortex to reach the extraosseous soft tissues including the nerves. It is this character which accounts for the considerable mass of extraosseous tumor before the underlying cortex gives roentgenographic evidence of permeation.

The author has seen a 16 cm. soft tissue tumor mass growing out from the medulla of the calcaneus without any roentgenographic evidence of bone involvement. Eventually the nutrient vessels are closed by the pressure of the finger-like processes of growing tumor tissue, and then the bone begins to show change. Where there is partial closure the bone becomes sclerotic, where closure is nearly complete there is rapid bone necrosis. It is this behavior which is responsible for the generally accepted idea that Ewing's tumor is highly lytic in nature. Actually, the process is very similar to that of infection with the inevitable thrombosis and formation of granulation that occur. The roentgenograms of the two conditions may be strikingly similar.

Two other characteristic features of Ewing's tumor, fever and leukocytosis, can be explained on the gross appearance and cytologic nature of the lesion. For some reason this tumor characteristically outgrows its blood supply, or perhaps it would be more accurate to say that the blood supply which sustains its growth does not remain to keep it viable. As a result large areas of the tumor degenerate; indeed it may be necessary to take samples from several levels in order to find one in which the cells have retained their morphologic character sufficiently for recognition. This fact probably accounts for the wide variation in morphology which is encountered by the microscopist. The nature of the degenerating cells, that is, their marrow origin, probably explains the fever and leukocytosis. These cells are closely related to pus cells and it is understandable that they should give rise to the same symptoms that one finds in suppurative infection. Indeed, it has been noted more than once that completely degenerated tumor tissue takes on the exact appearance of suppurative exudate. The signs and symptoms of Ewing's tumor are strong evidence for its origin from the marrow cells of the myelogenous series.

Abnormal temperatures range around 100 to 101° F. early in the disease. Later the fever may rise to 105°. The leukocytosis is usually moderate, often remaining under 20,000. Occasionally it may rise as high as 40,000. The sedimentation time is usually shortened.

ROENTGENOGRAPHIC MANIFESTATIONS

The most striking roentgenographic manifestation in Ewing's tumor is bone destruction. Classically, this first involves the medullary canal and then the cortex. Finally, the neoplasm elevates and penetrates the periosteum to produce a large soft tissue mass. The medullary destruction appears as mottled areas of intermediate density replacing the bony trabeculae. As cortical destruction occurs, the continuity of the cortex is interrupted or with less extensive destruction its outlines become indistinct. Opacification or sclerosis of bone may occur depending on the vascular involvement. The elevation of the periosteum results in the production of one or more layers of new bone (onion-skin appearance), and the extremes of the periosteal elevation form an angle with the cortex (Codman's triangle). This periosteal new bone is a response to the elevation of the periosteum. It is not neoplastic bone and is not specific for Ewing's tumor.

In a recent series, Sherman and Soong[19] report that approximately 25 per cent of Ewing's tumors present the classic appearance, i.e., a lesion in the medullary zone of the mid-shaft with cortical destruction and multiple layers of new periosteal bone. As might be expected, this radiographic appearance may be entirely compatible with osteomyelitis

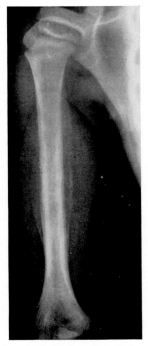

FIG. 325.   Ewing's tumor. The shaft is the site of the neoplasm. Irregular areas of bone destruction are evident as well as layers of periosteal new bone.

except for its location in the mid-portion of the shaft. These authors also noted that the metaphysis is frequently involved and the lesion may even arise in the epiphysis. Ewing's tumor may involve the cortex primarily and mimic an extraosseous lesion with secondary involvement of bone. At times, a large soft tissue mass may be evident with only minimal bony changes. The soft tissue mass of a Ewing's tumor may be evident on properly exposed films by virtue of displacement of more radiolucent muscle planes. Massive calcification within this mass is not common but spotty ossification, presumably of periosteal origin, may be seen.

Involvement of flat bones follows the same pattern of destruction with or without associated sclerosis. Sclerosis may produce a streaky appearance of the involved portion of the bone which is accentuated by contrast with areas of radiolucency produced by osseous destruction.

Radiographically, this neoplasm produces a response which is primarily that of a destructive process with a non-specific appearance. The pattern produced by this destructive process is modified by the extent of involvement, the location of the lesion and the degree of vascular involvement. Microscopic involvement is universally greater

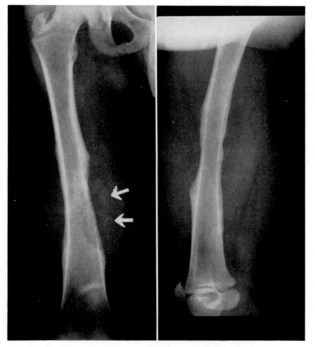

FIG. 326. Ewing's tumor. The lesion has destroyed the cortex medially and practically envelops the shaft. Calcification (arrow) is evident within the accompanying soft tissue mass. Involvement of the spongy bone of the medullary canal is not marked radiographically.

than are the macroscopic changes. The radiographic diagnosis, which can only be suggested rather than positively established, is dependent upon an understanding of the basic pathologic process coupled with a high index of suspicion.

GROSS PATHOLOGY

Ewing's tumor is a soft, pultaceous mass of cells with a pale color. Areas of degeneration mottle the white to gray color with patches of yellow or greenish brown. Hemorrhage is not usual but in the areas of degeneration there may be sufficient hemosiderin to give a dark red or brown color. Because the tumor causes thrombosis of and pressure on blood vessels it alters the blood supply of the involved bone and soft tissue. Reactive bone formation and collagen production are usual. As the periosteum is dissected away from the diaphysis (Fig. 327) it often produces a thin layer of mineralized bone along its inner layer. This is soon penetrated by the tumor and the periosteum is again lifted and again it forms a shell of bone. This may be repeated several times before the periosteum is destroyed and the tumor advances beyond its limiting influence. This mechanism accounts for the

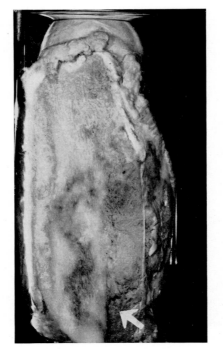

FIG. 327.   Ewing's tumor in the upper end of the femur. It arose in the shaft proximal to the metaphysis, infiltrated the cortex without destroying it and elevated the periosteum which laid down a thin shell of bone.

thickening of the cortex and the laminated "onion skin" appearance which often appears in the roentgenogram. If the periosteum is elevated by a rapidly growing tumor, the reactive bone may be laid down in strands about nutrient vessels which are perpendicular to the cortical surface. Thus the sunburst appearance which is so characteristic of osteosarcoma may also appear on the roentgenograms of Ewing's tumor.

When the nutrition of the affected bone falls below the level of viability, bone lysis occurs. The cortex becomes necrotic and fragmented. This appearance has given Ewing's tumor the reputation of being a bone-lysing neoplasm. Tumor tissue replaces the destroyed bone and advances out into the soft tissue. In turn its vessels are choked off and large areas of degeneration occur. These areas often become cystic and they may be filled with liquid debris which grossly resembles pus. This appearance sometimes convinces the surgeon that he is dealing with an infectious process.

MICROSCOPIC PATHOLOGY

Ewing described the morphology of the cells of this tumor as "monotonously uniform" and most text authors have borrowed this term in their accounts of it. Actually if one carefully evaluates these cells on the basis of their microscopic appearance, "monotonous" does not seem to be a very apt term. It is true that this tumor is very cellular, that the cells are quite undifferentiated and that there is little apparent supportive tissue, but if one examines the highly magnified fields one will note considerable variation between tumors and between areas of the same tumor.

Large areas of degeneration are as characteristic of Ewing's tumor as they are in Hodgkin's disease of lymph nodes. If the biopsy is small, one may have difficulty in finding enough intact cells on which to base an opinion. A second characteristic which has been inadequately emphasized is the considerable amount of bone and fibrous tissue which is found in the sections. The bone is largely reactive in type and one must be careful on frozen section not to conclude that it is being formed by the tumor cells,[20] thus suggesting a diagnosis of osteosarcoma.

The fields may be irregularly divided by bands of fibrous connective tissue of varying width. Some of this is doubtless invaded tissue but much of it appears indigenous to the tumor growth.

The appearance of the tumor cells themselves is also variable (Fig. 328). The nucleus ranges in size from one-half again to three times the size of the normal erythrocyte. The amount of chromatin

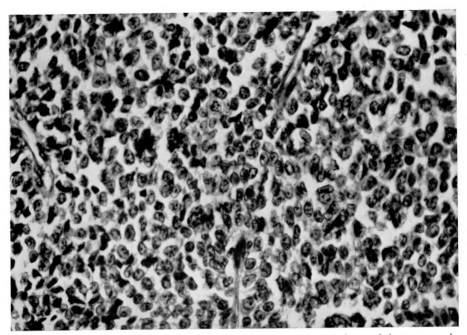

FIG. 328.   Section from a Ewing's tumor. In good preparations the nuclei vary some in
size and chromatin distribution. The cytoplasm stains poorly. (× 440.)

is variable but it is almost always finely divided and diffusely dispersed.
Mitotic figures in most tumors are inconspicuous but rarely they may
be abundant. In most lesions the nucleoli are small or lacking, in
others they may be prominent. The nucleus is usually ovoid, sometimes round, and though there may be variation in size the outline
is rarely irregular. This may be an important differential point in
distinguishing Ewing's tumor from reticulum cell sarcoma. The nuclear membrane is usually distinct.

The cell size is from two to three times that of the nucleus. The
cytoplasm is usually clear with whatever stain is used, but at times it
takes eosin and appears very similar to the cytoplasm of the macrophage. In either case the cell membrane usually remains intact, describing a fine tracery through the matrix. Sometimes no cytoplasm is
demonstrable and the nuclei appear naked.

The appearance of the tumor cells apparently depends greatly
upon the technique which is used in processing the sections. These
cells probably contain a higher water content than most and often the
dehydrating agents cause the cytoplasm to shrink to nothing and the
nuclei to appear heavily chromated and pyknotic. This may account
for the description that Ewing gave, one which seems so at variance
with what we now consider the typical Ewing's tumor.

If one examines this tumor closely, a fine meshwork of stromal fibers can be seen forming a net-like support for the tumor cells. These fibrils stain like collagen and one can often demonstrate spindled fibrocytes which apparently form them. In other areas no fibrocytes can be demonstrated and the grouping of the tumor cells suggests that they have a genetic relation to the intercellular substance. One must consider the possibility of shrunken reticulum elements. Silver stains are of no help since fine collagen fibers and reticulin fibrils are both argentophilic (Fig. 329).

The microscopic diagnosis on carefully prepared viable tissue should give the microscopist little difficulty except in excluding reticulum cell sarcoma, the rare neuroblastoma and the still rarer lymphosarcoma of bone. It is probable that metastatic neuroblastoma and Ewing's tumor cannot be differentiated by microscopy alone in many instances. When the rosettes of neuroblastoma are present they are most helpful, for though the cells of Ewing's tumor frequently form circles, these cells are usually arranged around blood vessels or nidi of degenerating cells. The fact that these two tumors may have an identical microscopy does not constitute proof that they are one and the same tumor or that one or the other does not exist, a hypothesis which has been offered by a few distraught writers who have had difficulty in making the distinction. If primary lymphosarcoma of bone occurs,

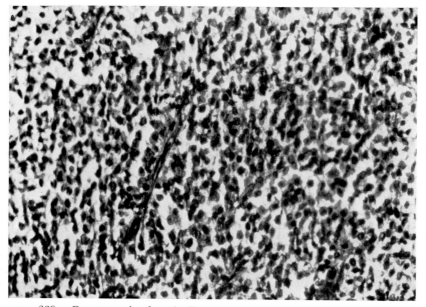

FIG. 329. Counterstained reticulin preparation of a section from a Ewing's tumor. In this case no reticulin fibrils are seen. They may be present, however, and the reticulin stain cannot be used as a dependable guide in differentiating Ewing's tumor from reticulum cell sarcoma. ($\times$ 300.)

it is a close relative of Ewing's tumor. The writer knows of no differentiating feature as long as bone alone is involved.

PROGNOSIS

Ewing's tumor is highly malignant because of its propensity to metastasize. Secondary deposits soon occur in the lungs and in other bones. Less frequently the lymph nodes, viscera and even the skin may be involved. The duration of symptoms before diagnosis ranges from three to nine months. Metastasis after diagnosis usually occurs within six months.

Multiple bone involvement has caused some to conclude that Ewing's tumor, like plasma cell myeloma, is multicentric. There is very little other evidence in support of this hypothesis. In the great majority of cases a single focus is present for some time before other bone lesions appear. About one-half the cases do not develop multiple bone lesions. Examination of the marrow removed from a site remote from the tumor has not revealed the presence of tumor cells, and to the writer's knowledge no case of Ewing's tumor has ever eventuated in leukemia. Pulmonary metastases are not as constant in Ewing's as in osteosarcoma, but death is caused in the majority of cases by this complication.

The over-all mortality of Ewing's tumor is exceedingly high. Some writers place it at 95 per cent even with early diagnosis and proper treatment. There is some evidence that the younger patient has a more rapid course and less hopeful outlook. This may be because reticulum cell sarcoma has a wider age range and better prognosis, and many pathologists refuse to make the distinction between Ewing's tumor and reticulum cell sarcoma.

The best method of treatment is still not definitely decided. At present the salvage rates for surgery and for x-ray are about the same. The optimum regimen of modern irradiation combined with chemotherapy needs more data before final decision is made.

RETICULUM CELL SARCOMA

In 1939, Parker and Jackson[21] reported 17 cases of what they called reticulum cell sarcoma of bone. The tumor occurred in all age groups, in both cylindrical and flat bones, caused extensive bone destruction and soft tissue growth and though often diagnosed late resulted in a very much better salvage than Ewing's tumor. This is the first reported account of this tumor as an entity in which the comparatively good response to therapy is associated with a specific tumor cell morphology. In 1928, Oberling published a paper in which he stated that the Ewing "group" of tumors arose not from endothelium but from the marrow reticulum. Since 1940, several series of 25 or more cases[22, 25] have been published and in 1957, Schwingen[26] reviewed the world literature and found 154 cases published under the name of reticulum cell sarcoma of bone. Despite this publicity there still are authors of eminence who state that they are unable to distinguish this lesion from other marrow tumors, particularly Ewing's tumor, and who thereby cast some doubt on the authenticity of the lesion as a separate entity.

Until recently the writer shared this lack of enthusiasm for reticulum cell sarcoma of bone, and then in evaluating the microscopic characteristics of a series of Ewing's tumors we found 4 which appeared to conform to the criteria laid down by Parker and Jackson. In examining the clinical records of these cases it was found that 39 cases classified as Ewing's tumor were all in patients under 30 years of age, whereas the four patients in question were aged 14, 46, 48 and 70. Because of this age difference, closer attention was paid to the nuclear detail as revealed on freshly cut sections. Today, though there are cases in which the microscopy appears to lie somewhere between the two classic concepts of Ewing's tumor and reticulum cell sarcoma, the author admits that, in the majority, the two lesions can be distinguished on the basis of cellular characteristics.

Why the reticulum cell sarcoma of bone is quite a different tumor in behavior from the reticulum cell sarcoma primary in lymph nodes and other soft tissue is a question which we cannot at present answer. Though the cells of the two tumor types are morphologically identical, the clinical courses are very different. Reticulum cell sarcoma of lymph nodes occurs about equally in both sexes. It affects patients generally over 40 years old. It is a fatal disease which metastasizes to the reticulum-bearing structures of soft tissue—lymph nodes, spleen and liver—and much less commonly to bones. Its response to irradiation is transient and its course is rapid. It is associated with a variety of forms—follicular lymphoma, lymphocytic lymphosarcoma, lymphatic leukemia and Hodgkin's disease. The behavior of reticulum cell sarcoma of bone as reviewed below will be seen to be quite different from that of the non-osseous reticulum cell sarcoma, suggesting that the two tumors are not the same despite their microscopic similarities.

The following account of reticulum cell sarcoma is drawn largely from the literature on the published cases. A review of the accounts turns up much contradictory data and many inconsistent statements, but today the records are sufficient to settle the controversy concerning its existence and to give us a fairly good concept of the behavior and morphology of this neoplasm.

Reticulum cell sarcoma of bone is probably less than half as common as Ewing's tumor. Most series stress the male predominance, usually calculated at about two to one. Whereas all but a very few patients with Ewing's tumor are under 30 years of age at the time of onset of their tumor, reticulum cell sarcoma is quite evenly scattered throughout the life span. Thus the age incidence of reticulum cell sarcoma of bone differs from that of both Ewing's tumor in the young age group and reticulum cell sarcoma of soft tissues in the older age group. There is a fairly widespread impression that reticulum cell sarcoma of bone is a tumor most often occurring after the age of 40. This is not supported by an analysis of the available case reports and probably is due to the frequently heard statement that reticulum cell sarcoma occurs in an older age group than does Ewing's tumor; this is true, but it also occurs in the Ewing's age group.

The skeletal distribution is apparently about the same for reticulum cell sarcoma as for Ewing's tumor and like the latter it may occur anywhere in the shaft rather than predominantly in the metaphysis. According to Ivins and Dahlin, reviewing a series of 49 cases, about one-half occur in the lower extremities, one-quarter in the shoulder and upper extremities and the remaining quarter in the bones of the head and the vertebrae. There is probably less tendency for the tumor to occur in the small bones of the hands and feet than there is in Ewing's tumor.

The symptoms of reticulum cell sarcoma of bone are minimal. In their original paper Parker and Jackson state "In no other bone tumor is the contrast between the comparative well-being of the patient and the size of the tumors so marked." Pain and, in about one-half the patients, a palpable tumor are the outstanding clinical features. Neither of these helps to differentiate the lesion from Ewing's tumor though the pain is apparently less severe than in the latter. Fever and leukocytosis have been lacking in most of the tumors though an increase in sedimentation rate has been reported in some. Characteristic alterations in the serum chemistry in relation to calcium, phosphorus, alkaline phosphatase, albumin and globulin have not been found.

Reticulum cell sarcoma apparently evolves more slowly than Ewing's tumor. If one averages the time from the reports in which this data is given, the duration of symptoms is usually between fifteen months and two years. In some cases it has been reported as ten years or longer.

Though this tumor grows quite slowly it eventually produces the same considerable bone destruction as does Ewing's tumor. Apparently because the process is more insidious, pathologic fracture is more common. It is said to occur in from one quarter to one third of the cases. Some reactive bone formation occurs in reticulum cell sarcoma. This may be sufficient to produce the picture of cortical expansion.

This tumor metastasizes much later than Ewing's tumor and its pattern of metastasis is somewhat different. Whereas approximately one half of the Ewing's tumors will eventually affect other bone sites and only occasional lymph node deposits are found, this pattern is reversed in reticulum cell sarcoma of bone. About 20 per cent have metastasized to lymph nodes and only occasionally are tumor deposits encountered in other bones. Both tumors kill by eventual metastasis to the lungs.

ROENTGENOGRAPHIC MANIFESTATIONS

Reticulum cell sarcoma is manifest roentgenographically by patchy destruction of bone, sometimes accompanied by opacification resulting from active new bone formation. The neoplasm arises from reticulum elements and hence first involves the medullary canal. Trabeculae of bone are destroyed and replaced by tumor tissue with the density of soft tissue. This destruction is patchy and irregular so that normal bone may be evident within the involved area. Areas of reactive new bone

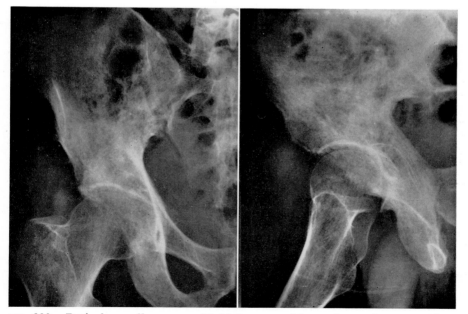

FIG. 330. Reticulum cell sarcoma. Multiple areas of bone destruction are evident within the ilium. Interspersed opacity reflects reactive bone formation.

which cast an opaque shadow contribute to the mottled density. Such reactive bone is probably a reflection of the slow growth of this tumor.

Periosteal new bone is usually not a feature of reticulum cell sarcoma, and even when present it usually is not lamellated as may be the case in Ewing's sarcoma. Soft tissue extension of the tumor is not common. As the medullary neoplasm grows the cortex is eroded and thinned, usually in a most irregular manner so that islands of normal cortex remain within the area involved by the neoplasm. Pathologic fracture through the involved area is frequent, particularly when the femur is involved.

MORBID ANATOMY

Reticulum cell sarcoma of bone usually has a pink or a pinkish gray color. It always begins in the medullary tissues and erodes bone from within. Sometimes the erosion is slow enough to permit the periosteum to lay down a shell of bone over it, causing cortical expansion. Pathologic fracture is reported more frequently and there is said to be less necrosis in reticulum cell sarcoma than in Ewing's tumor.

However slender the evidence for a difference in clinical behavior of these two tumors, the microscopic details of the cells concerned are sufficiently different in some cases at least to warrant separation. It will be remembered that the cells of Ewing's tumor are moderate in size, the nuclei are about half the mass of the cell, ovoid or round, and have a distinct, regular contour. The cells of reticulum cell sarcoma of bone are considerably larger than those of Ewing's tumor (Fig. 331). The cell membrane is usually not demonstrable and when it is, it is exceedingly irregular with processes which have been likened to pseudopods. The cytoplasm is smooth or moderately granular. Cytoplasmic volume in relation to nuclear volume is much greater than that of Ewing's tumor, in which it is approximately one to one or at most one to two. In some sections the cytoplasm appears more basophilic than most tissue cells.

The character of the nucleus is the most outstanding feature of the lesion. In the more mature forms it is large and reniform, in the younger cells it is frankly lobulated. In some the lobulation is so pronounced that the appearance is that of a cluster of small spheroid nuclei. Actually some cells are binuclear or even trinuclear. The nuclei are usually quite irregular in outline. As in the cells of Ewing's tumor the nuclear chromatin is sometimes finely divided and evenly dispersed, but more often it is coarsely clumped and quite irregular. Mitotic figures are much more common in reticulum cell sarcoma of bone than in Ewing's tumor. The nucleoli are apt to be quite

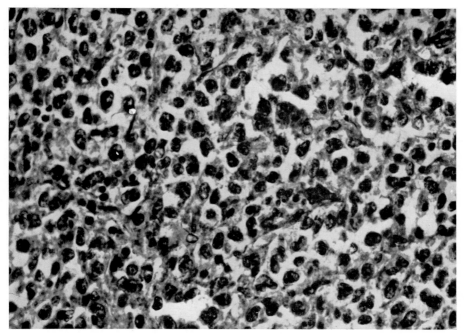

FIG. 331.   Reticulum cell sarcoma of bone. The cells are larger and more pleomorphic th n those of Ewing's tumor (Fig. 328). The nuclear outlines are reniform or frankly irregular. Sometimes the nucleus is lobulated or there may be more than one nucleus. (× 440.)

prominent. Thus, one gets the impression of quite marked cellular pleomorphism in reticulum cell sarcoma whereas in Ewing's tumor the cells are more uniform. Mixed in with the obvious tumor cells there is often a scattering of smaller round cells with scant cytoplasm which have the appearance of lymphocytes (Fig. 332). Some authors feel that these are an indigenous part of the tumor and represent the more mature components of reticulum differentiation.

The pattern and the supportive stroma of reticulum cell sarcoma are not of great differential help. There is probably less necrosis than in Ewing's tumor. Some sections show the tumor cells aligned along syncytial bands that are purported to be primitive reticulum. Actually, if these sections are carefully examined these bands may be seen to contain mature fibrocytes and at least some collagen. They appear to be a network of fibrous supporting fibers and the cellular arrangement is an artefact, a shrinking of the cells toward their scaffolding thus producing a reticulum pattern.

Special silver stains have been used to differentiate the reticulum cell sarcoma from the Ewing's tumor (Fig. 333). In the hands of the author, and admittedly in a very limited number of cases, this has been a futile exercise. In terms of the differentiation of these particular two

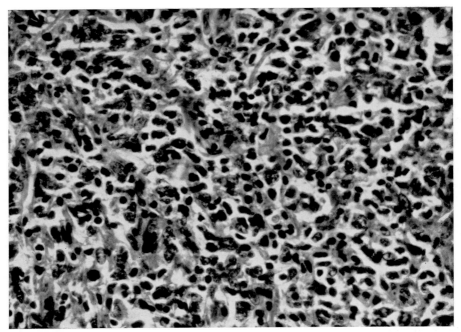

FIG. 332.   In some sections of reticulum cell sarcoma one can find small round nuclei resembling those of lymphocytes. Here they are quite densely infiltrating the reticulum cell elements. (× 440.)

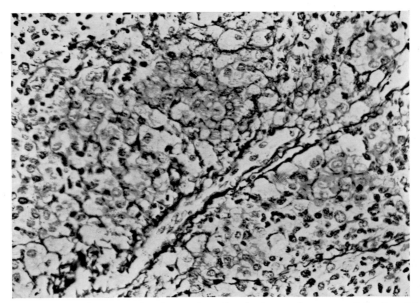

FIG. 333.   Reticulum stain of a section of reticulum cell sarcoma. The fine, black reticulin fibers are woven between the tumor cells. They are not always present in this tumor. (× 300.)

tumors, argentophilia is a property not of the cell but of the physical state of the intercellular substance. The intercellular material of many of the mesenchymal derivatives takes the silver stain to some extent. Broad bands of collagen stain a pale reddish brown, narrower bands stain more deeply. If the collagen fibrils are very fine they take an intense black stain similar to the neurofibrils in the central nervous system. The fine reticulin fibrils supposedly produced by the reticulum cells give the same staining reaction. If the cells of the reticulum cell sarcoma of bone produce reticulin fibrils they have not been helpful in distinguishing this tumor for the author. Indeed, the fine collagen fibrils of the Ewing's tumor have been more prominent in some cases. Some clinicians are under the impression that the reticulum stain has a special affinity for the reticulum cells, which it has not. Since it stains collagen fibrils exactly as it stains reticulin fibrils, a differentiation must be made on the basis of whether the fibrils surround single cells or groups of cells. To date there is lack of agreement on the character and arrangement of the intercellular fibrils of reticulum cell sarcoma of bone. Not until the properly prepared sections of large numbers of cases, proven by clinical behavior as well as by microscopy to be reticulum cell sarcoma of bone, have been studied and compared with those of Ewing's tumor can the virtue of reticulin staining be factually evaluated. Until then we must rely almost entirely upon the nuclear morphology to make the distinction between these two tumors. It is obvious that in cases with atypical morphology, mistakes in diagnosis will almost certainly occur.

PROGNOSIS

It is the definitely more cheerful outlook that makes the differentiation of reticulum cell sarcoma of bone from Ewing's tumor so important. Perhaps 50 per cent of reticulum cell sarcomas of bone can be cured by adequate irradiation therapy if the correct diagnosis is made reasonably early. Excellent results have been reported even after lymph node metastasis has occurred. It is becoming apparent that reticulum cell sarcoma grows more slowly, metastasizes later and is more vulnerable to x-irradiation than the other marrow tumors. It is now believed by those who have had the greatest experience with this tumor that x-ray therapy is as efficient as surgical ablation. It is often the only available means of treatment in cases in which the vertebral and pelvic bones are involved.

The mortality statistics of reticulum cell sarcoma of bone must be carefully evaluated in terms of years of survival. Recurrences and metastases have been reported as late as ten years after the original treatment. All cases of plasma cell myeloma and Ewing's tumor with five-year survival should be reevaluated with the possibility that they might represent reticulum cell sarcoma of bone with atypical microscopy. Therapeutic perseverance, even in the face of multiple site involvement, is probably warranted.

REFERENCES

PLASMA CELL MYELOMA

1. Wood, H., Quinlan, J. W., and Merrill, E. F.: Am. J. Roentgenol., 53:466, 1945.
2. Aegerter, E. E., and Robbins, R.: Am. J. M. Sc., 213:282, 1947.
3. Collier, F. C., and Jackson, P.: New England J. Med., 248:409, 1953.
4. Bell, E. T.: Am. J. Path., 9:393, 1933.
5. Blackman, S. S., Barker, W. H., Buell, M. V., and Davis, B. D.: J. Clin. Invest., 23:163, 1944.
6. Esposito, J. J.: Radiology, 40:195, 1943.
7. Toth, B. J., and Wintermantl, J. A.: Radiology, 41:472, 1943.
8. King, B. B.: J.A.M.A., 115:36, 1940.
9. Paul, L. W., and Pohle, E. A.: Radiology, 35:651, 1940.
10. Nadeau, L. A., Magalini, S. I., and Stefanini, M.: Arch. Path., 61:101, 1956.
11. Lowenhaupt, E.: A. J. Path., 21:171, 1945.
12. Schindler, J. A.: Ann. Int. Med., 19:140, 1943.
13. Johnson, L., and Meador, G.: Bull. Hosp. Joint Dis., 12:298, 1951.
14. Hellwig, C. A.: Arch. Path., 36:95, 1943.

EWING'S TUMOR

15. Ewing, J.: Proc. N. Y. Path. Soc., 21:17, 1921.
16. Stout, A. P.: Am. J. Roentgenol., 50:334, 1943.
17. Lichtenstein, L., and Jaffe, H. L.: Am. J. Path., 23:43, 1947.
18. McCormack, L., Dockerty, M., and Ghormley, R.: Cancer, 5:85, 1952.
19. Sherman, R. S., and Soong, K. Y.: Radiology, 66:529, 1956.
20. Garber, C. Z.: Cancer, 4:839, 1951.

RETICULUM CELL SARCOMA

21. Parker, F., and Jackson, H.: Surg., Gynec., & Obst., 68:45, 1939.
22. Shuman, R. S., and Snyder, R. E.: Am. J. Roentgenol., 58:291, 1947.
23. Jackson, H., Jr., and Parker, F., Jr.: Hodgkin's Disease and Allied Disorders. Oxford University Press, New York, 1947.
24. Ivins, J. C., and Dahlin, D. C.: J. Bone & Joint Surg., 35A:835, 1953.
25. Wilson, T. W., and Pugh, D. G.: Radiology, 65:343, 1955.
26. Schwingen, R. S.: Am. J. Surg., 93:41, 1957.

22

Tumors of Soft Parts

A heterogeneous group of tumors, hamartomas, choristomas and tumor-like processes affect those regions which are often referred to as "the soft parts," that is, those tissues exclusive of the skeleton and the viscera. Actually, these areas include the skin, the mediastinum and the retroperitoneal tissues. Since the orthopedist is not primarily concerned with these regions he has refined the term to mean the extremities, the shoulders, back, buttocks and pelvic regions exclusive of the skin. Since there are no glandular structures in these areas, these processes are all, with the exception of some of the peripheral nerve tumors, of mesenchymal origin. Some of the mesenchymal soft part tumors rarely occur in areas other than the skin, mediastinum and retroperitoneal regions and these need not be included in this discussion since the orthopedist is rarely called upon to diagnose and treat them. In brief, the lesions to be considered here are simply those mesenchymal masses of the non-osseous portions of the extremities and the regions to which the latter are attached.

Because the number of cell types is considerable and the terminology complex and often non-descriptive, many clinicians find great difficulty in organizing this group so that they can be remembered. For this reason an attempt will be made here to group them, hoping that by association the various entities will remain distinct in the minds of those who encounter these conditions.

In dealing with that class of lesions called tumors of bone, the writer went into considerable detail in attempting to differentiate between the true tumors, the hamartomas and those lesions which for lack of a better designation were called reaction to injury. Because in the mesenchymal soft part "tumors" there are transition forms between

559

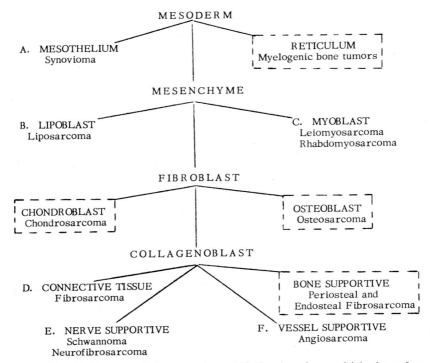

FIG. 334.   A diagram of the mesodermal derivatives from which the soft part tumors arise. The boxed derivatives represent the primary bone tumors discussed in previous chapters.

classes, such as the desmoid and fibromatoses, a simple classification becomes impossible. The best that can be offered is a division into cytogenic groups.

A glance at Figure 334, a diagram of the mesodermal derivatives, reminds us that we have already considered the lesions arising from four important tissue types in this class. They have been placed in rectangles to exclude them from the remaining mesodermal derivatives. Each of the latter contributes certain lesions to the soft part tumor group and we shall consider them in the progression of their designating letters. Only the malignant tumor representatives have been placed in the diagram though numerous related lesions will be discussed in association with the true neoplasms. The following is an outline of the soft part tumors which come to the attention of the orthopedist.

TUMORS OF SOFT PARTS

    A. Lesions of Mesothelial Origin
        1. Synovioma
        2. Benign synovioma (giant cell tumor of tendon)
    B. Lesions of Lipoblastic Origin
        1. Lipoma

       2. Hibernoma
       3. Liposarcoma
   C. The Muscle Tumor Group
       1. Leiomyoma
       2. Leiomyosarcoma
       3. Rhabdomyosarcoma
       4. Granular cell myoblastoma
       5. Alveolar soft part tumor
   D. Lesions of Connective Tissue Origin
       1. The Fibromatoses
       2. Desmoid
       3. Fibrosarcoma
   E. Lesions of Nerve Supportive Tissue Origin
       1. Neuroma
       2. Neurilemmoma
       3. Malignant schwannoma
       4. Neurofibroma
       5. Neurofibrosarcoma (neurogenic sarcoma)
   F. Lesions of the Supportive Structures of Vessels
       1. Hemangioma
       2. Hemangioendothelioma
       3. Hemangiopericytoma
       4. Hemangiosarcoma
   G. Mesenchymoma

A. LESIONS OF MESOTHELIAL ORIGIN

The mesothelium is that mesodermal derivative which is specialized for the lining of body cavities and fluid-conducting channels. The mesothelial cells are closely related to the fibroblasts. Indeed, when a fluid-filled cavity or channel is formed in collagenoblastic tissue there appears to be a transition in the lining collagenoblasts to the mesothelial structure, and in situations leading to mesothelial proliferation one can often find small amounts of collagen appearing in the cell aggregates. The mesothelial type which is pertinent to this discussion is the synovia. It lines the joint cavities except for the weight-bearing articular surfaces, the bursal walls and the sheaths of moving tendons and ligaments. It is concerned with the elaboration of hyaluronates which act as a lubricant for parts in motion where friction would otherwise cut down efficiency.

There are two lesions of the synovia which are commonly classified as tumors. The synovioma is a true malignant tumor. The benign synovioma is the end result of what appears to be proliferative inflammatory reaction.

SYNOVIOMA

This tumor rarely has been reported elsewhere than the extremities, and is more often in the legs than the arms. It is most commonly encountered in the vicinity of a joint and usually appears to arise from

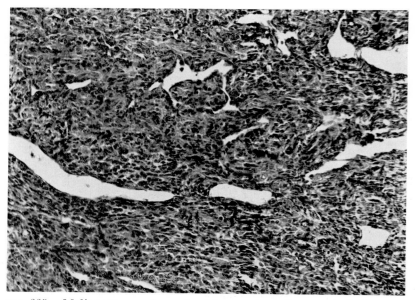

FIG. 335.   Malignant synovioma. In this type the cells are spindled, resembling collagenoblasts. The most characteristic feature is the formation by the tumor cells of irregular, elongated, empty spaces. These may have contained hyaluronate in the living tissue. (× 130.)

a tendon sheath, though in many instances it has been impossible to demonstrate an origin from a normal synovial structure. In some series there has been a preponderance in females, in others there has been a male preponderance. The tumor may develop at any age but usually occurs between the ages of eighteen and thirty-five.

The early accounts of synovioma were misleading because its slow growth led these writers to the conclusion that the tumor is benign. In the initial reports[1] many treated patients were thought to have been cured by conservative excision. Later these patients returned with recurrent tumor and many of them eventually succumbed to their disease after they had been reported as cures. Recurrence after excision is as characteristic as the slow growth. One patient in the material of the writer had eight such recurrences before the tumor metastasized widely.

In a small series of the author (14 cases) 10 were in females and only 4 in males. Thirteen of the 14 were located in the region of the knee or in the lower extremity distal to the knee. Eleven patients were under the age of twenty-six. Seven were treated by local excision with 6 deaths in from a few months to several years. Seven were treated by amputation with 5 deaths. It is obvious that the diagnosis of synovioma is associated with a very grave prognosis. The clinical and cytologic features are disarmingly innocent in character. Because of this, radical treatment is too often delayed until the tumor is no longer curable.

MICROSCOPY

The tumor is made up of two types of cells and cell patterns. In the commoner variety, the sarcomatous type, the cells are spindled or fusiform, quite uniform and have little fibrous supportive structure (Fig. 335). Slit spaces occur, usually lined by tumor cells. The channels

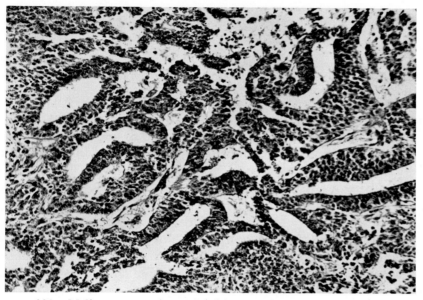

FIG. 336.   Malignant synovioma. In this type the spaces are lined with cells which suggest an epithelial origin. These tumors may be mistaken for metastatic adenocarcinoma. (× 130.)

may contain an eosin-staining material which is said to be hyaluronate. In the other variety, the carcinomatoid type, the cells are more cylindrical and often arrange themselves radially about the spaces to form a pseudoacinar pattern (Fig. 336). The cytologic characteristics appear to be unrelated to differences in behavior.

BENIGN SYNOVIOMA

This curious lesion is probably not a true tumor. In many instances it appears to be the final outcome of an idiopathic synovitis. It has been called giant cell tumor of tendon, tendon xanthoma, tendon fibroma and sclerosing hemangioma. It probably originates as a pigmented villonodular synovitis or tenosynovitis, and then by an

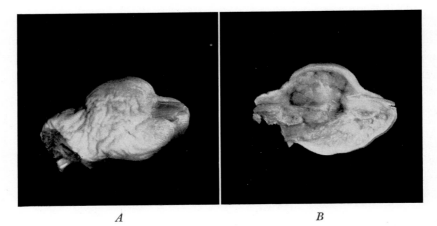

A   B

FIG. 337.   *A,* Benign synovioma on the dorsal aspect of an amputated finger. *B,* Sagittal section illustrating the well defined borders and erosion of the phalanx from without.

exaggerated proliferation of synovia-derived cells produces a solid tumor-like mass. In the tendon sheaths there is less evidence that it begins as a synovitis and it probably exhibits the proliferative phase from the outset.

The benign synovioma is a very common lesion in the periarticular soft tissues. It occurs much less frequently in the joint synovia, usually in the knee and less often the hip. It is somewhat more common in females. It grows slowly, reaching a size of from 0.5 to 2 or 3 centimeters, and occurs most commonly in the hands. When it rests against cortical bone it may cause erosion of the latter (Fig. 337), some times arousing the suspicion of malignant tumor. It has a tendency to recur after local excision,[2] probably because ramifications of the process are left behind.

When benign synovioma occurs within a large joint it may produce a bulky mass which gives the surgeon the impression that he is dealing with a sarcoma. If the biopsy material is unusually active and cellular, the pathologist also may overdiagnose the lesion. The tissue mass may break through the articular plate and invade the metaphysis, and in rare instances no perforation can be found, suggesting that the metaphyseal tissues are subject to the same proliferating stimulus as the synovia. Symptomless metaphyseal lesions have been discovered accompanying benign synoviomas in tendons, suggesting that this association may be more common than we have suspected. If such is the case, because the histologic appearance of benign synovioma and the more innocuous variety of benign giant cell tumor may be identical, it is probable that we have included this non-neoplastic entity in some of our series of giant cell tumors.

The term benign synovioma is an unfortunate one because it confuses this relatively innocent lesion with true synovioma, a highly malignant tumor. The only thing these lesions have in common is the genesis of the cells of which they are composed and, therefore, they are no more closely related than pulmonary tuberculosis and bronchiogenic carcinoma.

The writer analyzed a series of 49 cases. Nine-tenths of them were located in the hand, usually the fingers. Three were found in the knee and one in the hip joint. The ages varied from eleven to seventy-two years. The incidence was twice as great in females as males. One lesion was located in the ankle and recurred three times, causing considerable soft tissue destruction before it was controlled.

The cause of benign synovioma is unknown. Because at least some of the lesions are superimposed on a villonodular synovitis (the author has seen progression of one lesion into the other in a case with repeated biopsies), it appears to be a proliferative reaction to some inflammatory agent. Reaction to intercellular hemorrhage has been an attractive hypothesis since the cellular constituents include giant and xanthoid cells and hemosiderin is often a prominent feature, all of which factors are caused by extravasated blood. But the lesion is not common in hemophiliacs who commonly bleed into their joints, and some experimenters have been unable to produce the lesion in animals by injections of blood or blood and cholesterol. The process is not a part of systemic xanthomatosis and hypercholesterolemia has not been reported in a fairly large number of cases in which it has been looked for.

MORBID ANATOMY

Grossly the lesion is rarely large, seldom achieving a diameter greater than 3 centimeters. It is usually brown, reddish brown or yellow, the color contributed by the hemosiderin and cholesterol ester. It is usually ovoid and often definitely encapsulated with a smooth surface. Sometimes projections will extend from the main mass and dissect between nearby tendons, thus accounting for an unexcised residuum which may later give rise to recurrence.

When sections are viewed through the microscope the lesion is seen to consist of masses of spindled, cylindrical or less frequently polyhedral cells. Slit spaces and irregular channels are found in the younger lesions, suggesting the synovial origin of its cells (Fig. 338). In many of the spaces giant cells are seen. These vary considerably in size but usually they are not large and do not contain more than ten or twelve nuclei. They appears to be the product of the cells which line the spaces. As the process ages a network of collagen bands is

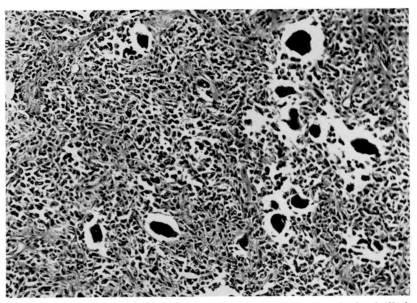

FIG. 338.   Benign synovioma. The cellular matrix is composed of spindled and polyhedral synovial cells. The giant cells are found in spaces. This lesion is often confused with the giant cell tumor of bone, particularly when it occurs within the metaphysis. (× 130.)

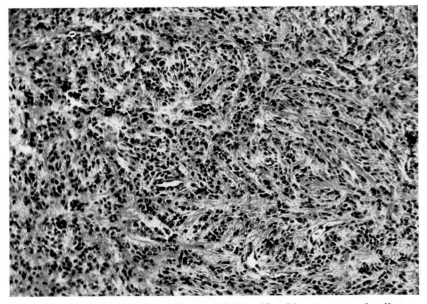

FIG. 339.   Benign synovioma. Eventually considerable amounts of collagen are formed, replacing both matrix cells and giant cells. One must use care in differentiating this from the Class III osteosarcoma. Spaces may be formed in either type, suggesting the possibility of malignant synovioma. (× 130.)

found, dividing the stromal cells into irregular fields. One gets the impression in looking at large numbers of these lesions that sclerosis progresses as the lesion ages (Fig. 339). Eventually it becomes a mass composed largely of collagen and scattered spindle cells. The xanthoid cells and hemosiderin granules are usually more prominent in the younger lesions.

B. LESIONS OF LIPOBLASTIC ORIGIN

Young fat cells and primitive fibroblasts cannot be differentiated until the former begin to accumulate lipid within their cytoplasm. Then the cell enlarges to many times its original size, the minute fat droplets coalescing to form a spheroid globule which stretches the cytoplasmic membrane about it and pushes the nucleus to one side, flattening it against the cell wall. Fields of these adult fat cells appear through the microscope as a network of delicate cell walls enclosing spaces from which the fat has been dissolved by the processing agents. When fat cells are injured, new fat cells may be formed from what appear to be primitive fibroblasts. As these enlarge their cytoplasm acquires a peculiar, ground glass opacity which gives them a characteristic appearance. These are called embryonic fat cells.

Physiologists have been able to tell us little about the reasons for and the mechanisms of intracellular fat accumulation. When the organism is exposed to an excess of lipids, it stores this material in certain depots. The distribution of these deposits is controlled, to some extent at least, by endocrine influence, being somewhat different in males than females. Excessive deposits of fat in abnormal places constitute the lipomas. Proliferation of the vestigial fat storage organ cells results in a hamartomatous mass known as a hibernoma. True neoplastic proliferation of fat cells results in the liposarcoma.

LIPOMA

The lipoma is a metabolic disturbance rather than a true neoplasm. In the extremities it is usually subcutaneous in location. It sometimes occurs within the muscles of the buttock. It produces a rounded, soft, poorly defined mass which may grow to considerable proportions. Masses of several pounds were frequently reported before access to surgical clinics was attainable by all. The accumulations may be multiple (lipomatosis) and sometimes symmetrical. Rarely they are painful.

The fat metabolism within the lipoma is governed by a different mechanism than that of normal fat depots. In the starvation state, fat

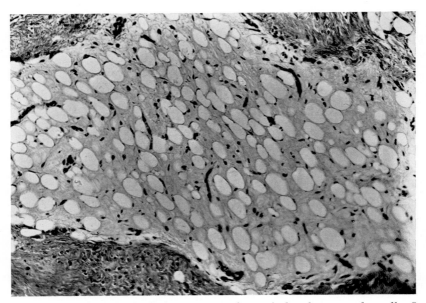

FIG. 340.   Lipoma. The lesion may consist entirely of mature fat cells. Some areas may contain numerous embryonic fat cells such as those seen here. They are smaller, the nuclei more central and the cytoplasm opaque. (× 130.)

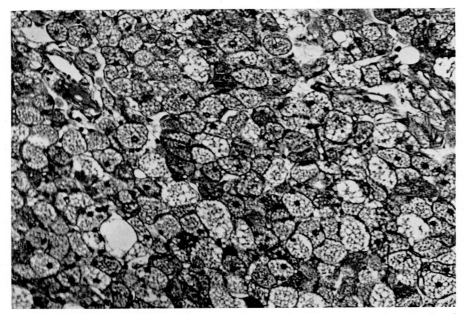

FIG. 341.   Hibernoma. The sections are composed of huge, coarsely vacuolated cells with small but central nuclei. (× 200.)

may completely disappear from the usual storage depots and still the lipoma may continue to grow. This is the only aspect of the lesion which is similar to true neoplasm.

Most of the common lipomas consist merely of aggregates of adult fat cells with a rather scant trabeculated fibrous support (Fig. 340) and a capsule so thin and delicate that it may be difficult to follow surgically, particularly when the lipoma lies within normal fat tissue. Admixtures of other mesenchymal derivatives are relatively common. When there is a considerable amount of proliferating fibrous tissue the lesion is sometimes designated a fibrolipoma, and when vascular channels are numerous it may be called angiolipoma. Often one can find fields in which embryonic fat cells predominate.

The hibernoma is a rare entity, usually occurring on the back or around the hips. It is thought by some to be a manifestation of a vestigial fat storage organ and comparable to the dorsal fat pads of hibernating animals. It has a striking microscopic appearance since it is made up of very large, polyhedral cells with a coarsely granular cytoplasm (Fig. 341).

LIPOSARCOMA

The liposarcoma is an important tumor from the standpoint of its incidence and its prognosis. It occurs most often in the fat-containing tissues of the buttock, the thigh and the lower leg but may be seen in the arm and shoulder region. It is often a bulky tumor and is usually invasive with very little evidence of border delineation. It almost always begins as a liposarcoma rather than a transition from a lipoma, but the writer has seen one perfectly characteristic, common, encapsulated lipoma of the leg in the center of which there was an undeniably obvious liposarcoma.

In its usual form the liposarcoma is not hard to diagnose on its microscopic appearance. It is composed of bizarre cells whose nuclei reveal all the characteristics of malignancy. Distorted giant cells are usual. The identifying features are the embryonic and even adult fat cells which are scattered among the more obvious tumor cells (Fig. 342). Sometimes the more mature forms are lacking and the tumor cells are quite uniform. Then evidence of fat-storing cells must be searched for. In these undifferentiated tumors a fat stain may be of little help since the tumor cells may contain no more fat than the tumors of other cytogenesis. Fat stains should always be done, however, if liposarcoma is suspected.

The liposarcoma must be removed widely or it will recur and often metastasize in the usual sarcoma pattern. Stout has described

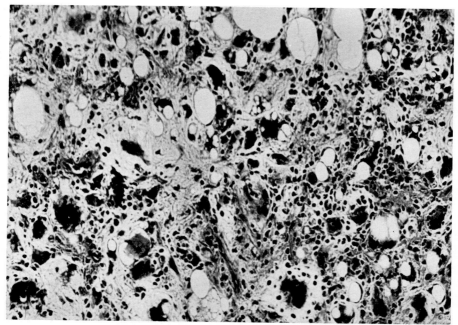

FIG. 342.   Liposarcoma. The sections have a pleomorphic appearance. There are many bizarre, multinucleated giant cells, primitive spindled lipoblasts, embryonic fat cells and mature lipocytes. ($\times$ 200.)

what he calls a "differentiated liposarcoma." Among lipoblasts and lipocytes one finds areas composed of stellate cells in a myxomatous ground substance. These tumors are apparently invasive but they do not metastasize.

C. THE MUSCLE TUMOR GROUP

This group contains several entities, the leiomyoma, the leiomyosarcoma and the rhabdomyosarcoma. The rhabdomyoma probably occurs only in the heart so is not considered here. Besides these lesions of known muscle origin there are two others, the granular cell myoblastoma and the alveolar soft part tumor, whose origins are actually unknown. Since the former was described as coming from the myoblast and this hypothesis has not been unequivocally disproved, and since the latter is thought by many to be the malignant analogue of the granular cell myoblastoma, both of these lesions will be discussed in this section.

LEIOMYOMA

The leiomyoma is an unusual lesion in the soft parts of the extremities, though it may occur in the skin and rarely in the deeper tissues. Its most common sites, of course, are in the uterus and gastro-intestinal tract. In the deep tissues of the extremities the leiomyoma is apt to occur in a purer form than in other tissues where it is apt to be mixed with a rich component of fibrous connective tissue and then is frequently designated a fibroid. Most of the leiomyomas of the extremity probably arise from the muscle sheath of vessels, though their exact origins are usually impossible to determine.

By many pathologists the leiomyoma is classified as a hamartoma rather than a true neoplasm. It is slowly growing and, though probably not truly invasive, its margins are usually difficult to determine either by gross or microscopic examination. It is made up of bluntly terminating, extending, fusiform cells with long oval nuclei. It may be exceedingly difficult to differentiate these cells from those of a fibroblastic proliferation, but careful study will usually make the distinction. The cells of leiomyoma have a tendency to arrange themselves in parallel rows, a feature which is called palisading. This arrangement is characteristic of neurilemmoma and sometimes the distinction between these lesions is not easy. Leiomyomas arising from the muscle sheath of vessels often form numerous vascular sinuses in their substance. These may be so prominent that they are apt to be classified as true angiomas. A Mallory stain for collagen may be of great help. A leiomyoma in an extremity usually takes very little of the blue color whereas the other tumor types which produce more collagen may stain predominantly blue.

It is important to note the number of mitotic figures in a leiomyoma. If there are more than one to the field, one may be dealing with a leiomyosarcoma.

LEIOMYOSARCOMA

The sarcoma of non-striated muscle rarely occurs in the deep tissues of the extremities. The writer has seen but one in the material from Temple Medical Center. These tumors occur somewhat more often in the skin and in the soft tissues of the trunk. A diagnosis is usually made by excluding leiomyoma, fibrosarcoma, liposarcoma and rhabdomyosarcoma. The greatest difficulty may arise in determining whether a smooth muscle tumor is benign or malignant. Gross evidence of invasion, hemorrhage and necrosis suggests malignancy. In the sections, mitotic figures and occasional irregular giant cell forms, when present, will make the distinction.

RHABDOMYOSARCOMA

The malignant tumor of striated muscle occurs often enough to be of real importance. Over half of these occur in the buttock, groin

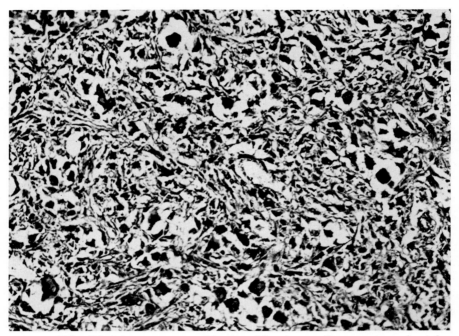

FIG. 343.   Rhabdomyosarcoma. Pleomorphic giant cells may occur but they are usually smaller than those of liposarcoma. Elongated (strap) forms are helpful features. The staining quality of the cytoplasm cannot be illustrated in this photograph. (× 200.)

or leg. They grow rather slowly to form a large mass. The mortality is over 50 per cent, and unless they are eradicated early they metastasize by way of the blood stream, usually to the lungs. They are usually found within the substance of the skeletal muscles and it may be impossible to determine the margins of the tumor. For this reason recurrence is usual unless a very wide excision is carried out. As in most malignant mesenchymal tumors, hemorrhage and necrosis are common. Usually, the tumor type is not suspected until sections are examined through the microscope.

Disparity in cell size and shape characterizes the rhabdomyosarcoma just as in liposarcoma. It is frequently difficult to differentiate the two. In the former, however, the cytoplasm of many or even most of the cells takes a deep rose eosin stain which is reminiscent of the sarcoplasm of normal muscle cells. This may be due to the presence of myoglobin. The less differentiated the cells, the less likely this staining characteristic is to appear. The next helpful diagnostic feature is the appearance of elongated strap-like forms (Fig. 343). When these appear they may contain more than one nucleus, sometimes arranged eccentrically beneath the sarcolemma. These appear in the better

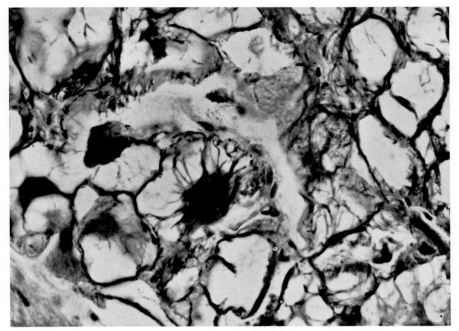

FIG. 344.   The "spider cell" of rhabdomyosarcoma. (×440.)

differentiated tumors. If one can find cross striations in these the diagnosis is certain. Phosphotungstic acid staining helps to bring out these
striations. Giant cells, often with numerous bizarre nuclei, are common
and these help to differentiate this tumor from fibrosarcoma and
leiomyosarcoma. Occasionally the nucleus and a narrow rim of cytoplasm are situated in what appears to be a large vacuole traversed by
thread-like processes radiating from the cell to the outer wall (Fig.
344). These forms have stimulated the imagination of certain microscopists to call them "spider cells." They occur more often in the
rhabdomyoma of the heart than in the rhabdomyosarcoma of soft parts.
Some writers contend that the clear portions of the cell contained
glycogen before the cell was processed. The appearance has suggested
to the author that the very large cell contained a considerable amount
of water and water-soluble substances which left the cytoplasm in the
course of dehydration, causing the residuum to shrink away from a
cell membrane which was held in shape by the more rigid surrounding
tissues.

GRANULAR CELL MYOBLASTOMA

This peculiar entity is uncommon but not rare. It has been reported in most tissues of the body but about one-half develop in rela-

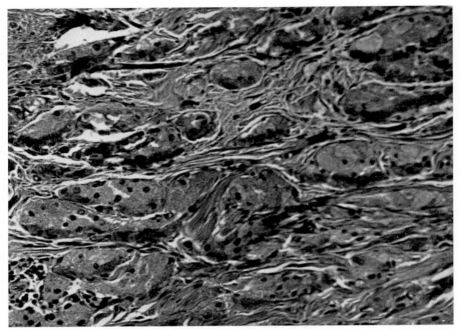

FIG. 345.   Granular cell myoblastoma. The cells are large, the nuclei relatively small and central, the cytoplasm granular. The cells are grouped in alveoli. (× 200.)

tion to striated muscle. Because of this relationship and the fact that the cells of which it is composed have a resemblance to the cross section of a young muscle fiber, it is said to be derived from the myoblast, hence the name. Actually, many granular cell myoblastomas are found in tissues where no normal muscle components exist, and embryologists claim that its cells do not resemble the rhabdomyoblast. Fust and Custer[3] analyzed a large number of these lesions and felt that all or most arose in the supportive cells of peripheral nerve filaments.

The tumor, if it be a tumor, grows slowly to form a small encapsulated mass, usually not greater than a centimeter in diameter. Though it may occur in almost any of the soft tissues, about one-third occur in the extremities, one-third in the trunk, neck and head and one-third in the tongue. Several have been reported recently in the vulva. They may be present for a year or much longer before they are brought to the attention of the physician.

Seen through the microscope they present uniformly similar fields of very large, polyhedral cells with relatively small nuclei. The cytoplasm is filled with rather coarse, moderately eosinophilic granules which give the tissue its outstanding characteristic (Fig. 345). The lesion, at least in this form, never demonstrates a malignant behavior.

ALVEOLAR SOFT PART TUMOR
(Malignant Granular Cell Myoblastoma, Granular Myoblastoma)

This tumor is less than one-quarter as common as granular cell myoblastoma. Many writers contend that it is unrelated to the latter. Others[4] feel that it is probably the malignant analogue of the benign granular cell myoblastoma. About half of these tumors run a rather benign course, at least for a number of years. They may invade and recur but seem to be controlled if completely excised. The other half have probably metastasized by the time the original tumor is discovered and removed. The patient will have an interim of several months' freedom of any signs of tumor and then a metastasis will appear. One patient in the author's material had eight such episodes before the tumor metastasized widely and caused death. The first four of these metastases occurred in striated muscle groups in various areas. Later the tumor went to lymph nodes and eventually ended as a sarcomatosis. Most alveolar soft part tumors arise within muscles of the extremities, though some appear to be derived from the sheath. They are usually obviously invasive from the beginning.

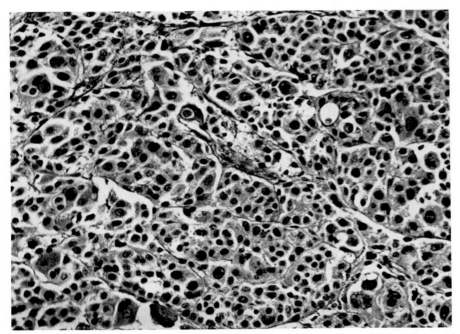

FIG. 346.   Alveolar soft part tumor. The cells are much more pleomorphic and the nuclei more irregular and hyperchromatic than those of granular cell myoblastoma. The alveolar grouping by thin partitions is the most characteristic feature. (× 200.)

Microscopically, they are made up of cells which are quite reminiscent of those of the granular cell myoblastoma. They are large and granular though they show much greater disparity in size, shape and staining quality. The most outstanding feature of the microscopy is the grouping of the cells in aggregates surrounded by narrow trabeculae of fibrous connective tissue (Fig. 346). This pattern has given rise to the term "alveolar" soft part tumor. The microscopist will experience the greatest difficulty in predicting the course this tumor will take. Some of the most innocent appearing will manifest the most malignant behavior.

D. LESIONS OF CONNECTIVE TISSUE ORIGIN

The collagenoblast, that is, that cell which as it matures is associated with the formation of an intercellular substance known as collagen, is the chore boy of the other body tissues. It supplies the support for the more highly specialized cells of the glands, the viscera, the nerves, the vessels and even the skeletal structures. This type we call simply "supportive collagenous tissue" (see Fig. 334). In each location its structure and pattern is modified to accommodate and complement the function of the tissue it supports. Another type binds each of the specialized units into a whole so that their function is organized for the welfare of the total organism. This we call "connective tissue." Recent emphasis on the study of collagen has revealed that it itself, in its subtle way, plays a very important role in body physiology, not only from the standpoint of association, support and protection but in the diffusion of most of the fluids and minerals which are so meticulously metabolized and so important to the parenchymal cells.

Abnormal proliferations, hamartomas and true tumors may develop from each collagenic type. They form a nebulous group difficult to classify, since one lesion merges imperceptibly into another without clear lines of distinction. In no other tissue type are the neoplasms and pseudoneoplasms so difficult to categorize.

These fall into four groups though the gross and microscopic characteristics of each may not be depended upon to distinguish it from members of another group. At times, only the behavior of the lesion may be relied upon to determine its exact nature. The term "fibroma" will be avoided since it connotes a benign tumor of connective tissue. If there is such a thing as a benign tumor of this tissue type it is the desmoid or the fibromatoses. The lesion which has been called a fibroma is probably nothing more than an abnormal proliferation of fibroblasts. It is not progressive since the cells mature and stop growing. It does not predispose to fibrosarcoma. In short, it may be likened to a spontaneous keloid which can occur elsewhere than in the skin. It is a most uncommon lesion in the deep soft parts of the extremities. Most of the so-called fibromas which affect the extremities occur in relation to the skin as congenital, localized overgrowths of the corium (true hamartomas), as the result of injury (keloids), as a part of neurofibromatosis (fibroma molluscum) or as a response to cholesterol-containing macrophages (xanthomas). None of these should be mistaken for a true tumor. There are three lesions which arise in proliferating connective tissue collagenoblasts which are either true tumors or whose behavior simulates that of tumor in some degree. These are the fibromatoses, the desmoids and the fibrosarcomas. Only the last kills by metastasizing.

THE FIBROMATOSES

In several regions of the body where normal fibrous connective tissue exists in considerable amounts, the fibroblasts, apparently spontaneously, begin to proliferate to form hard, bulky masses of collagenous tissue which interfere with the function of the part involved. These may occur in certain muscle groups such as those of the neck where they cause fibromatosis colli or congenital wryneck. Or they may be more diffusely scattered throughout several groups—progressive myositis fibrosa. They may develop in the supportive structure of parenchymal tissues as in penile fibromatosis (Peyronie's disease). The most important group involves the fasciae of the hands (palmar fibromatosis or Dupuytren's contracture) and the feet (plantar fibromatosis). As masses of connective tissue form and mature, considerable amounts of collagen are formed. Moving tendons become adherent and fixed. As the collagenous tissue ages it shrinks just as scar tissue does anywhere in the body, and the resulting contraction deforms the part and further inhibits function. The fibroblastic cells grow along cleavage planes and thus they dissect between and around tendons, vessels and nerves. Eventually, they involve the corium of the overlying skin. The result is a crippled, useless hand or foot and, tragically, the surgeon finds it impossible to completely dissect out this extraneous tissue. Any that is left behind may act as the seed of further growth unless the blood supply is reduced below the growth level by treatment with x-rays. Because of the appearance of the exuberant growth (Fig. 347), the appearance of invasion and the propensity for recurrence, these

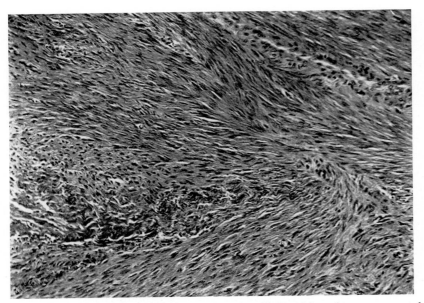

FIG. 347.   Plantar fibromatosis. Relatively mature collagenoblasts form a more or less
organized pattern of trabeculae. (× 120.)

lesions are frequently misdiagnosed as fibrosarcoma. Making the distinction between a well differentiated fibrosarcoma and a fibromatosis
in the proliferative stage is by no means an easy task. Metastasizing neoplasms do arise in the fasciae of the hands and feet but they are rare
and usually their microscopic features are florid enough to betray their
identity.

DESMOID

The desmoid was originally defined as a fibrosis of the rectus
abdominal muscles, usually following pregnancy. More recently it has
come to mean in many clinics a progressive fibroblastic proliferation in
the striated muscle of any part of the body and sometimes the same
process occurring in periosteum. This proliferation progresses slowly,
microscopic fingers of cells insinuating themselves between muscle
bundles and fibers. This gives the lesion the appearance of invasion.
In resecting the lesion it is difficult to make sure that all of the offending tissue has been removed. Recurrent growth apparently springs
from the remaining tags. Thus the lesion is characterized by slow
growth, progression and recurrence. If inadequately treated over a
long period it may eventually destroy large areas of normal tissue or,

gaining access to the trunk, surround and even infiltrate parenchymal organs. One such lesion beginning near the inner surface of the ischium in an adolescent female penetrated into the pelvic interior and infiltrated the bladder wall and distal ureter. Eventually, in order to control the process, it was necessary to do a hemipelvectomy. The author knows of two other such cases. All were in young women. Two followed pregnancy.

The insidious thing about the desmoid is the benign appearance of its cells (Fig. 348). In the early stages the lesion is relatively acellular, the nuclei are mature in appearance and considerable amounts of collagen are produced. The microscopist concludes that he is dealing with proliferating scar tissue following an injury or, if he is more concerned because of the clinical findings, he may suspect he has been given an area of collagenous reaction at the periphery of a more serious lesion. Sometimes it may take repeated biopsies to convince him that the innocent appearing cells in his sections constitute an invasive lesion. Blocks carefully taken from the periphery of the process usually reveal evidence of this invasion, and this feature alone may be the only clue to the exact nature of the disease. If a reasonably early diagnosis is made and the lesion completely excised, a cure is certain. Desmoids never metastasize.

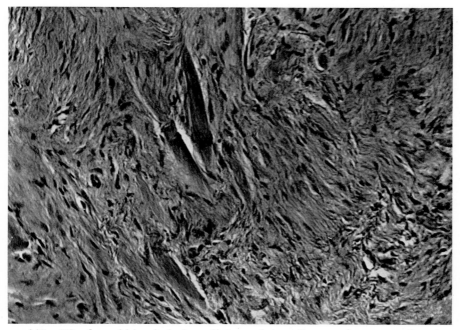

FIG. 348.   The desmoid is relatively acellular and the cells are quite mature. Invasion of muscle is quite characteristic. ($\times$ 200.)

FIBROSARCOMA

Fibrosarcoma occurs in the supportive structures of muscles, tendons, and ligaments, in fascia and periosteum, in subcutaneous tissue and in the corium. In the last area it is properly called dermatofibrosarcoma protuberans. It is rather uncommon in the soft parts of the extremities.

The great preponderance of fibrosarcomas are very slow growing. If they metastasize it is late. Perhaps the outstanding characteristic of fibrosarcoma is its history of recurrence or, to state it more exactly, its tenacious persistence after removal. This means simply that it is infiltrative and that fine ramifications of the tumor process extend farther than the unaided vision can appreciate, farther indeed than is expected. Since it rarely kills except by repeated recurrences and eventual invasion of vital structures, the surgeon is apt to decide on conservative measures of treatment. Such measures are often inadequate. A relatively small group of these tumors will manifest a moderately rapid and progressive growth with blood stream metastasis and death with deposits in the lungs and elsewhere. Once the diagnosis is unequivocally established, and this can be achieved only by biopsy, the excision should be designed, with the aid of frozen sections, to eradicate the entire process even though it necessitates mutilating surgery. The results of radiotherapy have not been encouraging.

MICROSCOPIC FEATURES

In general, there are two classes of fibrosarcomas. The common type is made up of spindled cells terminating in fine fibrils which take the silver stain. The more mature the cell type, the more tendency there is for the cells to grow in fascicles which interweave in undulating patterns (Fig. 349) or form whorls. Varying amounts of collagen are formed. In thread-like fibers it stains black with silver, in broader bands it stains brown. The nuclei are usually larger and more rounded than those of normal young fibroblasts but in some cases the distinction is exceedingly difficult to make. The number of mitotic figures is a fairly good indicator for the rate of growth. In general, the absence of trabecular or whorl pattern, the lack of collagen and the presence of nuclear pleomorphism suggest a more malignant behavior. It must be added, however, that tumors with the most innocent microscopic features occasionally will manifest a frankly malignant course.

A much less common variety is that which Stout prefers to call "myxoma" (Fig. 350). Its behavior is very much like that of the ordinary fibrosarcoma, that is, it is infiltrative and it recurs, but it probably

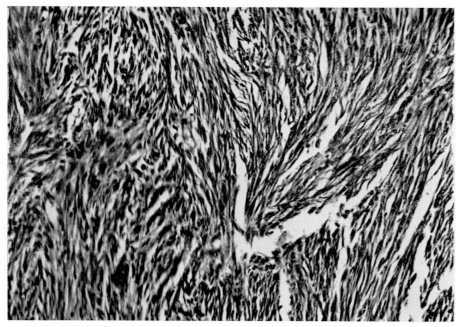

FIG. 349.   In the fibrosarcoma the nuclei are of neoplastic type. They form poorly defined trabeculae which weave through the section. ($\times$ 200.)

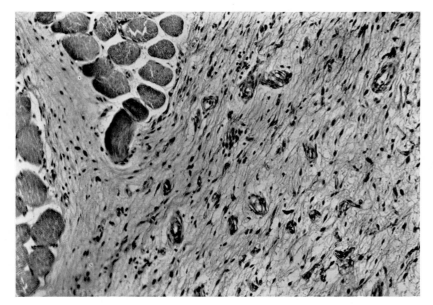

FIG. 350.   Myxoma. The cells are small, spindled or stellate in a myxomatous ground substance of hyaluronates. Invasion of muscle is highly characteristic ($\times$ 130.)

never metastasizes. The microscopic sections show it to be composed of stellate cells in a pale, acellular, myxomatous matrix. This material takes the mucopolysaccharide stains and is probably very closely related to the ground substance of normal collagen. For this reason it seems logical to consider the myxoma a type of fibrosarcoma, a type in which there is an increase in ground substance production. Since the myxoma does not metastasize, and since the more cellular varieties with little or no ground substance production quite often do metastasize, one might therefrom construct an interesting hypothesis.

E. LESIONS OF NERVE SUPPORTIVE TISSUE ORIGIN

The pseudoneoplastic and neoplastic lesions of the nerves of the extremities form a group about which there is considerable disagreement concerning cytogenesis. These lesions arise from the supportive cells of the nerve fibril, the latter playing little or no part in the production of the mass. The argument stems from the disagreement concerning the origins of these supportive cells. Some eminent writers believe that all structures within the outer nerve sheath are derived from the neural crest and are, therefore, ectodermal. Others believe they are all of mesenchymal derivation. Still others agree that the cells of the Schwann sheath are ectodermal but feel that the supportive cells between the ensheathed fibrils are collagenic. In order to avoid the involved polemics of one stand or the other it may be wiser to present the subject with a foot in each camp. Thus there can be four varieties of supportive tissue proliferation: (1) the neurilemmoma,* a benign growth from Schwann sheath cells, (2) the malignant schwannoma, its malignant counterpart, (3) neurofibroma from the endoneural fibrous connective tissue and (4) its malignant analogue, the neurofibrosarcoma. A fifth lesion is the traumatic neuroma which is a proliferation of all the supportive elements in an attempt to reestablish the continuity of a divided nerve.

NEUROMA

This term is now commonly used to designate the nodule of tissue which grows out from the proximal end of a nerve which has been severed by accident or surgery. It may be painful. It consists of a tangled mass of Schwann cells attempting to form sheaths for the growing nerve fibrils and the collagenic supportive cells. In cross sec-

* The term neurilemmoma is derived from the Greek "alifo" (to coat). The letter F when followed by M is changed to M for euphony. Neurilofmoma=neurilemmoma.

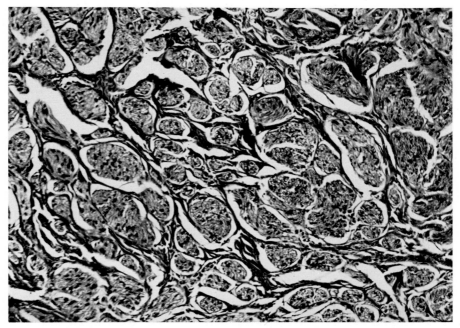

FIG. 351.   Neuroma. Cross section of the tangled mass of nerve filaments and their supportive tissue. (× 180.)

tion multiple tiny circles are found in which one can some times locate the nerve processes (Fig. 351). The lesion is non-neoplastic and warrants surgical intervention only when painful.

NEURILEMMOMA

A proliferation of cells which cover the myelin sheath produces a small mass attached to the nerve. It is usually encapsulated by a distended nerve sheath. The cells grow in palisaded groups of spindled cells (the Antoni type A) or as a patternless array of stellate forms in a clear, acellular substance (Antoni type B). For illustration see Figure 107. In the former, short rows of palisaded nuclei may oppose each other forming a vaguely delineated area called a Verocay body. The lesion probably never becomes malignant except perhaps in neurofibromatosis (see page 155).

MALIGNANT SCHWANNOMA

The malignant tumor of Schwann cell origin is rarely seen in the extremities except in neurofibromatosis. Its growth is said to be more rapid than that of neurilemmoma and it metastasizes widely through the blood stream. Since its cells are less mature than those of neurilemmoma, it may be impossible to differentiate this tumor from a fibro-sarcoma of nerve or other soft tissue structure. Cellularity and nuclear pleomorphism are the features on which the diagnosis of malignant tumor must depend. A palisaded pattern suggests its origin from the Schwann sheath.

NEUROFIBROMA

The term "neurofibroma" is usually applied to those nodular growths along the course of peripheral nerves in neurofibromatosis. They are poorly delineated and usually the edges merge into the surrounding fibrous tissues. Since they are non-progressive it is doubtful if they can be considered true tumors. It is probable that they are aberrations of growth with a hereditary background. Occasionally a solitary lesion may be encountered.

NEUROFIBROSARCOMA

It is this lesion which has been responsible for so much controversy among oncogeneticists. Most writers agree with Stout that it is usually impossible to determine whether a fibrosarcoma is arising in the supportive structures of a nerve or in extraneural connective tissue.

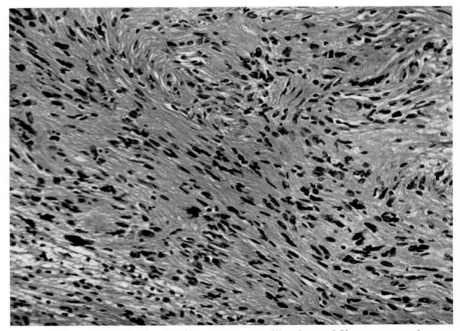

FIG. 352.   The cells of neurofibrosarcoma are like those of fibrosarcoma wherever it is found, except that there is a greater tendency for nuclear palisading. Some would call this a malignant schwannoma. ($\times$ 200.)

There is a tumor with a fairly constant microscopic appearance and clinical behavior which is believed by many pathologists to arise from nerve supportive tissue, whether the nerve is demonstrable or not. Its most common site of origin is the medial aspect of the thigh though it may occur elsewhere, usually within large muscle groups. It grows slowly, is infiltrative and has the same penchant for recurrence as does fibrosarcoma. It is set apart from the ordinary fibrosarcoma by a tendency for its cells to palisade (Fig. 352). When a tumor of this microscopic pattern is associated with a nerve, many microscopists would call it a malignant schwannoma. This particular tumor, however, tends to recur in the proximal nerve stump and it rarely metastasizes.

F. LESIONS OF SUPPORTIVE STRUCTURES OF VESSELS

In the embryonic formation of the finer ramifications of the vascular system the venous channels split off longitudinally from the arteries. Incomplete division may result in fistulous passages between the two systems. These have been called arteriovenous fistulas or arteriovenous aneurysms. They may occur in any tissue or organ and if they are large they may result in excessive work for the heart and eventual cardiac failure. When very small vessels are involved they are apt to be multiple. Microfistulae have been suggested as the cause of Paget's disease. They may cause hypertrophic osteoarthropathy. They have been named by some as the disturbance in the dynamics of blood flow which results in aneurysmal bone cyst.

Hamartomatous proliferations of small vessels are called angiomas. They may involve blood vessels (hemangiomas) or lymph channels (lymphangiomas). Neoplastic proliferation of various vessel components produces hemangioendotheliomas and hemangiopericytomas.

HEMANGIOMA

Hemangiomas occur in practically every body tissue. They are fairly common in the skeletal muscles. The vessels are distinctly formed and, depending upon the size of the lumina, they are called cavernous hemangiomas or capillary hemangiomas. They are congenital hamartomas since they grow in proportion to the structure they involve. A birthmark on the face grows during childhood and adolescence but at maturity it usually occupies about the same proportion of the face surface as it did at birth. Occasionally growth is excessive and these hamartomas produce a vermiform mass of tangled blood channels which may have an ominous appearance. In rare instances the hemangioma may sponsor a hemangiosarcoma. Arteriovenous fistulae and hemangiomas are commonly encountered in the gastrocnemius muscle. Occasionally they grow to immense proportion and constitute a challenge to the technical ability of the surgeon in accomplishing their removal.

HEMANGIOENDOTHELIOMA

If the proliferation is restricted to the endothelial lining cells in these vessel lesions, the result is a rather solid mass of large cells traversed by narrow blood channels about which the cells are arranged. The pattern may not be obvious, and since the cells resemble a number of the reticulum derivatives—serosal cells, synovial cells, histiocytes, epithelioid cells—the lesion is easy to misdiagnose on examination of microscopic sections. The hemangioendothelioma is a rare tumor occurring most commonly in young children. It is diagnosed much more often than it occurs. Several lymphangiosarcomas caused by a neoplastic proliferation of the endothelial lining of lymphatic channels of the arm, following occlusion of the latter by radical mastectomy, have been described.

HEMANGIOPERICYTOMA

Stout has described a tumor which apparently arises from the Rouget cells or pericytes of Zimmermann. These are elongated cells

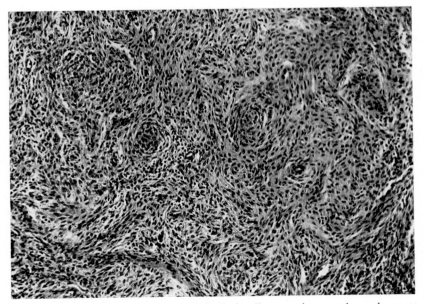

FIG. 353.   Hemangiopericytoma. Spindled cells grow in a perivascular pattern. With special stains the cells are found to be outside the endothelial basement membrane. (× 120.)

which are obliquely wrapped about the capillaries outside the basement membrane. They are modified muscle cells.

They produce tumors composed of spindled cells with a rich vessel network (Fig. 353). The nuclei are usually quite uniform and the sections may resemble those of a rather cellular, young fibrosarcoma. Sometimes they are arranged in rosette fashion about a vascular lumen. The hemangiopericytoma is related to the glomus tumor but it has no nerve elements like the latter.

The behavior of these tumors is erratic and unpredictable. Perhaps 50 per cent of them run a benign course. Others infiltrate deeply, recur and even metastasize.

HEMANGIOSARCOMA

Kaposi's disease is a neoplastic process which begins like an inflammatory reaction in vessels, usually of the skin. Poorly formed capillary channels leak blood into the surrounding supportive tissue. It is interesting to speculate upon the effect of this extravasated blood on the tissue which eventually leads to a malignant behavior. Early lesions may disappear spontaneously but eventually they progress, invade and ultimately metastasize (Fig. 354). Death may occur because of widespread metastatic deposits or hemorrhage from an eroded lesion within

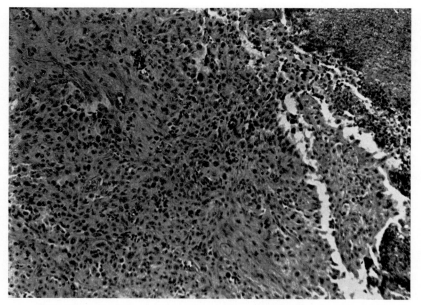

FIG. 354. Kaposi's disease. There is extravasation of blood at the right. Hemosiderin is scattered through the section. The tumor is composed of rounded or polyhedral endothelial cells, spindled collagenoblasts and a variety of in-between or transitional forms. ($\times$ 130.)

the intestinal mucosa.[5] A few cases have been primary in the pericardium. These lesions are probably true hemangiosarcomas though there is some debate concerning their exact nosologic position. Occasionally one is tempted to diagnose a hemangiosarcoma which cannot be included under the heading of malignant hemangioendothelioma, hemangiopericytoma or Kaposi's disease. Such tumors demonstrate more nuclear pleomorphism than any of the above and they are apt to have an explosively rapid and wide metastatic dissemination.

G. MESENCHYMOMA

Stout reserves the term "mesenchymoma" for a tumor which is composed of malignant components of two or more mesenchymal derivatives. Since fibrosarcomatous elements are commonly found in liposarcoma, rhabdomyosarcoma, chondrosarcoma and osteosarcoma, the second element must consist of some other than fibrosarcoma in these types. Areas of osteosarcoma or chondrosarcoma may be encountered in rhabdomyosarcoma or liposarcoma and various other combinations have been reported. This tumor runs a malignant course consistent with the types of tumor which are involved. Only a few bona fide mesenchymomas have been reported and most of these have occurred in the large muscles of the buttock and lower extremity.

REFERENCES

1. Smith, L. W.: Am. J. Path., *3*:355, 1927.
2. Wright, C. J. E.: Brit. J. Surg., *38*:257, 1951.
3. Fust, J. A., and Custer, R. P.: Am. J. Clin Path, *19*:522, 1949.
4. Christopherson, W. M., Foote, F. W., Jr., and Stewart, F. W.: Cancer, *5*:100, 1952.
5. Aegerter, E. E., and Peale, A. R.: Arch. Path., *34*:413, 1942.

Index